KINESIOLOGY
and
APPLIED ANATOMY

KINESIOLOGY
and
APPLIED ANATOMY

PHILIP J. RASCH, Ph.D., F.A.C.S.M.

Formerly Chief, Physiology Division,
Naval Medical Field Research Laboratory,
Camp Lejeune, North Carolina

With Contributions by:

Mark D. Grabiner, Ph.D.

Staff Scientist
Department of Musculoskeletal Research
Cleveland Clinic Foundation
Cleveland, Ohio

Robert J. Gregor, Ph.D., F.A.C.S.M.

Associate Professor
Department of Kinesiology
University of California at Los Angeles
Los Angeles, California

John Garhammer, Ph.D., F.A.C.S.M.

Associate Professor
Department of Physical Education
California State University at Long Beach
Long Beach, California

SEVENTH EDITION

LEA & FEBIGER

Philadelphia • London • 1989

Williams & Wilkins
Rose Tree Corporate Center, Building II
1400 North Providence Road, Suite 5025
Media, PA 19063-2043 USA

First Edition, 1959—Reprinted, 1960
Second Edition, 1963—Reprinted, 1964, 1965, 1966
Third Edition, 1967—Reprinted 1968, 1969
Fourth Edition, 1971—Reprinted 1972, 1973
Fifth Edition, 1974—Reprinted, 1975, 1976, 1977
Sixth Edition, 1978—Reprinted, 1980, 1983, 1984, 1985, 1986

First Spanish Edition, 1961
Second Spanish Edition, 1967
Third Spanish Edition, 1973

First Portuguese Edition, 1977

Library of Congress Cataloging-in-Publication Data

Rasch, Philip J.
  Kinesiology and applied anatomy/Philip J. Rasch; with
contributions by Mark D. Grabiner, Robert J. Gregor, John Garhammer.
—7 ed.
    p.   cm.
  Includes bibliographies and indexes.
  ISBN 0-8121-1132-X
  1. Kinesiology. 2. Physical education and training. 3. Anatomy,
Human. I. Grabiner, Mark D. II. Gregor, Robert J.
III. Garhammer, John. IV. Title.
  [DNLM: 1. Movement. 2. Muscles. 3. Physical Education and
Training. WE 103 R223k]
QP303.R33 1988
612'.76—dc19
DNLM/DLC
for Library of Congress   88-26649
                                      CIP

Printed in the United States of America

Print number: 5 4 3

Preface

In Tennyson's *Idylls of the King*, King Arthur recalls the events of his life and concludes, "The old order changeth, yielding place to the new." In 1959 such a changing of old order was marked when Philip J. Rasch and Roger K. Burke authored the first edition of *Kinesiology and Applied Anatomy*. The book represented an extensive revision of a text originally published in 1917 that had a history of seven editions.

The six editions of the Rasch and Burke text were based on a philosophy that an introductory text should present an overview of the subject and provide a point of departure for more in-depth study of specific topics. This seventh edition of *Kinesiology and Applied Anatomy* represents the most recent change of old order. The intent of the book remains as before, to serve as an introductory text for kinesiology, the biomechanics of human movement. Fundamental concepts and interactions of the biology and mechanics of human motion are presented as a springboard for the student's pursuit of more in-depth understanding.

The most visible changes in the text are in some of the chapters related to anatomy. Less emphasis has been placed on what is considered prerequisite basic knowledge of musculoskeletal anatomy. More important is the synthesis of the material on biomechanics and neuromotor considerations to elucidate simple biomechanical models of musculoskeletal systems. We present simplified methods of answering questions such as "What are the internal and external effects of a particular system of forces?" and "What are the biologic implications of the force systems?"

The new contributors, Mark D. Grabiner, Robert J. Gregor, and John Garhammer, wish to thank Philip J. Rasch and Roger K. Burke for the opportunity to take the first step toward the future of this work. Our goal for *Kinesiology and Applied Anatomy* is to maintain its introductory focus while reflecting the changes in the content areas prerequisite for the study of human movement. In kinesiology, though athletics will always provide an important avenue for study, the areas of orthopedics, rehabilitation, neuroscience, industrial biomechanics, and gerontology are also being emphasized. To a greater extent than ever, undergraduate programs in exercise science and kinesiology are attracting students preparing for medical school, dental school, and physical and occupational therapy. Future editions of this text will include topics specific to these areas necessary for an understanding of the biology and the engineering aspects of the human body and of how the human body adapts and maladapts to the movement environment.

San Pedro, California

Cleveland, Ohio
Los Angeles, California
Long Beach, California

PHILIP J. RASCH

Mark Grabiner
Robert J. Gregor
John Garhammer

v

Contents

I | FOUNDATIONS OF KINESIOLOGY

1 THE HISTORY OF KINESIOLOGY

PHILIP J. RASCH

The term *kinesiology* is a combination of two Greek verbs, "kinein," meaning "to move," and "logos," meaning "to discourse." Kinesiologists—those who discourse on movement—in effect combine anatomy, the science of structure of the body, with physiology, the science of function of the body, to produce kinesiology, the science of movement of the body.

The title "Father of Kinesiology" is usually given to Aristotle (384–322 B.C.), whose treatises, *Parts of Animals, Movement of Animals,* and *Progression of Animals,* described for the first time the actions of the muscles and subjected them to geometric analysis. He recorded such practical observations as the following:

. . . the animal that moves makes its change of position by pressing against that which is beneath it. . . . Hence athletes jump farther if they have weights in their hands than if they have not, and runners run faster if they swing their arms, for in the extension of the arms there is a kind of leaning upon the hands and wrists.[1]

Aristotle was the first to analyze and describe the complex process of walking, in which rotatory motion is transformed into translatory motion. His discussion of the problems of pushing a boat under various conditions was, in essence, a precursor of Newton's three laws of motion. For his time, Aristotle demonstrated a remarkable understanding of the role of the center of gravity, the laws of motion, and leverage.

Another Greek, Archimedes (287–212 B.C.), determined hydrostatic principles governing floating bodies that are still accepted as valid in the kinesiology of swimming. Some of them were used to develop means of space travel. The broad scope of his inquiries included the laws of leverage and problems related to determining the center of gravity. His treatises on the latter have been described as the foundation of theoretical mechanics.[2] Principles originally developed by Archimedes are still employed in determinations of body composition.

Galen (131–201 A.D.), a Roman citizen who tended the gladiators owned by the ruler of Pergamum in Asia Minor and who is considered to have been the first team physician in history, had a substantial knowledge of human motion. In his essay *De Motu Musculorum* he distinguished between motor and sensory nerves and between agonist and antagonist muscles, described tonus, and introduced terms such as diarthrosis and synarthrosis that even today are of major importance in the terminology of arthrology. The idea that muscles were contractile seems to have originated with Galen. He taught that muscular contraction resulted from the passage of "animal spirits" from the brain through the nerves to the muscles. Some writers consider his treatise the first textbook on kinesiology, and he has been termed "the father of sports medicine."[3]

Following Galen's myologic studies, kinesiology remained almost static for over 1000 years. It was not until the time of one of the most brilliant men in history, Leonardo da Vinci (1452–1519), that the science of kinesi-

3

ology was advanced another step. Artist, engineer, and scientist, da Vinci was particularly interested in the structure of the human body as it relates to performance, and in the relationship between the center of gravity and the balance and center of resistance. He described the mechanics of the body in standing, walking up- and downhill, rising from a sitting position, and jumping. Da Vinci was probably the first to record scientific data on human gait. To demonstrate the progressive action and interaction of various muscles* during movement, he suggested that cords be attached to a skeleton at the points of origin and insertion of the muscles. Although da Vinci was a prolific writer, his notebooks were designed to be unintelligible to the unauthorized reader. As a result, most of his writings were not published until 200 or 300 years after his death, and his influence during life was restricted principally to a small circle of acquaintances.

After studying medicine at the University of Pisa for 3 years, Galileo Galilei (1564–1643) became convinced that "nature is written in mathematical symbols," whereupon he turned to mathematics in search of the laws underlying physical phenomena. His demonstrations that the acceleration of a falling body is not proportionate to its weight and that the relationship of space, time, and velocity is the most important factor in the study of motion inaugurated classical mechanics and have been considered the introduction of experimental methodology into science. Galileo also proved that the trajectory of a projectile through a resistance-free medium is a parabola. His work gave impetus to the study of mechanical events in mathematical terms, which in turn provided a basis for the emergence of kinesiology as a science.

Alfonso Borelli (1608–1679), who studied under one of Galileo's pupils, endeavored to apply the master's mathematical formulae to the problems of muscular movement. In his treatise *De Motu Animalium*, published in 1630 or 1631, Borelli sought to demonstrate that animals are machines. The amount of force produced by various muscles and the loss of

force as a result of unfavorable mechanical action, air resistance, and water resistance were among the aspects of muscular movement he explored. It was Borelli's theory that bones serve as levers and that muscles function according to mathematical principles. Although he realized that the contraction of muscles involved complex chemical processes, Borelli's explanation of these processes was fanciful in the extreme. He suggested that the nerves are canals filled with a spongy material through which flow animal spirits (*succus nerveus*, sometimes translated "nerve gas"); that agitation of these spirits from the periphery to the brain produces sensation; and that agitation from the brain produces filling and enlargement of the porosities of the muscles, with resultant turgescence. Reaction of these spirits with a substance in the muscles themselves, said Borelli, initiated a process resembling fermentation, with subsequent contraction.[4] He distinguished between tonic and voluntary contractions and perhaps even vaguely perceived the principle of reciprocal innervation of antagonistic muscles. Steindler praised him as "the real founder of modern kinetics" and as "the father of modern biomechanics of the locomotor system."[4] Borelli is credited with having effectively founded and developed that branch of physiology that relates muscular movement to mechanical principles.

Borelli is also regarded as the founder of the iatrophysical school of medicine, which affirmed that the phenomena of life and death are based on the laws of physics. The tenets of this school were supported by Giorgio Baglivi (1668–1706), who in 1700 published *De Motu Musculorum*, which differentiated for the first time between smooth muscles, designed for long, sustained efforts, and striated muscles, designed for quick movements. Eventually, however, the iatrophysicists' neglect of the rapidly advancing science of chemistry caused their school to fall into disrepute and to disappear.

Borelli's theory of muscular contraction was attacked almost immediately. Among his critics was Francis Glisson (1597–1677), who contended that the muscle fibers contract, rather than expand, during flexion, as demonstrated by plethysmographic experiments. He sug-

*Before the eighteenth century few muscles had names. Galen used numbers and da Vinci used letters in their illustrations.

gested also that all viable tissue possesses the capacity to react to stimuli. This capacity he referred to as "irritability." Glisson's concept was later elaborated by Albrecht von Haller (1708–1777), the outstanding physiologist of the eighteenth century, into the theory that contractility is an innate property of muscle that exists independently of nervous influence.

The Italian Jesuit Francesco Maria Grimaldi was the first to report hearing sounds made by contracting muscles. Although his book, *Physicomatheis de lumine,* was published in 1663, 2 years after his death, techniques for studying these sounds were not available until 300 years later. In the last few years, the invention of the electronic stethoscope and computer analyses have made research in this field feasible. Oster has shown that the amplitude of muscle sound is directly proportionate to the weight used to maintain a constant contraction. These sounds appear to originate from the vibration of single muscle fibers, particularly the fast-twitch fibers. In the future it may be possible to use such sounds to determine which muscles are active in a given movement and how hard each is working.[5]

The circulation of the blood through the body was first demonstrated by William Harvey (1578–1657), although he erroneously attributed to the heart the function of recharging the blood with heat and "vital spirit."[6] Subsequently, Niels Stensen (1648–1686) made the then-sensational declaration that the heart was merely a muscle, not the seat of "natural warmth," nor of "vital spirit." This has been acclaimed as the greatest advance in our knowledge of the circulatory system since Harvey's discovery.[7] Three years later, Stensen, who has been credited with laying the foundation of muscular mechanics, wrote *Elementorum Myologiae Specimen,* an "epoch-making" book on muscular function. In this book he asserted that a muscle is essentially a collection of motor fibers; that in composition the center of a muscle differs from the ends (tendons) and is the only part that contracts. Contraction of a muscle, wrote Stensen, is merely the shortening of its individual fibers and is not produced by an increase or loss of substance.[8]

The word "orthopedics" was coined by Nicolas Andry (1658–1742) from the Greek roots "orthos," meaning "straight," and "pais," meaning "child." Andry believed that skeletal deformities result from muscular imbalances during childhood. In his treatise, *Orthopedics or the Art of Preventing and Correcting in Infants Deformities of the Body,* originally published in 1741, he defined the term "orthopedist" as a physician who prescribes corrective exercise.[9] Although this is not the modern usage, Andry is recognized as the creator of both the word and the science. His theories were directly antecedent to the development of the Swedish system of gymnastics by Per Henrik Ling (1776–1839).

In *Principia Mathematica Philosophiae Naturalis,* which is "perhaps the most powerful and original piece of scientific reasoning ever published,"[10] Isaac Newton (1642–1727) laid the foundation of modern dynamics. Particularly important to the future of kinesiology was his formulation of the three laws of rest and movement, which express the relationships between forces (interaction) and their effects:

I. Every body continues in its state of rest, or of uniform motion, in a right line, unless it is compelled to change that state by forces impressed upon it. (This is sometimes known as the law of inertia and was originally proposed by Galileo in 1638.)

II. The change of motion is proportional to the motive force impressed and made in the direction of the right line in which that force is impressed (law of momentum).

III. To every action there is always opposed an equal reaction; or, the mutual actions of two bodies upon each other are always equal and directed to the contrary parts (law of interaction).[11]

The application of these laws to muscular function may be demonstrated by the following analogy: While he is pivoting, a discus thrower must grasp the discus firmly (exert centripetal force) to prevent it from flying out of his hand. In accordance with the third law, the missile exerts an equal and opposite reaction (centrifugal force). When his grip is released and centripetal force no longer interacts with the discus, the implement flies off in a straight line tangential to its former circular path. The distance covered by the missile is proportionate to the motive force imparted to it, in accordance with the second law. The trajectory of the missile is affected by gravity, wind velocity, and other forces tending to alter its state of uniform motion, as predicted by the first law.

According to the Newtonian world view, changes of motion are considered as a measure of the force that produces them. From this theory originated the idea of measuring force by the product of mass and acceleration, a concept that plays a fundamental role in kinetics. The greater the speed with which the discus thrower whirls, the greater the acceleration applied to the mass of the discus, the farther it will fly before gravity returns it to earth, and the greater the force said to have been applied to the discus.

Newton is also credited with the first correct general statement of the parallelogram of force, based on his observation that a moving body affected by two independent forces acting simultaneously moved along a diagonal equal to the vector sum of the forces acting independently. By further analysis of the laws of movement as applied by the discus thrower, it can be demonstrated mathematically that the horizontal and vertical forces acting on the flying discus are equal. The diagonal, which is equal to the vector sum of the horizontal and vertical forces, is, therefore, 45°, and the missile should traverse the greatest distance when it travels at this angle. In practice, of course, other factors of lift, drag, shape, gyroscopic rotation, and so forth enter the situation, and it is possible that the most effective angle of release may not always be the one that is the theoretical optimum. Because two or more muscles may pull on a common point of insertion, each at a different angle and with a different force, the resolution of vectors of this type is a matter of considerable importance in the solution of academic problems in kinesiology.

Within the recent past, physicists have demonstrated that Newton's theories are valid only within the frame of reference in which they were conceived; they do not apply to relationships between forces in the Einsteinian world view. This discovery has little significance for the kinesiologist, however, since he deals primarily with the forces of

gross muscular movement, and these are governed by the laws of motion set forth by Newton.

In his studies of muscular contraction, James Keill (1674–1719) calculated the number of fibers in certain muscles, assumed that on contraction each fiber became spherical and thus shortened, and from this deduced the amount of tension developed by each fiber to lift a given weight. In *An Account of Animal Secretion, the Amount of Blood in the Human Body, and Muscular Motion* (1708), Keill drew the erroneous conclusion that a muscle could not contract to less than two thirds of its greatest length.

In *An Essay on the Vital and Other Involuntary Motions of Animals,* published in 1751, Robert Whytt (1714–1766) rejected Baglivi's theory of muscular action and contended that movement originates from an unconscious sentient principle, or soul. This idea brought him into disagreement with von Haller.[12] Possibly Whytt may not have comprehended the principle that movement may originate as reflex reaction to external stimuli; however, it appears that he was cognizant of the stretch reflex and the fact that a given stimulus may be adequate to excite one nerve ending but not another. Their differences of opinion arose from the fact that von Haller thought in terms of isolated muscle, and Whytt in terms of the reflex control of the movements of an organism.

The subject of anatomy, as taught prior to the time of Marie Francois Xavier Bichat (1771–1802), consisted of little more than dogmatic statements handed down through the ages. Through Bichat's efforts, anatomy became a science solidly founded on the systematic experimentation with the various systems into which he divided the living organism. Bichat observed that the organs of the body are composed of individual tissues with distinctive characteristics and was the first to describe the synovial membranes. Bichat is regarded as the author of the modern concept of structure as the basis of function, which led to the development of rational physiology and pathology. He distinguished between the cerebrospinal nervous system, which deals with the external relationships between the animal and its environment, and the autonomic nervous system, which controls the organs of internal function.

The six Croonian Lectures on Muscle Motion* delivered by John Hunter (1728–1793) in 1776, 1777, 1779, 1780, 1781, and 1782,[13] brought together all of this great anatomist's observations concerning the structure and power of muscles and the stimuli by which they are excited. Muscle, he declared, while endowed with life, is fitted for self-motion, and is the only part of the body so fitted. He emphasized that muscular function could be studied only by observations of living persons, not cadavers. In his lecture series, Hunter described muscular function in considerable detail, including the origin, insertion, and shape of muscles, the mechanical arrangement of their fibers, the two-joint problem, contraction and relaxation, strength, hypertrophy, and many other aspects of the subject. His lectures may be regarded as summarizing all that was known about kinesiology at the end of the eighteenth century, when, unwittingly, kinesiologists stood at the threshold of a discovery that was to revolutionize their methods of investigation.

About 1740 physiologists became excited over the phenomena produced by electrical stimulation of muscles. Haller summarized many of the early experiments in his treatise on muscle irritability, and Whytt reported clinical observations on a patient treated by electrotherapy. "Animal electricity" was proposed as a substitute for the "animal spirits" that earlier investigators had believed to be the activating force in muscular movement. During the summer of 1786, Luigi Galvani (1737–1798) studied the effects of atmospheric electricity on dissected frog muscles. He observed that the muscles of a frog sometimes contracted when touched by a scalpel, which led him to the conclusion that there was "indwelling electricity which proceeded along the nerve."[14] His *Commentary on the Effects of Electricity on Muscular Motion* (1791) is probably the earliest explicit statement of the presence of electrical potentials in nerve and muscle. Galvani is considered the father of experimental neurology.

The study of animal electricity at once became the absorbing interest of the physiologic world. The greatest name among the early students of the subject was Emil DuBois-Reymond (1818–1896), who laid the foundations of modern electrophysiology.

Fascinated by the prospect of investigating muscular response produced by electrical stimulation, Guillaume Benjamin Amand Duchenne (1806–1875) set out to classify the functions of individual muscles in relation to body movements, although he recognized that isolated muscular action does not exist in nature[15] (Fig. 1–1). His masterwork, *Physiologie des Mouvements*, appeared in 1865 and has been acclaimed "one of the greatest books of all times."[16]

The modern concept of locomotion originated with the studies of Borelli; however, very little was accomplished in this field prior to the publication of *Die Mechanik der menschlichen Gerverkzeuge* by the Webers in 1836. Their treatise, which still stands as the classical work accomplished by purely observational methods, firmly established the mechanism of muscular action on a scientific basis. The Weber brothers, Ernst Heinrich (1795–1878), Wilhelm Eduard (1804–1891), and Eduard Friedrich Wilhelm (1806–1871), believed that the body was maintained in the erect position primarily by tension of the ligaments, with little or no muscular exertion; that in walking or running the forward motion of the limb is a pendulum-swing owing to gravity; and that walking is a movement of falling forward, arrested by the weight of the body thrown on the limb as it is advanced forward. The Webers were the first to investigate the reduction in the length of an individual muscle during contraction and devoted much study to the role of bones as mechanical levers. They were also the first to describe in chronologic detail the movements of the center of gravity.

The study of animal mechanics was expanded by the talented and versatile Samuel

---

*William Croone (1633–1684), a professor at Gresham College, England, and author of *De Ratione Motus Musculorum* (1664), an important early work on muscle, left a will providing for annual lectures on the physiology of muscular motion. Fulton commented, "It is literally true that the history of muscle physiology in the Eighteenth, Nineteenth and Twentieth Centuries has been largely developed at these annual lectures." (*Muscular Contraction and the Reflex Control of Movement*, pp. 15–16.)

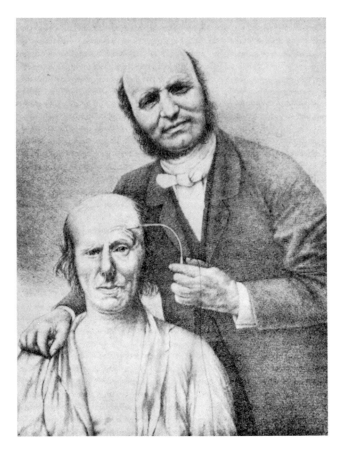

FIG. 1–1.   Guillaume Benjamin Amand Duchenne de Boulogne investigating the effect of electrical stimulation of the left frontalis muscle. (Jokl and Reich, courtesy J. Assoc. Phys. Ment. Rehabil.)

Haughton (1821–1897) in numerous papers bearing such titles as *Outlines of a New Theory of Muscular Action* (1863), *The Muscular Mechanism of the Leg of the Ostrich* (1865), *On Hanging, Considered from a Mechanical and Physiological Point of Veiw* (1868), and *Notes on Animal Mechanics* (1861–1865). However, advancement of knowledge concerning body mechanics was greatly impeded by lack of a satisfactory method of chronologic reproduction of movement. This advance was made when Janssen, an astronomer who had used serial pictures in 1878 to study the transit of Venus, suggested kinematographic pictures to study human motion. Eadweard Muybridge (1831–1904) produced his book *The Horse in Motion* in 1882, and in 1887 wrote his monumental *Animal Locomotion* in eleven volumes, an abridgment of which was reissued in 1955 under the title *The Human Figure in Motion*.[17] Etienne Jules Marey (1830–1904), who was

convinced that movement is the most important of human functions and that all other functions are concerned with its accomplishment, described graphic and photographic methods for biological research in *Du mouvement dans les functions de la vie* (1892) and *Le mouvement* (1894).

These photographic techniques opened the way for the experimental studies of Christian Wilhelm Braune (1831–1892) and Otto Fischer (1861–1917), which are still considered of major importance in the study of human gait. Even more famous than these investigations was Braune and Fischer's report of an experimental method of determining the center of gravity, published in 1889. An abridgment of this is available in an Air Force Technical Documentary Report.[18] Their major premise was that a knowledge of the position of the center of gravity of the human body and of the body's component parts was fundamental to an understanding of the resistive forces that the muscles must overcome during movement. Their observations were made on four cadavers, which, after having been preserved by freezing, were nailed to a wall by means of long steel spits. The planes of the centers of gravity of the longitudinal, sagittal, and frontal axes were thus determined. By dissecting the bodies with a saw and locating the points of intersection of the three planes, Braune and Fischer were able to establish the center of gravity of the body. The center of gravity of the component parts was determined in the same manner. Because one cadaver began to decompose and the investigators were not permitted to dissect a second cadaver, complete observations were made on only two of the four bodies. When the centers of gravity were plotted on a life-size drawing of one of the cadavers and compared photographically with those of a soldier having similar body measurements, the investigators observed a remarkable similarity. Braune and Fischer concluded that the original position of their frozen cadavers could be considered a normal one and referred to it as "normalstellung," which was intended to indicate only that it was the standard position in which their measurements were taken. Unfortunately, this term came to be understood as the ideal position, and generations of students were exhorted to imitate it. Their work with cadavers has recently been carried on and extended by Wilfrid Taylor Dempster.[19]

On the basis of subsequent studies, Rudolf A. Fick (1866–1939) concluded that the theory of "normalstellung" was not entirely valid, as the recumbent position of a cadaver could not be transferred to the vertical stance. The degree of lumbar lordosis is much less when the body is recumbent than when vertical; in the latter position the center of gravity shifts forward considerably more than Braune and Fischer assumed. Fick contended that no one posture is common for people of all races and cultures. Modern anthropological investigations have confirmed his opinion.

The late nineteenth and early twentieth centuries were most productive of physiologic studies closely related to kinesiology. Adolf Eugen Fick (1829–1901) made important contributions to our knowledge of the mechanics of muscular movement and energetics and introduced the terms "isometric" and "isotonic." The study of developmental mechanics was introduced by Wilhelm Roux (1850–1924), who stated that muscular hypertrophy develops only after a muscle is forced to work intensively, a point of view that was later demonstrated experimentally by Werner W. Siebert.[20] B. Morpurgo showed that increased strength and hypertrophy are a result of an increase in the diameter of the individual fibers of a muscle, not a result of an increase in the number of fibers. The theory of progressive resistance exercise is based principally on the studies of Morpurgo and Siebert,[21] but Morpurgo's work is now being questioned.

L. Ranvier, about 1880, discovered the difference in the speeds of contraction of red and white muscle. "The importance of this finding," says Granit, "is that it brought functional aspects into the focus of subsequent research."[22]

John Hughlings Jackson (1834–1911), "the father of modern neurology," made definite contributions to knowledge pertaining to the control of muscular movement by the brain. His conclusions* are summed up in these words:

. . . The motor centres of every level represent movements of muscles, not muscles in their individual character . . . the distinction between muscles and movements of muscles is exceedingly important all over the field of neurology. . . . The occurrence of convulsion of a muscular region which is already imperfectly and yet permanently paralyzed is unintelligible without that distinction. And without it we shall not understand how it can happen that there is loss of some movements of a muscular region without obvious disability in that region.[23]

Jackson mentioned postepileptiform aphasia and hemiplegia as practical examples of his dictum and coined the aphorism "nervous centers know nothing of muscles, they only know of movements." His ideas were cited approvingly by Charles Edward Beevor (1854–1908) in his 1903 Croonian Lecture on Muscular Movements.[24]

Beevor pointed out that the technique of

---

*Quoted by permission.

utilizing electrical stimulation employed by Duchenne demonstrated what a muscle *can* do, not what it *does* do; and since only the stimulated muscle responds, this method fails to show the action of associated muscles, some of which often and others of which always contract simultaneously in the natural situation, perhaps modifying the resultant movement. Beevor referred to James Benignus Winslow's* previous objection to the use of cadavers to demonstrate muscular action and the fallacious conclusions that had been based on these observations. After careful study of the muscular actions involved in the movements of certain joints, Beevor proposed that the muscles be classified as prime movers, synergic muscles, fixators, or antagonists. He was of the opinion that the antagonistic muscles always relaxed in strong resistive movements.

In this respect Beevor was influenced by the work of Charles Sherrington (1857–1952), who advanced the theory of the reciprocal innervation of antagonistic muscles in a number of papers published near the end of the nineteenth century and that he later incorporated into his book *The Integrative Action of the Nervous System* (1906), a monumental work in the history of kinesiology that has been republished many times. Contemporaneously, Henry Pickering Bowditch (1814–1911) demonstrated the treppe phenomenon (1871), the "all-or-none" principle of contraction (1871), and the indefatigability of the nerves (1890). The Sherrington theory and the "all-or-none" principle are considered "fundamental for an understanding of kinetic events in the human body."[25] Of inestimable value to the morale of kinesiologists, who at that time were insecure in their profession and depressed by the jibes of critics who contended that the study of the body was unworthy of man, was Sherrington's insistence that "the importance of muscular contraction to us can be stated by saying that all man can do is to move things, and his muscular contraction is his sole means thereto."[26] Actually, much the same thing had been said in 1863

by the famous Russian physiologist Ivan Mikhailovich Sechenov (1829–1905) when he declared, "All the endless diversity of the external manifestations of the activity of the brain can be finally regarded as one phenomenon—that of muscular movement."[27]

Karl Culmann (1821–1881), a German engineer, reviewed in *Die Graphische Statik* all that had been accomplished up to 1865 in the solution of static problems by graphic methods. Speaking at a meeting of scientists in 1866, he called attention to the fact that when the calcium phosphate was dissolved from the upper end of the femur, the internal architecture of this bone coincided with graphostatic determinations of the lines of maximum internal stress in a Fairbairn crane, which he assumed resembled the femur in shape and loading. Although his basic assumption has been severely criticized, his analysis forms the basis of the trajectorial theory of the architecture of bones.

The trajectorial theory was supported by Roux and became the basis for his interpretation of the trajectory system of other bones. In 1892 this theory was classically expressed by Julius Wolff (1836–1902) in the famous Wolff's law: "Every change in the form and function of a bone or of their function alone is followed by certain definite changes in their internal architecture, and equally definite secondary alteration in their external conformation, in accordance with mathematical laws." He believed that the formation of bone results from both the force of muscular tensions and the resultant static stresses of maintaining the body in the erect position, and that these forces always intersect at right angles. Wolff's law also applies to the healing of skin wounds.

Bassett has proposed a restatement of Wolff's law in modern terms: "The form of the bone being given, the bone elements place or displace themselves in the direction of the functional pressures and increase or decrease their mass to reflect the amount of functional pressure."[28] The probable mechanism is biochemical—a piezoelectric effect of the bone crystal or from a diode with collagen and mineral components.

In his paper "Laws of Bone Architecture,"[29] which has been proclaimed "the most thor-

---

*Winslow (1669–1760) was the author of *An Anatomical Exposition of the Structure of the Human Body.* Originally published in 1749, it was translated into several languages.

ough study of stress and strain in a bone by mathematical analysis of cross sections,"[30] John C. Koch concluded that the compact and spongy materials of bone are so composed as to produce maximum strength with a minimum of material and that, in form and structure, bones are designed to resist in the most economical manner the maximum compressive stresses normally produced by the body weight. Because the stresses from body weight are so much greater than the tensions that are normally produced by the muscles, reasoned Koch, the effect of muscular action is of relatively little importance in determining the architecture of the bones and, therefore, could be ignored in his analysis. In endeavoring to draw practical applications from his theoretical studies, Koch commented that alterations in posture increase the stress in certain regions and decrease it in others, and that if postural alterations are maintained, the inner structure of the affected bones is altered. The proper mechanical means of counteracting these alterations, said Koch, was to impose new mechanical conditions by the use of braces, jackets, or other suitable devices to reverse the transformative process and restore the original structure.

Murk Jansen's monograph *On Bone Formation* (1920) disagreed with many of Wolff's premises, including the "dualistic" doctrine that bone formation is dependent on both tension and pressure. Wolff's hypothesis that these forces intersect at right angles in the trabeculae of cancellous bone constituted a fatal flaw in the theory, contended Jansen, since the major trabecular systems do not always cross at right angles. Jansen insisted that the jerking action of a contracting muscle, combined with gravity, is the chief mechanical stimulus for the formation of bone and, moreover, is a determinative factor in the structure of cancellous bone.

Eben J. Carey[31] also criticized Koch's denial of the role of muscular tension in the formation of bone and asserted that the dominant factors affecting the growth and structure of bone are the powerful back pressure vectors produced by the forces of muscular contraction. He rejected Koch's emphasis on static pressure. The body, he said, is sustained in the upright posture by mutual interaction between the skeleton and the muscles, and he expressed the opinion that the dynamic action of the muscles may exceed the static pressure of body weight. He contended that the normal growth and structure of mature bone is the result of this dynamic muscular activity and of the intrinsic capacity of skeletal cells to proliferate centrifugally against extrinsic centripetal resistances.

F. Pauwels endeavored to demonstrate that muscles and ligaments act as traction braces to reduce the magnitude of stress in the bones. His work was criticized by F. Gaynor Evans on the grounds that it was concerned only with the stresses produced by loads placed on solid models shaped like bones. It is possible that Wolff and Roux overemphasized the importance of mechanical stresses without proper consideration for biological factors, which sometimes exceed mechanical influences. Nevertheless, the theory of functional adaptation to static stress remains a major hypothesis in the study of skeletal development. J. H. Scott[32] has reviewed the material in the field in an effort to construct a working hypothesis of the developmental and functional relationships between the skeletal system and the neuromuscular system.

Prior even to the time when the development of bone became a subject of heated debate, even more highly controversial hypotheses were introduced into the scientific world. Charles Darwin (1809–1882) published two books, *The Origin of the Species* (1859) and *The Descent of Man* (1871), which have become classics and have revolutionized man's ideas concerning the human body. Darwin's conception of man as a "modified descendant of some pre-existing form" whose framework is constructed on the same model as that of other mammals, and whose body contains both rudimentary muscles that serve useful functions in the lower mammals and modified structures that resulted from a gradual change from quadrupedal to bipedal posture, was at first bitterly opposed. Now generally accepted, his concepts have clarified many questions pertaining to kinesiology that might otherwise have remained obscure and have attracted to the study of kinesiology many physical anthropologists whose contributions have been of great value.

Yet another scientist of the nineteenth century, Angelo Mosso (1848–1910), made an important contribution to the study of kinesiology, the invention of the ergograph in 1884. This instrument, now available in an endless array of specialized forms, has become a nearly indispensable tool for the study of muscular function in the human body.

The first extensive compendium on body mechanics, *The Human Motor*, by Jules Amar, was published in 1914. Inspired largely by the increase in work productivity achieved by Frederick Winslow Taylor's[33] application of scientific principles of body mechanics to industry, Amar (1879–?) sought to bring together "in one volume all the physical and physiological elements of industrial work."[34] Since its publication, countless industrial studies based on Amar's principles have been published, perhaps the best known of which are the numerous reports of the British Industrial Fatigue Research Board and of Frank B. (1868–1924) and Lillian M. (1878–1972) Gilbreth.

This type of kinesiologic research initiated studies in the unexplored areas of time and motion. Investigations in this field have been greatly accelerated as a result of rapid advances in engineering and the development of machines so complex that the physical abilities of the human operator become a limiting factor in their use. Scientists have brought together massive collections of data pertaining to the application of scientific principles of body mechanics to industry, now known as human engineering, or the science of ergonomics—"the customs, habits, or laws of work." Attempts to solve the problems of space flight have provided further impetus to studies of this nature.

Kinesiology of the Human Body Under Normal and Pathological Conditions, by Arthur Steindler (1878–1959), was an important contribution to our understanding of body mechanics. Information has continued to accumulate, and some of the facts and theories that have been presented are both curious and instructive. As an example, men frequently sustain femoral fractures as a result of automobile accidents, whereas women are more likely to incur dislocations of the hip. This difference is attributed to the social conditioning of women to sit with their knees or legs crossed, whereas men are conditioned to sit with their legs spread apart. An impact on a person sitting with the knees or legs crossed tends to drive the head of the femur out of the acetabulum, but a similar impact on an individual sitting with his legs apart tends to drive the head of the femur further into the acetabulum until the femur buckles and breaks.

As early as 1880, Wedenski demonstrated the existence of action currents in human muscles, although practical use of this discovery had to await the invention of a more sensitive instrument. This became available when W. Einthoven developed the string galvanometer in 1906. The physiologic aspects of electromyography were first discussed in a paper by H. Piper, of Germany, 1910–1912; however, interest in the subject did not become widespread in the English-speaking countries until publication of a report by E. D. Adrian in 1925.[35] By utilizing electromyographic techniques, Adrian demonstrated for the first time that it was possible to determine the amount of activity in the human muscles at any stage of a movement. The development of the electromyograph represents one of the greatest advances in kinesiology. By means of this instrument many generally accepted concepts of muscle action have been proved erroneous and new theories have been brought forth. In this area the work of John V. Basmajian has been of particular value to students of kinesiology and is frequently cited in this book.[36]

The brilliant studies of Archibald V. Hill (1886–1977) in the oxygen consumption of muscle won him a share in a Nobel Prize in 1922. Hugh E. Huxley's (1924–   ) work in the ultrastructure of striated muscle and Andrew F. Huxley's (1917–   ) studies in the physiology of striated muscle distinguish them as leading authorities in their respective fields.[37–39]

Interest in the subject of posture has declined among kinesiologists in the United States during the last few years. In part, this decline may have resulted from general acceptance of the dictum that "the physiological benefits obtained from correction of common postural defects are mostly imaginary"[40]; in part, it may reflect the growing realization that individual differences almost preclude valid generalizations. Perhaps much of the effort that in earlier times was devoted to the study of static posture is now directed to research concerning dynamic locomotion. Wallace Fenn (1893–1971), Plato Schwartz, Verne Inmann, Herbert Elftman, Dudley Morton, and Steindler should be listed among the scientists who have made important contributions to knowledge concerning this phase of kinesiology.

The use of cinematography for kinesiological studies of athletes and industrial workers has become commonplace. An important recent development in the study of human motion is the use of cineradiographic techniques. In time, advances in technique may make it possible to record the complete sequence of musculoskeletal movements rather than only a fraction of them. A fascinating new parameter was opened up with the invention of the electronic stroboscope by Harold Edgerton. This instrument, which is capable of exposures as short as one millionth of a second, can record in a series of instantaneous photographs an entire sequence of movement. This apparatus seems particularly promising for analysis of the various sequences of skilled movement. In a somewhat related field, the science of aerodynamics has greatly increased our knowledge of the movement of objects in space through investigations involving the use of wind tunnels and other specialized research tools and artificially produced environments.

Psychologists, psychoanalysts, psychiatrists, and other social scientists have become interested in investigating the psychosomatic aspects of kinesiology. The studies of J. H. Van Den Berg, Edwin Straus, and Temple Fay may be cited as representative analyses that have contributed significantly to our knowledge concerning the "why" of human movement.[41–43]

According to the old psychologic stimulus→response theory, the individual is merely a communication channel between the input and the output. This view fails to consider the contribution that the individual makes to the circuit. In information theory it is recognized that through experience man accumulates certain knowledge about his external environment, such as how an object travels through space, and that the signals he receives from his kinesthetic proprioceptors reveal to him how his body is responding to the external presentation. The individual is viewed as a limited-capacity channel, receiving and responding to signals originating from internal sources as well as from the external display. The relative importance of these two types of stimuli in determining individual response appears to vary with practice and with the ease or difficulty of the required response. One of the chief difficulties confronting a performer is to separate one signal from another when they are presented in rapid succession. Perception of essential data is usually obscured by competing signals that create "noise" on the input circuits. A distinguishing characteristic of a skilled performer is his ability to select, integrate, and respond only to those signals that are germane to the situation; that is, in effect, to filter out signals that are mere noise. The fact that stimuli may be correlated with each other may enhance the difficulty for the performer.

Engineering theory treats communications systems as organisms. Because the two are operationally equivalent (Table 1–1), the insights of the cyberneticians (scientists who postulate that the processes of control are similar in the animal, the machine, and an organizational structure) and the psychologists are also equivalent and may be used interchangeably (Fig. 1–2).

The modifications that a man makes in his environment cause a change of input from that environment into his organism. Feedback from these functional alterations affect his structure. Alterations of structure affect the relationship between the various components and result in changes in function. Thus man to some extent is his own architect.

Since the appearance of the first edition of this book, the physiologically motivated researchers largely have concerned themselves with the waveforms of electrical activity in the nerves or brain or in the transmission properties of nerve tissue. Psychologically oriented investigators have tended to search for

Table 1–1.   Operational Relationships of Communications Systems and Biological Organisms

Communications Systems	Biological Organisms
Source of input	Environment
Transmitter	Sensory organs
Communications network	Peripheral nervous system
Receiver	Central nervous system
Communication controls	Kinesthetic processes
Feedback	Learning

regular descriptions of the input-output of the human organisms. For example, the neuro-geometric theory holds that the receptor and the motor systems are linked by space-time organized feedback mechanisms. These are multidimensional. Motion is made up of posture, transport, manipulation, and tremor movements, each controlled by its own sensory feedback. The brain coordinates and regulates these feedbacks. Learning is thus based on the brain's integration of the anatomic and

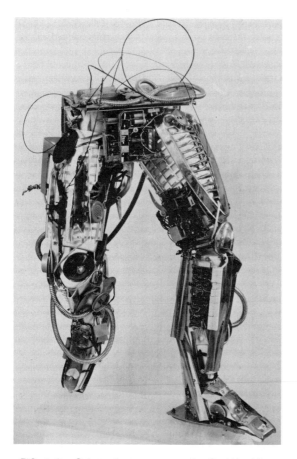

FIG. 1–2.   Cybernetic man, as seen by Paul Van Hoey-donck. (Reproduced by special permission of the artist and the Museum of Contemporary Art, Chicago.)

physiologic relations between the efferent and the afferent systems.

Such new insights have rich import for kinesiology, but also introduce new complications. The advanced student must now become accustomed to such explanations as the suggestion that a smooth landing after a drop is due to the release of a "complete preprogrammed open-loop sequence of neuromuscular activity virtually unaided by myotatic feedback."[44]

While further use of the electromyograph will continue to refine our understanding of how the body functions, it seems unlikely that additional major surprises will emerge from this technique. Probably, the next important advances will result from computer simulation studies, particularly of situations in which it would be impossible to use human subjects (Fig. 1–3).

In the second half of the twentieth century, kinesiology has gradually emerged as a distinct entity in the family of scholarly scientific disciplines. Like all disciplines, its origins have been in discrete human needs and practical problems; its organized form has become much more comprehensive and theoretically integrated. As a discipline, the focus is on the movement behavior of living organisms.

The Society for Behavioral Kinesiology has defined behavioral kinesiology as "the science of the structures and processes of human movement and their modification by inherent factors, by environmental events, and by therapeutic intervention." Although definitions such as this have done much to expand the concept of kinesiology beyond the historical constraints of "applied anatomy," the limitation of a discipline to the study of human phenomena and applications is inappropriate and has not been characteristic of other biologically based disciplines. For one thing, such limitation excludes the impressive body

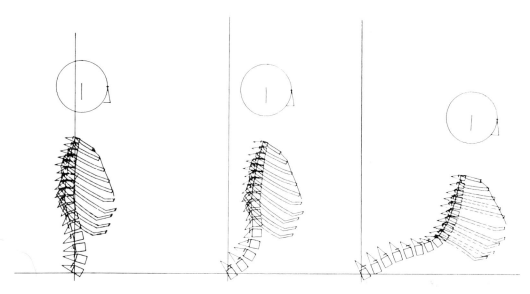

NORMAL SPINE   30 MPH CRASH SIMULATION 20 MSEC   30 MPH CRASH SIMULATION 40 MSEC

FIG. 1–3. Quite possibly, the next major advances in kinesiology will result from computer simulation studies. The above figures illustrate the effect of a 30-mph automobile crash on the human spine as shown by drawings derived from a computer. Such methods will provide the researcher with data it would be impossible to obtain from actual subjects. (Courtesy Albert B. Schultz, University of Illinois at Chicago Circle.) A PC program that reads radiographic data simulates the spine on which they are based, and compares that spine with the "normal" spine for persons of the patient's physical characteristics is already available but is very expensive.

of knowledge pertaining to the movement of nonhuman organisms and therefore tends to ignore the pervasive theoretical generalizations that emerge from comparative phylogenetic and ontogenetic data.

A vivid example is seen in the work of Kortlandt,[45] whose study of chimpanzees led him to conclude that living in the forest encourages peaceful living and walking on all fours, whereas living in the open grasslands favors aggressive hunting and the use of weapons, which demand walking on two limbs in order to free the other two. Although his interpretations have been challenged, they serve to illustrate the scope of the problems that kinesiologists may consider.

Kinesiologists of the future may find themselves concerned with the entire range of living organisms, and they may be required to integrate a number of disciplinary subdivisions, such as Structural-Functional Kinesiology, dealing with interactional relationships between the structure and movement functions of organisms; Exercise Physiology, which examines the physiology and biochemistry of homeostatic adjustments and disruptions of organisms under various conditions

of movement stress; Biomechanics, the investigation of movement phenomena through the concepts of physics and by means of engineering techniques; Developmental Kinesiology, relating movement to growth, development, nutrition, aging, and similar phenomena; Motor Behavior, encompassing systems analysis of motor control, motor learning, and neuromotor behavior; and Symbolic or Psychological Kinesiology, the study of the mutualities of movement and meaning, as implied in such topics as body image, self-image, aesthetic expression, cultural communication, personality, motivation, and self-realization.

At this point a warning is in order. A narrative history of this kind gives the student the impression that a science develops in a linear fashion by a series of independent discoveries by scientists; each has supplied a concept, a theory, a fact, or a law. But, as Kuhn has demonstrated in his invaluable *The Structure of Scientific Revolutions*,[46] this is not the way a science develops. Each generation has its own paradigms and its own instruments and concepts for working with them. As new and unexpected phenomena are uncovered by scientific research, these paradigms are found to be unable to explain them. A crisis arises, and new theories are devised to explain these anomalies. In effect, a scientific revolution occurs.

The next generation of scientists has a new world view and poses questions that were not even conceivable under the old theories. Rather than being a linear progression in which each step brings mankind closer to "the truth," scientific development is a process of evolution whose successive stages are characterized by an increasing understanding of nature. It is, Kuhn suggests, evolution from what we know to evolution toward what we wish to know. Unfortunately space here is insufficient to discuss this further. Students who wish to *understand* how the developments described in this chapter actually occurred will find Kuhn's booklet an essential guide.

REFERENCES*

1. Aristotle: Progression of Animals. English translation by E.S. Forster. Cambridge, Harvard University Press, n.d., p. 489.
2. Heath, Thomas Little: Archimedes. Encyclopaedia Britannica, Vol. II, 1972, pp. 298–299.
3. Snook, George A.: The father of sports medicine. Am. J. Sports Med., 6:128–131, 1978.
4. Steindler, Arthur: Mechanics of Normal and Pathological Locomotion in Man. Springfield, Charles C Thomas, 1935, pp. 1–9.
5. Oster, Gerald: Muscle sounds. Sci. Am., 250:108–114, March 1984.
6. Harvey, William: An Anatomical Disquisition on the Motion of the Heart and Blood in Animals. *In* Classics of Medicine and Surgery, collected by C.N.B. Camac. New York, Dover Publications, 1959, pp. 24–113.
7. Miller, William Snow: Niels Stensen: Bull. Johns Hopkins Hosp., 25:44–51, 1914.
8. Fulton, J.F.: Muscular Contraction and the Reflex Control of Movement. Baltimore, The Williams and Wilkins Co., 1926, pp. 3–55.
9. Andry, Nicolas: Orthopaedia. Facsimile Reproduction. Philadelphia, J.B. Lippincott Co., 1961.
10. Taylor, F. Sherwood: A Short History of Science and Scientific Thought. New York, W.W. Norton & Company, Inc., 1949, p. 118.
11. Sir Isaac Newton's Mathematical Principles of Natural Philosophy and His System of the World, July 5, 1668. English translation by Andrew Motte, 1729; revision by Florian Cajori. Berkeley, University of California Press, 1946.
12. French, R.K.: Robert Whytt: The Soul and Medicine.

London, Wellcome Institute of History of Medicine, 1969, pp. 63–92.
13. The Works of John Hunter. Edited by James F. Palmer. London, Longman, Rees, Orme, Brown, Green, and Longman, 1837, 4:195–273.
14. Galvani, Luigi: Commentary on the Effects of Electricity on Muscular Motion. Translated by Margaret Glover Foley. Norwalk, Conn., Burnaby Library, 1953.
15. Duchenne, G.B.: Physiology of Motion. Translated and edited by Emanuel B. Kaplan. Philadelphia, W.B. Saunders Co., 1959.
16. Jokl, Ernst, and Reich, Joseph: Guillaume Benjamin Amand Duchenne de Boulogne. J. Assoc. Phys. Ment. Rehabil., 10:154–159, 1956.
17. Muybridge, Eadweard: The Human Figure in Motion. New York, Dover Publications, 1955.
18. Human Mechanics. AMRL-TDR-63-123. Wright-Patterson Air Force Base: Aerospace Medical Research Laboratories, 1963.
19. Dempster, Wilfrid Taylor: Space Requirements of the Seated Operator. Washington, D.C.: U.S. Department of Commerce, 1955.
20. Siebert, Werner W.: Investigation of hypertrophy of the skeletal muscle. Translated by Robert Kramer. J. Assoc. Phys. Ment. Rehabil., 14:153–157, 1960.
21. Steinhaus, Arthur H.: Strength from Morpurgo to Muller—A half century of research. J. Assoc. Phys. Ment. Rehabil., 9:147–150, 1955.
22. Granit, Ragnar: The Basis of Motor Control. New York, Academic Press, 1970, p. 1.
23. Selected Writings of John Hughlings Jackson. Edited by James Taylor. Vol. 1. London. Hodder & Stoughton, 1931, pp. 420–421.
24. Beevor, Charles: The Croonian Lectures on Muscular Movements Delivered Before the Royal College of Physicians of London, June, 1903. London, Macmillan and Co., Ltd., n.d.
25. Steindler, Arthur: Kinesiology of the Human Body Under Normal and Pathological Conditions. Springfield, Charles C Thomas, 1955, p. 7.
26. Sherrington, Charles: Man on His Nature. 2nd Ed. Garden City, Doubleday & Co., Inc., 1953, p. 110.
27. Cited in Ruch, Theodore C., and Patton, Harry D.: Physiology and Biophysics, 19th Ed. Philadelphia, W.B. Saunders Co., 1965, p. 114.
28. Bassett, C.A.L.: Biologic significance of piezoelectricity. Calcif. Tissue Res., 1:252–272, 1968.
29. Koch, John C.: The laws of bone architecture. Am. J. Anat., 21:177–298, 1917.
30. Evans, F. Gaynor: Stress and Strain in Bones. Springfield, Charles C Thomas, 1957.
31. Carey, Eben J.: Studies in the dynamics of histogenesis. Experimental, surgical and roentgenographic studies in the architecture of human cancellous bone, the resultant of back pressure vectors of muscle action. Radiology, 13:127–168, 1929.
32. Scott, J.H.: Muscle growth and function in relation to skeletal morphology. Am. J. Phys. Anthropol., 15(NS):197–234, 1957.
33. Taylor, Frederick W.: Principles of Scientific Management. New York, Harper & Brothers, 1915.
34. Amar, Jules: The Human Motor. Reprinted. Dubuque, Brown Reprints, 1972.
35. Adrian, E.D.: Interpretation of the electromyogram. Lancet, 2:1229–1233, 1925; 2:1283–1286, 1925.
36. Basmajian, J.V., and MacConaill, M.A.: Muscles & Movement: A Basis for Human Kinesiology. Revised Edition. Huntington, N.Y., Krieger, 1977.

*When possible, citations are usually to an edition that the student may readily secure, rather than to the original edition. In the cases of prolific authors, only the item most important or most typical of their work is cited.

37. Hill, A.V.: First and Last Experiments in Muscle Mechanics. London, Cambridge University Press, 1970.
38. Huxley, H.E.: The Croonian Lecture, 1970. The structural basis of muscular contraction. Proc. R. Soc. Lond., *B178*:131–149, 1971.
39. Huxley, A.F.: The Croonian Lecture, 1967. The activation of striated muscle and its mechanical response. Proc. R. Soc. Lond., *B178*:1–27, 1971.
40. Karpovich, Peter V.: Physiology of Muscular Activity. 6th Ed. Philadelphia, W.B. Saunders Co., 1965, p. 253.
41. Van Den Berg, J.H.: The human body and the significance of human movement. Philosophy and Phenomenological Res., *13*:159–183, 1952.
42. Straus, Edwin: The upright posture. Psychiatry, *26*:529–561, 1953.
43. Fay, Temple: The origin of human movement. Am. J. Psychiatry, *111*:644–652, 1955.
44. Watt, D., and Jones, G. Melville: On the functional role of the myotatic reflex in man. Proc. Canad. Fed. Biol. Soc., *9*:13, 1966.
45. Kortlandt, Adriaan: Chimpanzees in the wild. Sci. Am., *206*:128–138, 1962.
46. Kuhn, Thomas S.: The Structure of Scientific Revolutions. 2nd Ed. Enlarged. Chicago, University of Chicago Press, 1970.

RECOMMENDED READING

Atwater, Anne E.: Kinesiology/Biomechanics: perspectives and trends. Res. Q. Ex. Sport, *51*:193–218, 1980.
Clein, Marvin J.: The early historical roots of therapeutic exercise. JOHPER, *41*:89–91, 1970.
Jokl, Ernst: Motor functions of the human brain. A historical review. Medicine and Sport, Vol. 6. Biomechanics II, 1–27. Basel: Karger, 1971.

2 THE FRAMEWORK AND COMPOSITION OF THE BODY

PHILIP J. RASCH

The adult skeleton contains approximately 206 bones. The use of dried bones as skeletal demonstration materials frequently generates the impression that the skeleton is a hard, rigid, static structure comparable to steel girders in a skyscraper. One purpose of this chapter is to show that skeletal structures are dynamic, living, developing, growing tissues whose metabolism influences function and is influenced by function.

THE COMPOSITION AND STRUCTURE OF BONES

Constituents of Bone Tissue. About 25 to 30% of bone is water. The remainder is what engineers describe as a "two-phase" material. Approximately 60 to 70% is composed of mineral (calcium phosphate and calcium carbonate), which gives bone the ability to resist compression; the balance is made up of collagen (a protein), which provides its ability to resist tension. Generally speaking, a bone can withstand about six times the stresses to which it is subject in ordinary activities. After maturity, the proportions of fluid and organic material gradually decrease with age. For these and other reasons, the bones of aged people are brittle and healing becomes more difficult.

The exterior of bone is composed of cortical or trabecular (compact, dense) tissue; the interior is composed of cancellous (spongy, lattice-like) tissue (Fig. 2–1). These two tissues differ in their amount of solid material and their amount of open space but can be con-

sidered as one material. The relative quantity of each varies in different bones and in different parts of a single bone, depending on the functional needs.

The fact that bones are a tissue means that they can hypertrophy as a result of exercise but are also vulnerable and may be damaged by overly severe training or repeated stress, especially in immature athletes. This problem is especially serious in the case of young female gymnasts.

Kinds of Bones. *Long bones,* such as the humerus and tibia, are found in the limbs. *Short bones* are roughly cubical and are represented by only the carpal and tarsal bones. *Flat bones,* represented by the sternum, ribs, some of the skull bones, ilium, and scapulae, have outer layers of compact bone with an interior of spongy bone and marrow. They are designed to serve as extensive flat areas for the attachment of muscles and ligaments, and, except for the scapulae, to enclose cavities. They are usually curved, thick where tendons and fascia sheets attach, and thin to the point of translucence where the fleshy muscle fibers attach directly to the bone. *Irregular bones,* such as the ischium, pubis, maxilla, and vertebrae, are adapted to special purposes.

Structure and Functions of the Long Bones. Evolutionally, the long bones are adapted for weight-bearing and for sweeping, speedy excursions. They serve these purposes admirably because of their tubular form, their broad and specialized articular surfaces and shapes at their ends, and their great length.

18

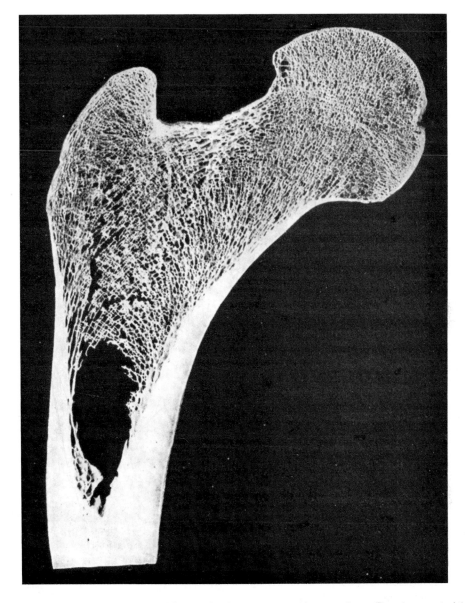

FIG. 2–1. Frontal longitudinal midsection of femur, showing compact and spongy bone. The placement of the curved lines of the trabeculae is exquisitely suited to bear the stresses shown in Fig. 2–2, while keeping bone mass at a minimum. Evidence suggests that trabecular bone in the lower limbs of cross-country runners can hypertrophy and that the amount of cancellous bone is reduced during aging. (Gray's Anatomy. 30th Ed. Philadelphia, Lea & Febiger, 1985, p. 3).

Both the proximal and distal ends typically display protrusions called condyles, tubercles, or tuberosities, which serve as attachments or "pulleys" for tendons and ligaments. The shapes of the articular surfaces are commonly specialized to enable the bone to fit securely into the conformations of its neighbors and to determine or limit the kind of action possible at the joint. Each articular surface has a cap of hyaline cartilage, which functions to increase the smoothness of fit, prevent excess wear, absorb shocks, and prevent dislocations of the joints.

Toward the ends of long bones, the medullary cavity gives way to *spongy* or *cancellous bone* within the external layers of compact bone. Spongy bone is as hard as compact bone but is arranged in a complex grillwork.

These bars of latticework are called *cancelli* or *trabeculae* (from Latin, meaning lattice bars or little beams). The basic tubular structure of long bones conserves weight, at the same time providing great resistance to stress and strain (Figs. 2–1 and 2–2). The tensile strength of compact bone is 230 times greater than that for muscle of a similar cross section.[1]

Membranes of Bone. The *periosteum* is a connective tissue that covers the outside surface of bones, except at articular surfaces, where it is replaced by the articular hyaline cartilage. It has two layers, an outside layer of collagenous fibers, and a deep layer that is osteogenic (that is, capable of producing *osteoblasts*, which in turn may develop into osteocytes). Periosteum is supplied with blood vessels and nerve branches. It is extremely sensitive to injury, and from it originates most of the pain of fractures, bone bruises, and "shin splints." It adheres to the outer surface of compact bone by sending tiny processes, similar to small roots, into the bone. Muscles are attached to periosteum, not directly to the bone.

Effects of Bone Function on Bone Structure. The term "bone remodeling" refers to the ability of bone to respond to the mechanical demands placed on it by changing its size, shape, and structure in accordance with Wolff's law (see Chapter 1). It remodels by laying down bone where needed and by reabsorbing it where not needed. However, Wolff's law of bone transformation was an overstatement. Bone forms in response to many factors, including hereditary tendencies, nutrition, disease, and hormonal and biochemical influences. Yet functional stress is certainly significant. Bone growing in tissue culture, isolated from a living organism, has been known to adapt to artificial forces present. Normal bone repair and growth after fractures is found to be suited to the stresses received. Constant irritative pressures, such

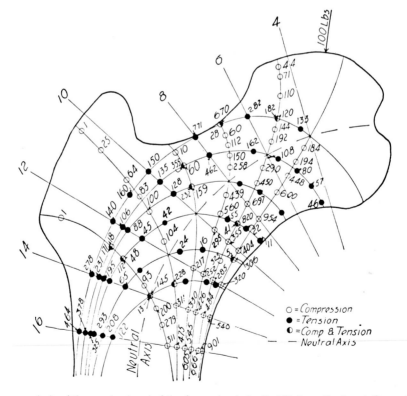

FIG. 2–2. Stress analysis of the proximal end of the femur, loaded with 100 lb on the head. Curved lines show the directional paths of maximum tensile and compressive forces and their magnitude in lb/sq in. These forces should be multiplied by 1.6 for walking and by 3.2 for running. The femoral neck will fail at approximately 2000 lb load. (Koch, Amer. J. Anat., 21:249, 1917.) One result of the recent surge of interest in jogging and marathon running is reported to be an increase in the incidence of stress fractures of the femoral neck.

as occur in postural deformities, cause bone to atrophy, but the intermittent stresses of normal muscular activity produce significantly increased cross-sectional areas and allow the bones to carry a greater load and absorb more energy before failure occurs.[2]

A confirmation of Wolff's theory is seen in the effects of the lack of stress. Bones atrophy or cease to grow when muscular and functional forces are negated by paralysis. Even a few weeks of encasement in a plaster cast are accompanied by noticeable atrophy. Bones lose substance during prolonged spaceflights, just as they do in encasement. In both cases urinary calcium is significantly increased. The greatest changes occur in weight-bearing bones, suggesting that reductions in mechanical loading are important, although vigorous exercise by spaceflight crews does not eliminate bone loss. Soviet scientists have found that rats subjected to prolonged spaceflight develop significantly larger adrenal glands. This affect reflects an increase in corticosterone content, which has been shown to decrease bone formation and the number of osteoblasts. If the hypercalciuria and decrease in bone formation were to continue for an extended period, osteoporosis might result.[3]

Osteoporosis is a major public health problem. It is defined as an age-related disorder characterized by decreased bone mass and by increased susceptibility to fractures.[4] Women are at a higher risk than men because men have 30% more bone mass than women; whites are at a higher risk than blacks because blacks have approximately 10% more bone mass than whites.

In women, early menopause is one of the strongest predictors of osteoporosis. Numerous studies have shown that the low estrogen states associated with early menopause are also associated with low levels of skeletal bone mass. Treatment includes estrogen replacement and calcium supplementation. Exercise involving weight-bearing may reduce bone loss and increase bone mass, but the optimal type and amount of physical activity have yet to be determined.[4] Drinkwater et al. comment that "numerous questions remain to be answered regarding the long-term effect of amenorrhea on the skeletal integrity of female athletes."[5]

GROWTH AND DEVELOPMENT OF BONES

Ossification of Bones. *Ossification* means the depositing of bone salts in an organic matrix. It must be preceded by the differentiation and proliferation of the cells that will lay down the collagenous matrix, and this may occur either in an existing connective tissue membrane, producing *intramembranous ossification*, or in hyaline cartilage, producing *endochondral* or *intracartilaginous ossification*. The clavicle and most skull bones ossify intramembranously, the short bones intracartilaginously, and the long bones by both methods.

Ossification of Long Bones. In the embryo, hyaline cartilage models of the bones appear. Well before birth, a primary center of ossification, known as a *diaphysis*, arises near the center of the future shaft of long bones. Ossification progresses in all directions from these primary centers. At the same time, a *bone collar* ossifies intramembranously in the periosteum around the shaft, defining its outside diameter. One or more secondary centers of ossification, called *bony epiphyses*, develop at the ends of the long bones. The time of such development is specific for each center, some appearing before birth and some as late as adolescence. This epiphyseal ossification also progresses circumferentially, and finally all the original cartilage has been replaced except for a comparatively thin *epiphyseal cartilage*, *epiphyseal plate*, or *epiphyseal disk* that separates the shaft or diaphysis from the end or epiphysis. The most recently formed bone at the end of the diaphysis is called the *metaphysis*.

Growth of Long Bones. Growth in diameter occurs most rapidly before maturity, but can continue during nearly all of the life of the individual. The periosteum produces concentric layers of bone on the outside, while a more or less proportionate resorption of bones takes place in the medullary cavity, enlarging its diameter.

Growth in length is a continuation of ossification of the diaphysis toward the epiphysis. However, the epiphyseal cartilage continues to proliferate and keep the diaphysis and epiphysis separated. At an age that is specific for each epiphysis, varying from middle childhood to adulthood, the epiphyseal cartilage ceases to proliferate, and bony union (*closure*) takes place between diaphysis and epiphysis, usually leaving an elevated ridge called the *epiphyseal line* on the surface of the matured bone.

Theoretical considerations have led some writers to suggest that chronic intense work, such as weight training or distance running, during youth may damage the articular cartilages or overload the epiphyses and result in growth disturbances. Earlier closure, for instance, would result in a failure to attain one's potential stature. These considerations signal a need for caution in such activities; however, defining the line between training and overtraining is very difficult, and scientific evidence on the subject is lacking. The possibility of such trauma requires that the cause of pain in weight-bearing joints be carefully diagnosed and treated.

Physical educators often pay attention to the size of the bones, as seen at the wrist, ankles, and hips, in order to get a better estimate of an individual's capacity for bearing weights and stresses. In general, the bones of black individuals are denser than those of white individuals, and those of the male are denser than those of the female. One investigator reported that the bone densities of black females were 15 to 20% higher than those of white females, which, he suggested, explained the relatively few occurrences of fractures in the former group.[6] Most right-handed people have greater bone density in the right phalanges than in the left, whereas the relationship is reversed in left-handed people.

Growth of Short Bones. A short bone usually grows as if it were an epiphysis, except that it maintains its independent identity.

Influence of Trauma. Numerous factors affecting bone growth were mentioned earlier in this chapter in the discussion of Wolff's law. In addition, bone growth may be affected adversely by trauma. Either a single catastrophic force or repeated severe insults can stop bone growth or dislocate the growing parts at the epiphyseal cartilage. Interrupted growth is often considered to be more serious than a clean fracture in a fully ossified area

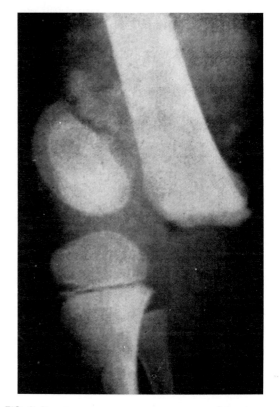

FIG. 2–3.   Dislocation of the distal femoral epiphysis of a high school football player. The patient suffered considerable shortening of this leg as a result of premature closure of the epiphysis and subsequently required a shortening of the good leg. (Courtesy Leonard F. Bush, M.D.)

of the same bone, partly because pain and deformity are less obvious at the time of injury, resulting in the delay of corrective measure until an irremediable defect has resulted. The strength of the fibrous capsule and ligaments surrounding a joint is two to five times greater than the strength of the metaphyseal-epiphyseal junction. Consequently, "sprains" in children must be carefully evaluated to rule out possible injury to the epiphyses (Fig. 2–3).

Most of the major epiphyses do not close until 17 to 19 years of age. Therefore, many orthopedists regard football, wrestling, and other stressful contact sports as undesirable during the period of bone immaturity. From the kinesiologic point of view, the following questions are pertinent:

How serious is the danger of anatomic injury?

Is it greater in the organized sports programs than in the unsupervised sandlot activities that it replaces?

Can the rules be modified to minimize the danger of trauma?

Is adequate protective equipment available and used?

Is there adequate medical supervision of injuries?

Are medical examinations required of participants?

Are the managers, teachers, coaches, and officials aware of anatomic physiologic factors in growth and development, and do they use their prestige and authority in such a manner as to protect the safety of the participants?

Ossification Dates. The statement that the age at which epiphyseal fusion takes place is specific for each epiphysis should not be interpreted too literally. It is true that the fusion ages at various centers provide an amazingly accurate physiologic time clock, but the clock can run slow or fast according to the state of endocrine secretion, health, and nutrition of the individual. Undoubtedly there are racial, geographic, and hereditary differences, although these have not as yet been adequately determined. On the average, a given epiphysis will ossify and growth in the length of the bone will cease from 1 to 3 years earlier in a female than in a male. Trauma or overstrain may cause premature closure, but illhealth and malnutrition are likely to delay the date. None of the epiphyses of the limbs fuse before puberty, but all of the epiphyses will normally be fused before age 21.

A youngster who is larger than average or who is obese is often subjected to unwarranted epiphyseal stresses. His bulk may give a false impression of the degree of his bony maturity. For this reason, age should be a factor in athletic classification indices, and sports leaders should not (for example) always put the biggest boy on the bottom of a pyramid in gymnastic lessons. Radiographs of the degree of ossification of carpal bones provide a precise estimation of skeletal and physiologic maturity of preadolescents.

THE ARCHITECTURE OF JOINTS

Types of Joints. The junction of two bones is called a *joint* or *articulation*. There are three classes of joints, the *synarthrodial* or immovable, the *amphiarthrodial* or slightly movable, and the *diarthrodial* or freely movable. The first two classes have no true joint cavity; the third class has a joint cavity and is subdivided into seven types. The classification and terminology of joints are presented differently by various authors. A reasonably complete listing of types and terms is presented in Table 2–1 with descriptive explanations, but students are cautioned to be alert for small differences in classification when consulting other source books. Each specific joint of the body has its own peculiarities.

Diarthrodial Joints. The diarthrodial, freely movable, or synovial joints are of greatest interest to students of human motion. The typical structural aspects are shown in Figure 2–4. The weight-bearing or articular surfaces of the bones are covered with a layer of hyaline cartilage known as *articular cartilage*. Being resilient but not especially brittle, this cartilage absorbs shocks and prevents direct wear on the bones to ensure a better fit. It has no nerve or blood supply of its own. In some joints, the articular cartilages show specialized modifications and are given distinct names, as is the case with the *glenoid labrum* of the shoulder joint and the *semilunar cartilages* or *menisci* of the knee. The joints must not be thought of as a hard surface. They should be considered as resilient bearings, with the articular cartilage having characteristics somewhere between those of a solid and of a liquid. Under pressure the cartilage appears to exude lubricant in advance of the point of pressure, but the mechanics involved are not well understood.

A ligamentous sleeve called the *capsule* or *capsular ligament* is attached firmly to both bones of the joint, enclosing it completely. This capsule is lined internally by a thin vascular *synovial membrane*, which secretes *synovial fluid* or *synovia* into the *joint cavity*. The synovial fluid provides nourishment to the articular cartilages, lubricates the joint, and converts the compressive stress, which would otherwise harm the high spots, to hydrostatic stress, which is much less damaging to the material of the joint. Normally, only 2 ml or less of synovial fluid is present, and there is a slight negative pressure (suction) in the joint

Table 2–1. Classification of Joints by Structure and Action

Kind	Class	Type — Common Name	Type — Technical Name	Explanation and Examples
Without a joint cavity	I. Synarthrosis (immovable)	A. Fibrous	Suture*	Two bones grow together, with only a thin layer of fibrous periosteum between. E.g., sutures of the skull.
	II. Amphiarthrosis (slightly movable)	B. Ligamentous	Syndesmosis*	Slight movement permitted by meager elasticity of a ligament joining two bones, which may be distinctly separated. E.g., coracoacromial "joint"; mid-radioulnar joint; mid-tibiofibular joint; inferior tibiofibular joint.
		C. Cartilaginous	Synchondrosis or symphysis	Bones are coated with hyaline cartilage, separated by a fibrocartilage disk, and joined by ligaments. Motion is allowed only by deformation of the disk. E.g., between bodies of vertebrae; symphysis pubis; between manubrium and body of sternum.
Having a joint cavity	III. Diarthrosis (freely movable)	1. Gliding joint	Arthrosis or plane joint	Nonaxial. Allows gliding or twisting. E.g., intercarpal and intertarsal joints.
		2. Hinge joint	Ginglymus	Uniaxial. A concave surface glides around a convex surface, allowing flexion and extension. E.g., elbow joint.
		3. Pivot joint	Trochoid joint	Uniaxial. A rotation around a vertical or long axis is allowed. E.g., atlantoaxial joint; proximal radioulnar joint.
		4. Ellipsoid joint	Ellipsoid joint	Biaxial. An "oval" ball-and-socket joint, allowing flexion, extension, abduction, adduction, and circumduction, but not rotation. E.g., carpometacarpal (wrist) joint.
		5. Condyloid joint	Condyloid joint	Biaxial. A spheroidal ball-and-socket joint with no muscles suitably located to perform rotation, which otherwise could take place. E.g., 2nd to 5th metacarpophalangeal joints (but not of the thumb).
		6. Ball-and-socket joint	Spheroid, or enarthrosis	Triaxial. Spheroidal ball-and-socket allows flexion, extension, abduction, adduction, circumduction, and rotation on the long axis. E.g., shoulder and hip joints.
		7. Saddle joint	Saddle joint	Triaxial. Both bones have a saddle-shaped surface fitted into each other. Allows flexion, extension, abduction, adduction, circumduction, and slight rotation. E.g., carpometacarpal joint of the thumb.

*Some classification systems include both sutures and syndesmoses under the heading of fibrous joints. Both sutures and syndesmoses tend to ossify completely in later life, in which case the union is known as a *synostosis*.

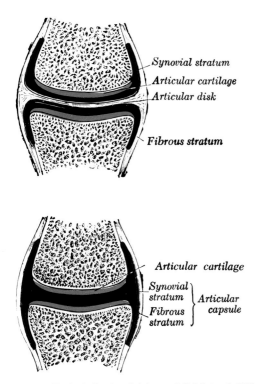

Synovial stratum

Articular cartilage

Articular disk

Fibrous stratum

Articular cartilage

Synovial stratum ⎫
Fibrous stratum ⎭ *Articular capsule*

FIG. 2–4. Typical diarthrodial (synovial) joints. *A*, With an articular disk. *B*, Without an articular disk. (Gray's Anatomy, Philadelphia, Lea & Febiger.)

cavity. Thus, the "cavity" is difficult to find and explore in dissection, unless it has previously been injected to expand it. Injury or irritation, however, causes profuse secretion of synovial fluid, sometimes resulting in evident swelling.

Some diarthrodial joints have an intra-articular *fibrocartilage disk* that partitions the joint cavity into two parts. This sectioning makes it resemble a synchondrosis or cartilaginous articulation (Table 2–1), except that the later has no cavity or synovial membrane. The sternoclavicular and distal radioulnar joints are diarthrodial joints having fibrocartilage disks. The attachments of these disks have peculiarities that enable them to assist in holding the bones together.

The ligamentous capsules sometimes have definite thickenings on one or more aspects, and these are sometimes named as separate ligaments. In addition, typically several other ligaments join the two bones and are discrete from the capsule. Ligaments are tough and practically nonelastic. Their function is to bind bones together and to limit range of movement. Tensile stresses, if constantly applied, may result in their gradual lengthening—even to the point of destroying their function of maintaining the integrity of the joint.

Every synovial joint contains at least one male and one female articular surface. There is only a single position in which they are fully congruent. In this position the two surfaces fit point for point, and gravity or muscular force causes the principal ligaments of the joint (especially hinge joints) to become so taut that they screw the articular surfaces together in such a way that the two bones function as a single unit. This is known as the *close packed* position. In all other positions the male and female surfaces are not fully congruent. The ligaments tend to be slack, and the joint is said to be in the *loose packed* position.

Numerous factors contribute to the stability and integrity of synovial joints. Suction in the joint cavity can be a powerful inhibitor of traction-dislocation. Depth of fit of the male and female surfaces may (as in the acetabulum) or may not (as in the shoulder joint) provide stability. Ligaments bind adjacent bones together tightly when the joint is close packed or at the extreme of its range of motion. Contracting muscles can exert tremendous stabilizing forces. Injuries and habitually sagging postures can permanently overstretch the ligaments; when coupled with weak muscles, this condition predisposes a joint to easy dislocation.

Tendons and sheets of fascia cross most joints. Although their function is usually considered to be the transference of muscle tension to cause movement, the fact that they hold bones together should never be overlooked. Because most muscles insert at very small angles, a large component of muscular force is usually directed along the bone toward the joint, tending to reinforce the joint by pulling the bones together.

Bursae and Tendon Sheaths. Wherever soft structures are frequently submitted to frictional rubbing on a bony protuberance, the friction is reduced by the appearance of tough connective tissue and some form of synovial sac. Even tendons cannot withstand constant friction on a bone without further protection. Frequently tendons are surrounded by a cylindric sac consisting of two layers of connective tissue, the interior of which is firmly attached to the tendon and the exterior of which is attached to the surrounding tissue. The cavity of this *tendon sheath* is lined with synovial membrane, secreting a small amount of lubricating fluid into the cavity and preventing solid tissues from rubbing directly against each other. Nontendinous soft structures are similarly protected. Thus, the fascia and skin at the back of the elbow are separated from the olecranon process by a simple synovial sac called a *bursa*. Bursae occur in many other places. For example, as the supraspinatus muscle passes under the acromion process, it is separated from that hard structure by the *subacrominal bursa*; similarly, the patellar ligament is protected from the head of the tibia by the *deep infrapatellar bursa*. Bursae and tendon sheaths are not parts of joints in a technical sense, but may be regarded as associated structures.

JOINT MOTION TERMINOLOGY

Description of joint movement, whether movement of only one joint or of a number of joints, follows a generalized system based on planes and axes and related directional terms. The planes and axes are defined with respect to the anatomic position, which places the body standing erect with the feet together, arms at the side, and the palms facing forward. The *sagittal* plane divides the body into left and right parts. Joint actions in the sagittal plane occur about a horizontal axis, which, like all axes, lies orthogonal to its associated plane, and include flexion and extension. The *coronal* or *frontal* plane divides the body into *anterior* (ventral) and *posterior* (dorsal) parts. Movements in this plane, which occur about an anteroposterior (AP) axis, include abduction and adduction. The *transverse* plane, associated with the *vertical* axis, divides the body into *superior* (cranial) and *inferior* (caudal) parts. Motion about the long axis of a bone such as medial-lateral rotation and pronation-supination occur in this plane.

Other anatomic directional terms include *medial* and *lateral*, which refer to landmarks either closer or further from the midline, respectively; *superficial* and *deep*, referring to the depth from the surface; and *proximal* and *distal*, indicating a direction toward or away from the center of the body, respectively.

Flexion at any joint takes place when any body segment is moved in a plane so that its anterior or posterior surface approaches the anterior or posterior surface, respectively, of an adjacent body segment. Thus, moving the left limb from anatomic position to scratch the back of the left shoulder blade involves flexion of the arm at the shoulder joint, of the forearm at the elbow, of the hand at the wrist, and of the fingers at the metacarpophalangeal and interphalangeal joints. Bringing the front surface of the thigh toward the abdomen is hip flexion. Bringing the calf of the leg toward the back of the thigh is knee flexion. Curling the toes is toe flexion. *Extension* is the reverse—the moving from a flexed position back toward the anatomic position, and even past it, if that is possible.

Abduction means moving a segment away from the center line of the body. Once started, the movement is called abduction throughout its entire range, even though, as in the case of abducting the arm at the shoulder joint, the part seems to be coming back toward the center line of the body during the second 90° of its excursion. *Adduction* is the reverse of abduction—the moving from a position of abduction back toward the anatomic position, and past it, if this is possible.

Rotation around the long axis of a bone can take place, for example, at the shoulder, hip, and knee joints. *Medial rotation* occurs when the anterior surface turns inward; *lateral rotation* is the reverse of this, when the anterior surface turns outward. With regard to rotation, the anatomic position is often regarded as the *neutral position*; thus, from a position of inward rotation, the thigh may be rotated outward to the neutral position and then further rotated outward.

Circumduction is a movement in which a body part describes a cone, with the apex at the joint and the base at the distal end of the part. There is no term to distinguish circumduction around a base of small radius from that around a base of large radius. Circumduction does not involve rotation; therefore, it may occur in biaxial joints like the metacarpophalangeal joints by a combination of flexion, abduction, extension, and adduction.

Hyperextension means a continuation of extension past anatomic position, usually. Thus, from the normally extended anatomic position of the elbow, slight further extension is possible in some people. This is characteristically seen in gymnasts. In no case does the prefix "hyper" indicate a different motion, but only an exceptional continuation of the movement involved.

In the tremendously varied activities of athletics, aquatics, combatives, gymnastics, dance, and recreational and vocational pursuits, the joint actions can become complex indeed. Confusion in terminology must be carefully minimized. For this reason, it is perhaps better to describe a joint action as (for example) "hip flexion" or "shoulder joint abduction" rather than "thigh flexion" or "arm abduction," although both usages are correct. If the term "thigh flexion" is employed, beginning students are sometimes confused when it is used to refer to a motion of the pelvis forward onto the thigh, as in doing sit-ups. The word "thigh" seems to indicate to some that the thigh must be the moving part, whereas there is no such connotation if "hip flexion" is used because attention is centered upon the joint rather than on the body part. The preference is strictly pedagogic.

MOBILITY OF JOINTS

Range of motion may be limited by ligaments (including the joint capsule), length and extensibility of muscles and fascia, tendons, occlusion of soft-tissue masses, or impingement of bone against bone. The transient state of voluntary muscular contraction, as well as the autogenic stretch reflex regulated by muscle spindle mechanisms, may also influence range of motion.

Flexibility (the common synonym for range of joint motion) is not usually a general factor, ordinarily being highly specific to each joint. Even the two joints of a bilateral pair in one person may vary markedly. Hypermobility of a joint, which is considered to result from a ligamentous laxity, represents one extreme in the normal variation in joint mobility.

A generalized pattern of hypermobility associated with musculoskeletal complaints in otherwise normal subjects is termed hypermobility syndrome. Such individuals are often said to be "double-jointed" and may suffer growing pains as children. As they mature they may experience osteoarthritis, joint pains, degenerative joint changes, recurrent dislocations, injury to ligaments, or rheumatic disease. Many such persons have poor muscular development. British physicians encourage them to swim as a regular exercise.[7]

"Benign hypermobility" indicates a generalized pattern of hypermobility not associated with an increased incidence of musculoskeletal complaints. Benign hypermobility is found in about 5% of the healthy adult United States and British populations and is more common in women than in men. Possibly this difference is due to the fact that the heavier musculature of men may restrict free joint movement[8] (but see Fig. 2–6).

The extent of hypermobility and the particular joints involved may affect performance in nearly every activity. Ballet dancers, for instance, often show a generalized joint hypermobility, and this may favor their selection for training. The dancer is taught to prevent by muscular control hyperextension of joints producing unaesthetic motions.

Successful participants in different sports demonstrate flexibility patterns typical for each sport. These patterns are significantly different from those of nonathletes. An overview of the experimental evidence supports the conclusion that flexibility correlates with habitual movement patterns for each person and each joint, and that age and sex differences are secondary rather than innate. Linear measurements of flexibility, such as the sit-and-reach test, are crude and unsatisfactory for comparisons of individuals.

In general, flexibility decreases gradually from birth to old age.

Habitual postures and chronic heavy work through restricted ranges of motion lead to adaptive shortening of muscles. Over a period of years, inflexibility tends to become permanent and irreversible, especially as the usual development of osteoarthritis invokes calcification of tissues near the joints. Thus, the foot of a baby shows remarkable flexibility, while the foot of an adult tends to be rigid

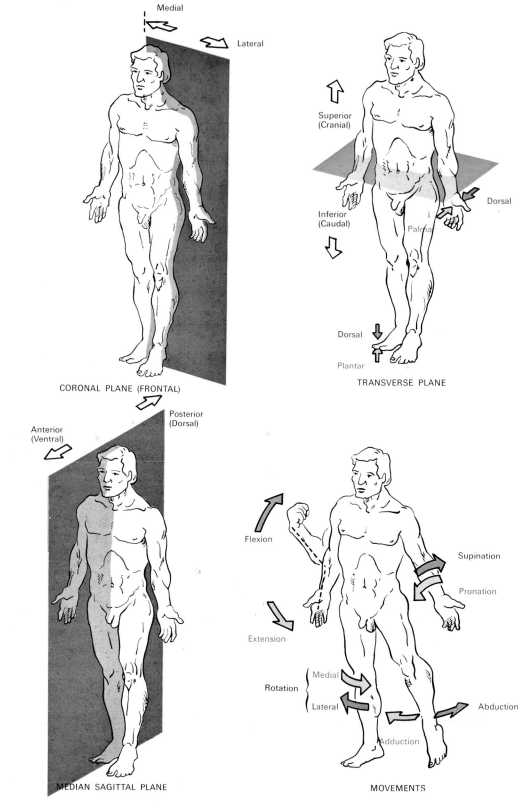

FIG. 2–5.   Diagrams illustrating the planes of the body and the terms of position and direction. (From Gray's Anatomy. 30th Ed. Philadelphia, Lea & Febiger, 1985, p. 3.)

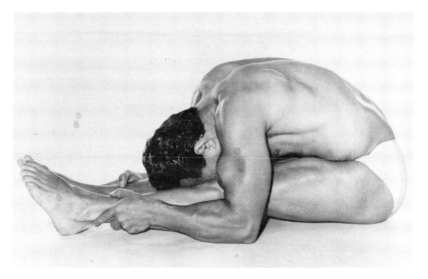

FIG. 2–6.   Walt Baptiste demonstrating that muscular strength and hypertrophy resulting from the practice of progressive resistance exercises are compatible with flexibility. (Courtesy Strength and Health.) Relationships between static tests of strength and ranges of flexion and extension of the lumbar spine are generally not statistically significant.

after years of encasement in shoes. A rounded program of progressive resistance exercise is likely to increase flexibility beyond normal ranges, when the movements are carried through a complete range of motion and when exercises are selected to include both members of antagonistic muscle groups (Fig. 2–6). Lack of normal flexibility may be responsible for bad posture, compression of peripheral nerves, dysmenorrhea, and other ailments.

Tables of normal ranges of motion are available but are remarkable for their lack of agreement. Discrepancies arise from unreliable instruments, lack of standardized measurement procedures, the shifting axis of rotation during movement in some joints, and a startlingly wide range of individual differences. Furthermore, average flexibility is not necessarily synonymous with optimum flexibility. An excellent review by Clarke provides a starting point for a more detailed knowledge of this subject.[9]

BODY COMPOSITION

Physical performance is related to body composition. Knowledge of a subject's weight alone is of limited usefulness. The most common approach to analysis of body composition has been to consider the body as made up of a fat component with a density of about 0.9007 and of a fat-free component with a density of 1.100. The total density of the body (D_b) is taken as the resultant of the densities of these two components. It is usually obtained by determining the following measurements: the mass of the subject in the air (M_a), the mass of the subject under water (M_w), the density of water at a standardized temperature (D_w), and the residual air volume of the lungs and respiratory passages (R_v). These are substituted in the formula

$$D_b = \frac{M_a}{\left(\dfrac{M_a - M_w}{D_w}\right)} - R_v$$

Once the D_b has been determined, the percentage of body fat (% F_b) can be calculated by the formula

$$\%F_b = 100 \left(\frac{4.570}{D_b} - 4.142\right)$$

Obviously, the lower the D_b, the higher the fat content.

There are two serious problems with the use of such formulae. First, in many cases they violate the rule that investigators must use equations that have been cross-validated on populations of similar characteristics. These equations were established on a young adult white male population. The fat-free density of a young black population has recently been found to be 1.113, and that of children ages 8 to 10 years is about 1.083. As a result, the actual body fat of black athletes has been seriously underestimated and that of children has been overestimated. Use of the equation

$$\%F_b = 100 \left(\frac{4.374}{D_b} - 3.928 \right)$$

has been recommended when dealing with black subjects.[10]

Second, it is becoming increasingly evident that the distribution of body fat may be as important as the total body fat.[11] Consequently, the student must be cautious when dealing with reports of earlier findings on these two populations.

Sophisticated methods involving the use of scintillation counters, electrical impedence, gas displacement techniques, nuclear magnetic resonance (NMR), computer-assisted tomography (CT), and other expensive high-technology instrumentation promise to produce more accurate data in the future. These methods are expensive and require the assistance of highly trained technicians. Because it is usually not possible to employ such equipment under field conditions, epidemiologic researchers often estimate body com-

position by using the Body Mass Index (sometimes called the Quetelet Index), where

$$BMI = \frac{\text{weight in kg}}{(\text{height in m})^2}$$

The BMI is a standard measure in the study of such epidemiologic problems as whether larger joggers/runners are more subject to injury than smaller ones are.

The relationship of the center of gravity (see Chapter 6) and body composition to success in women's gymnastics has received a great deal of attention. Most champion female gymnasts are very young. As they grow older and develop a more mature figure their bodies change shape and their centers of gravity shift. They must then relearn their skills. As they become heavier there is also an unfavorable shift in the strength/weight ratio. It has been alleged that Eastern European coaches have sought to prevent these developments by keeping the fat content of their gymnasts' bodies at less than 3% of their body weights in the belief that this will postpone both the onset of puberty and undesired changes in the strength/weight ratio. Natalia Shaposhnikova, for example, is said to have weighed only 79 lbs at age 17. The immature appearance of these gymnasts has suggested to many Western observers that a drug acting on the pituitary gland may have been used to slow their physical development.

STUDY QUESTIONS

1. Which bones are the most useful to physical anthropologists and detectives in determining stature from skeletal material? (Suggestion: See Mildred Trotter and Goddine C. Gleser: A re-evaluation of estimation of stature based on measurements of stature takes during life and long bones after death. Am. J. Phys. Anthropol., *16* N.S.:79–123, 1958.)

2. Karate students practice striking a board called a *makiwara* in order to toughen their fists. In the December 1968 issue of Black Belt a practitioner of the art explained: "Pounding a makiwara gradually powders and slowly crushes the knuckle, rounding it off and depositing a calcium mold into a solid mass." Evaluate this statement from the standpoint of the kinesiology of bones and joints.

3. Read Chapter IV, "Skeletal Adaptions," of Bones, Bodies, and Disease, by Calvin Wells. (New York: Frederick A. Praeger, 1964.) In it the author discusses some modifications found in various bones of the skeletons of earlier men as a result of their working or living habits. What, if any, comparable changes might anthropologists of the future find in the skeletons of contemporary man?

REFERENCES

1. Koch, J.D., cited in Martz, C.D.: Studies on stress

and strain in treatment of fractures. J. Bone Joint Surg., *46-A*:409, 1964.

2. Woo, D.L.-Y., et al.: The effect of prolonged physical

training on the properties of long bone: a study of Wolff's law. J. Bone Joint Surg., *63-A*:730, 1981.

3. Morey, E.R., and Baylink, D.J.: Inhibition of bone formation during space flight. Science, *201*:1138, 1978.
4. Osteoporosis. National Institute of Health Concensus Development Conference Statement, Vol. 5, No. 3, 1984.
5. Drinkwater, B., et al.: Bone mineral content of amenorrheic and eumenorrheic athletes. N. Engl. J. Med., *311*:277, 1984.
6. Albanese, A.A.: Nutritional aspects of bone loss. Food Nutr. News, *47*:1, 1976.
7. Kirk, J.A., et al.: The hypermobility syndrome: musculoskeletal complaints associated with generalized joint hypermobility. Ann. Rheum. Dis., *26*:419, 1967.
8. Jessee, E.F., et al.: The benign hypermobile joint syndrome. Arthritis Rheum., *23*:1053, 1980.
9. Clarke, H.H.: Joint and body range of movement. Phys. Fit. Res. Digest, Series 5, 1975.
10. Schutte, J.E., et al.: Density of lean body mass is greater in blacks than in whites. J. Appl Physiol., *56*:1647, 1984.
11. Body Composition Assessment in Youth and Adults. Edited by Alex F. Roche. Report of the Sixth Ross Conference on Medical Research. Columbus, Ross Laboratories, 1985, p. 20.

RECOMMENDED READING

Adrian, M.J.: An introduction to electrogoniometry. Kinesiology Review. Washington, D.C.: AAHPER, 1968, pp. 12–18.

Caine, D.J., and Lindner, K.J.: Growth plate injury: a threat to young distance runners. Phys. Sportsmed., *12*:118, 1984.

Caine, D.J., and Lindner, K.L.: Overuse injuries of growing bones: the young female gymnast at risk? Phys. Sportsmed., *13*:51, 1985.

Falls, H.B.: Coed Football: Hazards, Implications, and Alternatives. Phys. Sportsmed., *14*:207, November 1986.

Jones, H.H., et al.: Humeral hypertrophy in response to exercise. J. Bone Joint Surg., *59-A*:204, 1977.

Revicki, D.A., and Israel, R.G.: Relationship between body mass indices and measures of body adiposity. Am. J. Public Health, *76*:992, 1986.

Rigotti, N.A., et al.: Osteoporosis in women with anorexia nervosa. JAMA, *311*:1601, 1984.

Round Table: Body composition. Phys. Sportsmed., *14*:144, 1986.

Thornton, M.L.: Pediatric concerns about competitive preadolescent sports. JAMA, *227*:418, 1974.

3 THE STRUCTURE AND FUNCTION OF SKELETAL MUSCLE

ROBERT J. GREGOR

TYPES OF VERTEBRATE MUSCLE

The muscles of the body are the generators of internal force that convert chemically stored energy into mechanical work. Three different types of contractile tissue with certain similar characteristics are found in the body. All three tissues are affected by the same kind of stimuli; produce an action potential soon after stimulation; possess the ability to contract, with the force of the contraction (within physiologic limits) depending on their initial length and the velocity of contraction; have the ability to maintain muscle tone; will atrophy as a result of inadequate circulation; and will hypertrophy in response to certain types of overload training. In other respects they may show marked differences.

Smooth Muscle. Smooth, or involuntary, muscle forms the walls of the hollow viscera, such as the stomach and bladder, and the walls of various systems of tubes, such as are found in the circulatory system, the alimentary tract, the respiratory system, and the reproductive organs. These muscle cells possess myofibrils but do not have cross-striations and have only one nucleus. Smooth muscle contains pain sensors but no proprioceptors. Compared to skeletal muscle, it displays a slower contraction time, greater extensibility, the potential for a more sustained and rhythmic contraction, greater sensitivity to thermal and chemical stimuli, and a longer chronaxy.

Cardiac Muscle. Cardiac muscle has structural and functional resemblances to both skeletal and smooth muscle. Its contractile elements are transversely striated, and the A, I, and Z bands can be observed in the myofibrils. The sarcoplasm is more abundant, the sarcolemma is much finer, and the striations are less distinct. The most characteristic features of the fibers are their branches, which furnish a means of communication between adjacent fibers for the conduction of the neural impulse for contraction. These structures led to the belief that cardiac muscle was an anatomic syncytium, that is, that the cells themselves were connected. Recent evidence using electron microscopy, however, shows that they are actually separated. The cardiac muscle can be considered a functional syncytium, however, because the whole tissue acts electrically as if it were a single cell.

Striated Muscle. Striated muscles are composed of thread-like fibers displaying alternating dark and light bands. Each fiber is actually a greatly elongated, multinucleated cell. It may be over 30 cm in length and have a diameter of 0.01 to 0.1 mm. Each cell is separate. According to one estimate, the body contains about 270 millon striated muscle fibers,[1] innervated by motor neurons and under voluntary control. This type of muscle contains both pain endings and proprioceptors; its principal functions are body movement and maintenance of posture. Because this is the type of muscle with which kinesiologists are primarily concerned, the following discussion of muscle will deal with the structure and function only of striated skeletal muscle.

GROSS STRUCTURE
OF STRIATED MUSCLE

Numbers and Shapes of Muscles. The muscles make up approximately 40 to 45% of adult body weight. While the voluntary muscular system includes approximately 434 muscles, only about 75 pairs are involved in the general posture and movement of the body and will be considered in this text. The other muscles are smaller and concerned with mechanisms not directly related to whole body movement (e.g., voice control and the act of swallowing). Some muscles, like the trapezius, are arranged in flat sheets; some, like the sartorius and the peroneus longus, are long and slender; some, like the biceps brachii and the pronator teres, are spindle shaped; and some, like the pectoralis major, are fan shaped. Most of them are of such irregular shape that a classification based on form is not practicable. Each is named, some of the names indicating the muscles' forms, as in the case of the rhomboid and teres major muscles; some indicating their actions, as with the levator and supinator muscles; some indicating their location, as with the intercostal and supraspinatus; and some indicating the bones that they join, as the brachioradialis and the sternomastoid muscles.

Attachment of Muscle. Units of 100 to 150 muscle cells or fibers are bound together with a connective tissue called perimysium to form a bundle termed a fasciculus. Several fasciculi are in turn bound together by a sheath of perimysium to form a larger unit. These units are enclosed in a covering of epimysium to form a muscle. The soft, fleshy, central part of a muscle is called the belly. Toward the ends of the muscle, the contractile cells disappear, but their investment of connective tissue (the perimysium and epimysium) continues in order to attach the muscles to the bones. If the site of the bony attachment is distant from the belly of the muscle, these extensions of the connective tissue sheaths merge to form either a cordlike tendon or a flat aponeurosis. The fibers of the tendon or aponeurosis are braided with one another, so that tension in any part of a muscle is usually distributed more or less equally to all parts of the attachment to the bone. Because a tendon collects and transmits forces from many different muscle fibers onto a small area of bone, the site of the tendinous attachment is normally marked by a rough tubercle on the bone. Likewise, an aponeurosis gives rise to a skeletal line or ridge at its attachment.

The structure of the insertion of the tendon onto the bone and the tendon's behavior under mechanical loading is very similar to that of a ligament. The size and shape of a tendon and the speed of loading on it are two main factors that determine its strength. The tendon is a very important link between muscle and bone, the stress on it increasing as its muscle contracts. Large muscles usually have large tendons. During normal activity a tendon usually experiences only 25% of the maximal stress it can withstand; very rapid, unexpected stretches of a tendon are common conditions for tendon rupture. For example, having your heel unexpectedly drop into a hole in the ground could cause rupture of the Achilles tendon.

The thickness and strength of the external muscle sheath will vary greatly, depending on the location of the muscle. The sheath is usually very heavy if the muscle is situated near the distal end of a limb where the muscle might be exposed to blows and abrasions. Ordinarily additional fascia covers the muscle to give further protection. A muscle situated deep within the body and consequently well protected, such as the psoas, has a minimum of connective tissue in the various sheaths.

These sheaths form a sort of structural framework for the muscle. This structure is tough and somewhat elastic and will return to its original length even after having been stretched as much as 40%. The fact that the relative amounts of connective and contractile tissue vary greatly from muscle to muscle has at times been disregarded and has led to great discrepancies when experimental physiologists have reported the physical properties of muscle.

The fleshy fibers of some muscles do not give way to tendons at their attachments, but continue almost to the bone, where the individual sheaths of the contractile tissues make the attachment over an area as large as the cross section of the muscle belly. In these cases, the skeleton will be smooth, as on the

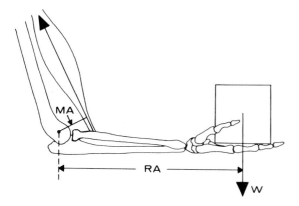

FIG. 3–1. Example of a third-class lever system in the human upper extremity.

surface of the scapula, because tensile forces are widely distributed across the attachment.

Muscle Insertions and Levers. When a muscle contracts strongly, it tends to move both of the bones to which it is attached, but to simplify the problem it is usually assumed that the bone moving least is stationary. The point at which the muscle joins the stationary bone, which is usually the more proximal bone, is called the proximal attachment of the muscle, and its point of attachment to the distal, moving bone is called its distal attachment. The muscle insertion (whether proximal or distal) is the place where the force is applied to the bone.

Muscles attach to the bone at some distance from the joint (e.g., the distal attachment of the biceps muscle of the arm on the radius). The resistance, however (e.g., a weight in the hand), is usually applied some distance further away from the joint axis. The muscle force lever and weight resistance lever then typically form a third-class lever system in the body (Fig. 3–1). The advantage of this system is speed and range of motion at the expense of a great deal of force generated by the muscles involved (i.e., because the muscle lever arms are smaller than the resistance lever arms they are required to move).

Longitudinal and Penniform Muscles. The musculoskeletal machine is basically an arrangement providing relatively large forces for the rapid manipulation of long lever arms. This mechanical system possesses a low mechanical advantage, with the result that high speeds of motion are made possible only at the price of great exertion. While the human body may be said to be specialized more for speed than for strength, the forces required for various movements are relatively large. For example, 300 lb of tension in the deltoid may be needed to raise an arm and hand holding a 10-lb weight to an 80° angle of abduction.

The internal structure of muscles—that is, the arrangement of their fibers—bears an important relation to the force and distance of their contraction. While there are two main types of muscle structure, longitudinal (or fusiform) and penniform, there are many variations from each basic type. The longitudinal is the simpler of the two forms and consists of parallel fibers possibly running the length of the muscle. In general, muscle that is long and slender has a small physiologic cross-sectional area and therefore is not capable of producing large forces. However, it can shorten through a relatively large distance and typically has higher shortening velocities. Muscle that is short and broad has greater force production capability but usually exerts it through a proportionately shorter distance and has lower velocities. The sartorius, for example, is a narrow band of extremely long fibers, well suited to contract with little force through a relatively great distance, whereas the intercostals, consisting of a great number of very short fibers, are constructed to contract with considerable force through a very short distance. Fusiform muscles are very common in the extremities.

Fully three fourths of all the muscles in the human body are situated so that they are required to exert more strength than a longitudinal muscle would afford. As a consequence, we find penniform muscles rather than longitudinal muscles. Because their muscle fibers are arranged diagonally to the direction of pull, the actual force they contribute to the total force along the pulling axis of the muscle is reduced slightly, but more fibers can be brought into play, resulting in a greater total cross-sectional area.

Penniform muscles come in several different arrangements (Fig. 3–2):

Unipennate—Muscle to one side of the tendon, as in the semimembranosus muscle.

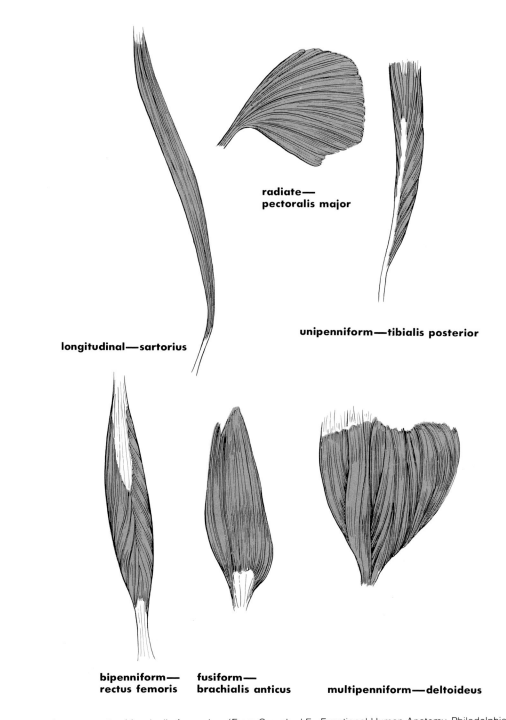

FIG. 3–2. Arrangements of fasciculi of muscles. (From Crouch, J.E.: Functional Human Anatomy. Philadelphia, Lea & Febiger, 1985, p. 197.)

Bipennate—Muscle converges to both sides of a tendon, as in the rectus femoris.

Multipennate—Muscle converges to several tendons, giving a herringbone effect, as in the deltoid muscle.

MICROSTRUCTURE OF VERTEBRATE STRIATED MUSCLE

Organization of Muscle Fibers. A muscle fiber is an elongated cell enclosed in sarcolemma, a thin, structureless, selectively permeable membrane that adheres to an outer network of reticular fibers termed endomysium. The sarcolemma keeps adjacent fibers from merging into a single jellylike mass, isolates them so that they can act as separate units, and mediates the passage of ions and molecules, admitting some and excluding others. Each muscle fiber may run for the entire length of the fleshy part of a muscle, and its endomysium becomes continuous with the other connective tissue sheaths. Within each muscle cell is a specialized but undifferentiated protoplasm termed sarcoplasm. This is a protein sol (a liquid solution of colloids) of relatively low viscosity.

Embedded within the sarcoplasm are myofibrils, semicrystalline gels (firm solutions of colloids) in which the actual contractile activity takes place. It is here that metabolic energy is transformed into mechanical energy and potentially into work. The basic structural unit of the muscle fiber is the sarcomere. Sarcomeres appear to be compartments lying between two Z (zeischenscheibe, or intermediate) lines (Fig. 3–3) in which certain processes are believed to occur during contraction. The Z lines themselves adhere to the sarcolemma, stabilize the structure and localize damage. When an electrode is applied to a Z line, a contraction of the two adjacent half-sarcomeres results.

Myofibrils run parallel to each other and to the long axis of the muscle fiber, merging into the sarcolemma at each end of the cell. Seen under polarized light, they consist of alternating anisotropic (light) and isotropic bands (Fig. 3–3). Under plain light or with different settings of the microscope this coloring is reversed.

The A bands contain thick, rough filaments composed primarily of myosin, each surrounded by six thin, smooth filaments composed primarily of actin. The H (after Hensen, who discovered them, or hell, meaning clear) zones, located in the center of the A bands, contain only thick filaments. The I bands contain only thin filaments, which extend into the A bands as far as the H zones (Figs. 3–4 and 3–5). When a muscle actively shortens, the Z bands are drawn in toward the A bands. No change occurs in the width of the A bands, but the I bands narrow. As a result, the A bands come closer together. The H zone is obliterated in full contraction but reappears as an area of lesser density when the length of the muscle increases. If the muscle goes into a state of rigor, forcible attempts to stretch it will result in a tearing of the filaments, usually in the I bands.

Projections on the myosin filaments, termed cross-bridges, furnish a mechanical linkage between the actin and myosin filaments. Some believe that the force required for muscle contraction is developed by direct physical contact between these cross-bridges and the actin filament. When a muscle shortens, the length of the filaments remains essentially constant (some slight conformational changes may occur), but the thin filaments, which extend from each end of a sarcomere, slide toward each other. The tetanic force, the rate of chemical energy dissipation, or both are proportionate to the number of interactions between the cross-bridges and the actin filaments.

The M (mittelscheibe, or intermediate) band is so called to indicate its position in the middle of the sarcomere. Its function is not understood. The N (nebenscheibe, or next to) bands may be sites of intracellular calcium concentration.

Within the cell are units known as mitochondria (Fig. 3–6), often located opposite the I and Z bands. About 95% of the adenosine triphosphate (ATP) that furnishes the energy necessary for contraction is produced in them, and their main function is to provide this substance to the myofibril. For this reason they have been described as the "power plants" of the cells. There are wide variations in mitochondrial content in muscle fibers Muscles respond to training by increasing the

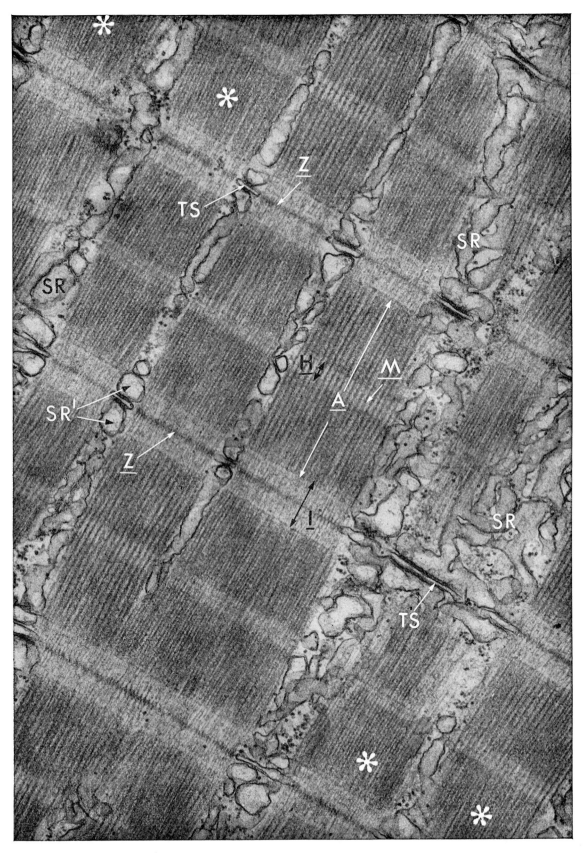

FIG. 3–3. Photomicrograph of skeletal muscle and the sarcoplasmic reticulum (SR). Fibrils (*), A band (A), H band (H), I band (I), M line (M), dilated sacs of endoplasmic reticulum (SR′), T system (TS), and Z band (Z). (Porter and Bonneville: Fine Structure of Cells and Tissues, 4th ed. Philadelphia. Lea & Febiger. 1973.)

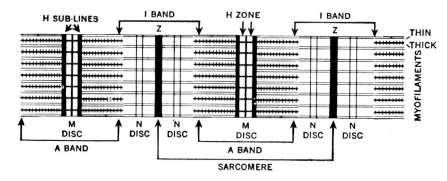

FIG. 3–4.   Schematic representation of the myofibril from skeletal muscle.

number of mitochondria, the size of the mitochondria, or both.

Surrounding the myofibrils is a complex network of two different types of tubules, the T (or transverse tubular) system and the sarcoplasmic reticulum (SR). In most mammalian muscles the transverse tubules are located near the end of the A bands. Apparently an excitation wave proceeds from the surface membrane into the center of the fiber along these tubules. The SR tubules are arranged parallel to the fibers and surround each fibril. Near the end of each sarcomere a pair of terminal cisternae, or sacs, flank each T system tubule. This tripartite structure is called a triad. These terminal sacs are thought to contain calcium ions, which are released with depolarization, thus initiating a contraction. Relaxation occurs when calcium is reaccumulated by the SR.

Because the two systems do not appear to have direct connections, much remains to be learned regarding how depolarization of the T system produces the release of calcium ions from the sarcoplasmic reticulum. Constituents of some major cellular components of muscles are summarized in Table 3–1. A great deal more is to be learned about the physiologic and anatomic functions of muscle contraction. In the words of Peachey, it seems that the concepts presently formulated at best "can be taken as a first approximation to the real mechanism."[2] The effort here has been to give no more than an extremely brief description of the constituents most intimately concerned with the processes of muscular contraction.

Since the investigations of Morpurgo it has been believed that an increase in hypertrophy resulted from an increase in the cross section of the muscle fibers and not from an increase in the number of muscle fibers. However, some cytological evidence indicates an increase in fiber number during rapid hyper-

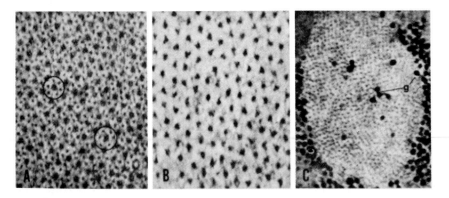

FIG. 3–5.   Human quadriceps femoris tissue under high magnification. *A*, Cross section through an A band, showing both thick and thin myofilaments. Six thin filaments appear to surround each thick filament. (× 130,000.) *B*. Cross section of an H zone. Only thick filaments are present. (× 130,000.) *C*, Cross section of an I band. Only thin filaments are present. g = glycogen granules. (× 80,500.) (Prince, courtesy Am. J. Med.)

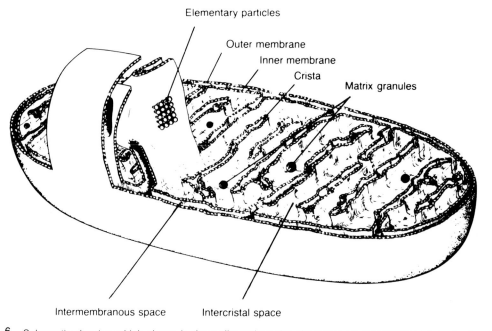

Elementary particles
Outer membrane
Inner membrane
Crista
Matrix granules
Intermembranous space   Intercristal space

FIG. 3–6. Schematic drawing which shows in three dimensions the ultrastructural organization of a mitochondrion. (From Geneser, F.: Textbook of Histology. Munksgaard, Copenhagen, 1986.)

trophy.[3] Much more research is needed before final conclusions can be made.

Components of Muscle. If muscle were a relatively simple mechanism like a spring, and some investigators have modeled it that way, a direct relationship would exist between the tension it could develop at different lengths and the amount of work it could accomplish. Actually, muscle appears to consist of three interdependent elements: a contractile component, a series elastic component, and a parallel elastic component.

The contractile component actively develops tension and shortening, which is transmitted to the muscle tendon through the series elastic component. This component can lie in part in the tendinous filaments into which the muscle fibers insert, and in part in the muscle itself (e.g., Z bands). Its function is related to tension development in the whole muscle-tendon unit, most importantly when the muscle shortens from a previously stretched position. The parallel elastic component is believed to come into action only when the muscle is stretched. It is thought to be largely connective tissue and to be responsible for the resting tension of a muscle. This physical arrangement has practical consequences. During standing posture and at low-speed locomotion (3 mi/hr), the contractile component of the muscle appears responsible mainly for the mechanical work and power output. At higher speeds (12 mi/hr), shortening contractions (positive work) are im-

Table 3–1. Constituents and Function of Some Major Muscle Cellular Compartments

Compartment	Pertinent Biochemical Constituents	Function
Sarcoplasm	Enzymes	Glycolysis
Mitochondria	Enzymes of oxidation and phosphorylation	Steady-state aerobic activity or recovery from oxygen debt
Fibrils	Actin and myosin	Contraction
Sarcotubular system	Concentration and release of calcium ions	On-and-off control of active state
Membrane	Lipoprotein structure with variable selective permeability for ions	Excitation and impulse conduction

(After Pearson et al., Ann. Intern. Med., *67*:615, 1967.)

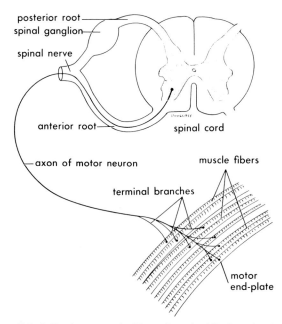

FIG. 3–7. A motor unit. (From Crouch, J.E.: Functional Human Anatomy. Philadelphia, Lea & Febiger, 1985, p. 187.)

mediately preceded by a lengthening contraction (negative work) during which the active muscles are stretched and mechanical energy is stored in the muscle's elastic and viscoelastic components. This energy is then released during the shortening contraction that immediately follows and results in enhanced work and power output. This "stretch-shorten" cycle commonly seen in skeletal muscle during moderate and high-speed movements results in a very efficient use of muscle resources and enhanced work output by the musculoskeletal system.

Comparative Sizes of Structures. Whole muscle fibers are from 10 to 100 μ in diameter (1 μ = 1/1000 mm). Myofibrils range from 0.5 to 2 μ in diameter. The diameter of the thick myosin filament is about 0.01 μ; that of the thin actin filament is about 0.005 μ.

INNERVATION OF MUSCLE

The muscles not only are penetrated and served by the vessels of the circulatory system, but they are also well supplied with nerves. One or more nerves containing both motor and sensory fibers enter each muscle from the central nervous system. As the nerve enters the muscle it divides into a number of

terminal branches (Fig. 3–7), each of which has a motor end plate embedded into a single muscle fiber. The number of muscle fibers innervated by a single motor nerve fiber may vary from three to several hundred. Under normal conditions, the group of muscle fibers innervated by a single motor nerve constitute what is typically referred to as a motor unit. These motor units then become the functional unit of tension development in the muscle. A graded increase in muscle tension is accomplished either by recruiting more motor units and therefore more fibers, or by increasing the rate of firing of motor units already active. Estimates have been made of the number of muscle fibers and motor units in human muscles[4] (Table 3–2).

In the hand, where not only strength but the ability to do delicate and accurate work is required, each motor unit is composed of relatively few muscle fibers. Because of this structure, forces exerted by the fingers can be changed by relatively small increments. In contrast, heavy postural muscles have many fibers per motor unit and have large increments in tension increase. The smallest motor units are to be found in the muscles that control movements of the eye (e.g., 3 or 4 fibers), where great precision is required.

ROLES MUSCLES PLAY

What is the function of a given muscle-tendon unit? If it is activated, what will happen? Such questions cannot be answered directly because many factors can influence the results of muscular contraction. Depending on the circumstances, a muscle may act in one of several ways. Before discussing these various possible roles, it will be helpful to list some basic axioms.

1. A muscle fiber can do only one thing: develop tension within itself.
2. When a muscle fiber or a whole muscle is activated by its motor neuron it will tend to shorten. Whether the muscle will shorten or produce any joint movement depends on the amount of tension developed, the amount of internal or external resistance, the mechanical leverage of the muscle-tendon-bone system, its angle of pull with respect to the bone,

Table 3–2.   Estimated Number of Muscle Fibers and Motor Units in Selected Human Muscles

Muscle	Mean Diameter of Muscle Fibers (Microns)	No. of Muscle Fibers	No. of Large Nerve Fibers	Calculated No. of Motor Units	No. of Fibers per Motor Unit
Platysma	19.8 ± 0.3	27,100	1,826	1,096	25
Brachioradialis	34.0 ± 0.8	129,200	525	315	410
Tibialis anterior	56.7 ± 0.2	250,000	742	445	657
Gastrocnemius, medial head	54.1 ± 1.2	1,120,000	965	579	1,934

and other factors. A major consideration is the related influence of other muscles that also may be activated.

3. When a muscle contracts, it tends to do all of its possible actions. Some muscles are mechanically situated so that they tend to produce more than one movement in a joint. For example, when Part IV of the trapezius muscle shortens, it tends to cause adduction, depression, and upward rotation of the scapula. There is no intramuscular mechanism to determine which of the several possible joint movements will occur. The muscle can exert only a pulling force. Some muscles cross more than one joint, and potentially they can produce movements in all of those joints. Again, because the muscle can only pull its ends toward its center, its contraction will always tend to produce all of its possible joint movements.

4. What a muscle can do or could do is no indication of what it will do. Sometimes the motor programs in the nervous system do not activate a muscle that could help with a given movement. When the gluteus maximus contracts, one of its tendencies is to cause hip extension, yet it is not ordinarily "turned on" during hip extension in walking. Also, the force exerted by another muscle may prevent a muscle from performing one or all of its possible joint movements.

The Role of Mover or Agonist. If a muscle undergoes a shortening contraction it is said to be a mover or agonist for the joint actions that result. For example, the triceps brachii is a mover for elbow extension. Some muscles are movers for more than one action in a given joint; many may have one or many actions on

each of two or more joints that they happen to traverse. The biceps brachii, for instance, is a mover for both elbow flexion and radioulnar supination, and in addition it is a mover for several shoulder joint actions, because of its two-headed proximal insertion on the scapula.

The Role of Prime Mover and of Assistant Mover. In a particular set of circumstances, the muscles most effective in causing the observed joint movement are said to be prime movers for that joint movement, and the muscles that help but that are less effective are said to be assistant movers. In borderline cases, the designation of a muscle as prime or assistant mover is unclear.

When the same joint movement takes place but under a different set of circumstances, sometimes the classification of muscles as prime or assistant movers may have to be changed; the designation always depends on the circumstances. Some kinesiologists have questioned the practice of designating a muscle as a prime or assistant mover for a joint movement in general; other kinesiologists have argued about which classification should be assigned. In this textbook, individual muscles are designated as prime or assistant movers for particular joint movements. This designation is essential in the orientation of beginning students. As one becomes familiar with the experimental literature of electromyography and with the intricacies of exercise analysis, exceptions to the classifications will become apparent.

The term emergency muscle may be used to designate an assistant mover that is called into action only when an exceptional amount of total force is needed. The long head of the biceps brachii, for example, is not often called into action in the performance of shoulder joint abduction, but it may assist that action in times of great need. Some therapists claim to have taught patients with paralyses of the deltoid and supraspinatus muscles to abduct the shoulder joint by contraction of the long head of the biceps.[5]

Some kinesiologists have stated that every muscle must have at least one prime-mover function. This rule appeals to one's sense of orderliness but does not appear to have a clear biologic basis. The subclavius muscle, for example, does not appear to be able to do any joint action very well, and it is usually listed only as an assistant mover for shoulder girdle depression.

The Role of Antagonist. An antagonist is a muscle whose contraction tends to produce a joint action exactly opposite to some given joint action of another specified muscle. An extensor muscle is antagonistic, potentially, to a flexor muscle. Thus, the biceps brachii is an antagonist of the triceps brachii with respect to elbow extension, and to the pronator teres muscle with respect to radioulnar pronation. The biceps is not an antagonist of the brachialis muscle, because it cannot oppose any motion for which the brachialis muscle is a mover.

The Role of Fixator or Stabilizer. A fixator or stabilizer is a muscle that anchors, steadies, or supports a bone or body part in order that another, active muscle may have a firm base on which to pull. If a person reaches forward to pull open a resistant door, he must stabilize his body part if he is to overcome the resistance. To open the door, elbow flexion may be needed, and if the scapula, for example, is not stabilized, the contraction of the biceps may cause a pulling forward of the shoulder girdle rather than an opening of the door. When a muscle contracts, it tends to pull both of its ends toward its center with equal force. Typically a person wants to cause motion only at one end of the muscle. Therefore, he attempts to stabilize the bone to which the opposite end of the muscle is attached.

In the ideal case a fixator or stabilizer muscle will be in an isometric contraction, although in practice, there is a slight motion in the "stabilized" part to continuously adjust the stabilization to the requirements of the desired motion; this condition may be called

moving fixation or a guiding action. Sensory organs constantly update the fixator regarding the changing demands on the system, and the fixator adjusts itself accordingly to make the most efficient use of its efforts.

A good example of fixation or stabilization occurs in the floor push-up exercise. The abdominal muscles contract isometrically during push-ups to prevent an undesirable sagging of the body in the hip and trunk region. In this example, the fixation is necessary not so much to provide a firm base for the action of other muscles as to counteract the action of gravity on the hip and vertebral column. Another example is the isometric contraction of the neck extensors to fixate the cervical spine to provide a firm base for the action of the sternocleidomastoid muscles on the anterior surface of the neck. This fixation allows the sternocleidomastoid muscles to assist in lifting the rib cage during forced breathing after exhaustive exercise. Without such fixation, the head may curl forward on the chest, interfering with deep breathing.

The Role of Synergist. The term synergist has been used with so many different connotations, both historically and in contemporary works, that its meaning has become very generalized, if not actually ambiguous. Some writers define synergist as a muscle that acts along with some other muscle or muscles as a part of a team; others use the term in a more restricted sense, but there is little agreement among these viewpoints.

Two specific kinds of synergy may be identified: helping synergy and true synergy. In these usages, synergy is defined as a counteracting of undesired action by other active muscles. Helping synergy occurs during the action of two muscles that share a joint action and have their own second action antagonistic to that of the other. As both of these muscles contract simultaneously, they act together to produce the desired common action, and they act as helping synergists to each other as they counteract or neutralize each other's undesired secondary action. An example occurs in the sit-up exercise from the supine position. Several abdominal muscles cooperate in producing vertebral flexion in this exercise, but we may for the moment consider only the right and left external oblique abdominal muscles. Both of these muscles co-operate in flexing the spine, since each is a prime mover for this action. The right external oblique is also a prime mover for right lateral vertebral flexion and for left vertebral rotation, however, while the left external oblique is a prime mover for left lateral vertebral flexion and for right vertebral rotation. The lateral flexion and the rotation tendencies, in opposite directions, are mutually counteracted, or neutralized, and the resultant motion is pure vertebral flexion.

True synergy occurs when one muscle contracts statically to prevent any action in one of the joints traversed by a contracting two-joint or multijoint muscle. According to the axiom that a muscle tends to perform all of its possible actions when it contracts, a two-joint muscle will tend to cause movement at each joint it crosses. Sometimes, however, action at only one of the joints is desired and another muscle must contract in order to prevent an undesired action from occurring at the other joint. For example, when the fist is clenched, the extensors of the wrist act as true synergists. If the wrist were not held extended, the long flexors of the fingers would produce wrist flexion as well as finger flexion. Flexion of the wrist added to flexion of the fingers stretches the tendons of the long finger extensors until they can yield no more, at which point continued wrist flexion causes the fingers to open out and the grip to slacken.

The Role of Neutralizer. A neutralizer is a muscle that contracts in order to counteract, or neutralize, an undesired action of another contracting muscle. Thus, the term neutralizer describes the role played by a helping synergist or a true synergist as defined in the preceding section. As a technical term, it has the distinct advantage of avoiding the several different meanings that have been attached to the general term "synergist" by various kinesiologists.

Tonus and Relaxation. The term relaxation may refer to the process of relaxing (the stage during which the force of contraction is diminishing) or to the state of inactivity. Even a relaxed muscle has a residual low-level turgor or feeling of firmness, however. At the lowest levels, this is known as tonus or muscle tone. Muscle tone is a function of the natural fullness (turgor) of the muscular and fibrous tissue and of the response of the nervous system to stimuli.

Muscles that are used much are apt to have more tone than those used less. When the tone in two antagonists is different, the segments upon which they act may deviate from their normal position. This inequality may be the cause of certain types of postural defects.

The fact that muscle groups can be made to develop increased tonus and that certain muscles can be shortened by exercise within a limited range of motion is used in some phases of therapeutic exercise. Through such procedure certain muscles of the dorsal aspects of the shoulder girdle may be shortened and their tonus increased, adducting the scapula, with resultant stretching and temporary change of tone of certain antagonistic muscles of the ventral aspect. This change will result in a shifting of the relative position of the shoulders, causing them to be pulled back more than previously. Still another factor to be considered in this connection is that when a muscle is used when habitually held in a shortened position, in time the muscle will shorten and accommodate itself to the new length with the restoration of normal tonus; the joint affected will then have a new resting position. This situation implies, of course, that the antagonistic muscle group will be correspondingly stretched, and that it also will accommodate itself to the new length and re-establish its normal tone. This readjustment is a common experience of children who wear shoes in winter, go barefoot in the summer, and then revert to wearing shoes with the advent of cold weather. When footwear is discarded, the soleus and gastrocnemius are stretched and the antagonistic muscles shorten. When shoes are again worn, the reverse process occurs.

Residual Tension. Generalized residual tension may result from central nervous system irritation, pain or other forms of severe stimulation, local muscular fatigue, and persistent use of small accessory muscles in tasks requiring fine manipulation.

SPURT AND SHUNT MUSCLES

Mathematic analysis led MacConaill to conclude that skeletal muscles act as spurt or shunt muscles. Spurt muscles have their proximal attachments at a distance from the joints about which they act, while their distal attachment is near the joint. They direct the greater part of their force across the bone rather than along it and provide the force that acts along the tangent to the curve traversed by the bone during movement. Shunt muscles have their proximal insertions near the joints on which they act and their distal insertions at a distance from them, so that the greater part of their contractile force is directed along the bones. This arrangement tends to pull the joints together, making these muscles largely stabilizers. The muscles do, however, provide the increase in centripetal force required in rapid or resisted movements. The pronator quadratus muscle, for example, a spurt muscle, is the prime mover in pronation of the forearm. When rapid or resisted action is involved, the pronator teres, a shunt muscle, is called in to assist.

When a muscle acts on two joints, it is usually a shunt muscle to one and a spurt to the other. The biceps brachii is a shunt muscle for the shoulder joint and a spurt muscle at the elbow. In some cases, the role of the muscle may be changed when the direction of contraction (lengthening or shortening) is reversed. Some muscles may combine both types; for instance, the posterior fibers of the adductor magnus muscle are shunt muscles and the anterior fibers are spurt muscles.[6]

KINDS OF MUSCULAR CONTRACTION

To the kinesiologist, the term contraction refers to the development of tension within a muscle. It does not necessarily imply that any visible shortening of the muscle takes place.

Static or Isometric Contraction. When a muscle develops tension that is insufficient to move a body part against a given resistance and when the net external length of the muscle remains unchanged, the contraction is said to be static or isometric. Recent studies show that muscle fibers may shorten and lengthen the tendon slightly, but the total muscle-tendon unit usually remains at a fixed or constant length.

Shortening or Concentric Contraction. When a muscle develops sufficient tension to overcome a resistance, so that the muscle visibly shortens and moves a body part in spite of a given resistance, it is said to be in concentric contraction. For example, the biceps brachii contracts concentrically when a glass of water is lifted from a table toward the mouth. In this case, the resistance is the combined weight of the forearm, the glass, and the water, and the source of resistance is the force due to gravitational acceleration.

Lengthening or Eccentric Contraction. When a given resistance overcomes the muscle tension so that the muscle actually lengthens, the muscle is said to be acting eccentrically. For example, when a heavy weight is slowly lowered to the top of a table, the biceps brachii acts eccentrically. If the muscles were simply relaxed, gravity would extend the elbow joint and lower the weight with little or no control from the arm. Another way of lowering the weight would be to contract the triceps brachii concentrically, thus adding to gravitational force and extending the elbow with greater speed. Such an action might be appropriate in driving nails with a hammer, but not during the controlled movement in the example cited.

Both concentric and eccentric contraction are known to physiologists as isotonic contractions.

Identification of an eccentric contraction is a persistent and crucial problem in performance analysis. In performing floor push-ups, it is clear that the up-phase involves elbow extension and shoulder girdle abduction. The resistance is the weight of the body, which tends to flex the elbow and adduct the shoulder girdle. Therefore, the elbow extensors and the shoulder girdle abductors must contract concentrically, overcoming the force of gravity, to perform the movement. When analyzing the down-phase of push-ups, beginning students do not always find the problem so simple. It is easy to see that elbow flexion and shoulder girdle adduction take place, and it is tempting to believe that the elbow flexors and shoulder girdle adductors are contracting concentrically. Such is not the case. Gravity is quite sufficient to energize the movement; if muscle force were added to it, the body would hit the floor hard enough to cause injury. Instead, the elbow extensors and the shoulder girdle abductors must develop enough tension to modify the gravitational force ("put the brakes on") and lower the body to the floor at a reasonable speed. In doing push-ups, the same muscles act throughout the exercise, contracting concentrically on the up-phase, statically during the momentary held position between phases, and eccentrically during the down-phase.

Some professionals not trained in kinesiology have advocated the following exercise for conditioning the abdominal muscles: from a position of standing with arms raised overhead, bend forward downward and touch the toes on count 1; return to starting position on count 2. While the abdominal muscles may receive some passive squeezing during this exercise, it is obvious that the vertebral extensors are the active muscles, contracting eccentrically on the way down and concentrically on the way up. The abdominal muscles can remain relaxed during both motions.

In exercise analysis it is always necessary to consider the external forces that may be operative. The most important of these is gravity, but it is by no means the only one. Muscular forces exerted by opponents in such contact sports as football and wrestling, the force of moving objects such as balls and other sports implements, the force of waves, tides, and currents in swimming—all of these must be carefully evaluated in the analysis of muscular action of bodily movement.

KINDS OF GROSS BODY MOVEMENT

Preceding sections on the roles muscles can play and on kinds of muscular contraction can now be generalized further by means of a classification of kinds of gross body movement. This classification provides a necessary starting point for any formal analysis of coordinated movement, because the categories typify unitary movements such as lifting, batting, holding a "scale" on the balance beam, and performing elementary dance movements. More complex sequential movements, such as serving a tennis ball or fielding a bounding ball and throwing to first base, must be broken down into phases before an orderly analysis can be delineated.

Sustained Force (SF) Movement. Sustained force movements may be fast or slow, strong or weak. Sustained force is applied against a resistance by contracting agonists while relaxing their antagonists. If a weight is to be lifted, for example, the agonists contract concentrically and overcome the resistance (SF+). If a weight is to be lowered, the resistance overcomes the force of the agonists as they contract eccentrically (SF−). Holding a weight stationary requires that the sustaining force be equal to the resistance (SFO). Other examples of SF movement are an armstroke in swimming, initial leg thrust in a sprint start, forcing a wrestling hold, pressing up to a handstand, and sustaining a slow body extension in contemporary dance.

Passive (PAS) Movement. Any body movement, however originated, that takes place without continuing muscle contraction can be categorized as passive. Three major subdivisions of passive movement may be identified.

Manipulation (MAN). The motive force for manipulation is another person, or an outside force other than gravity. Examples: being lifted or swung, while relaxing, by a partner in ballet dancing or skating; unresisted limb movements performed by a therapist on a completely relaxed patient; and body movement resulting from unresisted collision. Therapists distinguish passive or manipulative exercise from assistive and resistive exercise, in which the patient is active and the therapist either assists or resists the movement.

Inertial (INER) Movement, or Coasting. Inertial movement is a continuation of pre-established movement, with no concurrent motive muscular contraction. For convenience and practicality, inertial movement is considered to include frictional influences—air resistance, tissue viscosity, residual tension in ligaments and stretched muscles, and other deceleratory elements. Examples: the glide phase of the elementary breaststroke in swimming; sliding into a base; and the horizontal component of the free flight of a jump or racing dive. Although a football fullback, plunging through the line, attempts to use sustained force by continuing to drive with his legs, he also depends strongly on the inertial movement resulting from his previously established momentum.

Gravitational (GRAV) Movement, or Falling. Although gravitational movement is actually a special case of manipulative movement, it is given consideration here because it results from acceleratory force that is constant in direction and magnitude, in all practical terrestrial problems. Examples include free fall, the vertical component of the free flight of a jump, and relaxed pendulum movements of limbs in contemporary dance or of the whole body in gymnastic stunts.

Ballistic (BAL) Movement. Ballistic movement is a compound movement. The first phase is a sustained force movement (SF+), with body parts accelerated by concentric contraction of agonists, unhindered by contraction of antagonists. The second phase is an inertial, or coasting, movement (INER), without muscular contraction. The final phase is a deceleration resulting from eccentric contraction of antagonists (SF−) or from passive resistance offered by ligaments and stretched muscles. The three phases overlap only at the transition stages, where one kind of movement blends smoothly into the next. Examples include batting a baseball, smashing a badminton bird, stroking a tennis ball, and many movements typical of vigorous sports.

Guide (GUI) Movement, or Tracking. When great accuracy and steadiness but not force or speed are required, the muscles antagonistic to the movement as well as the principal movers are active. When one attempts to hold some instrument as steady as possible, both members of a pair of antagonistic muscle groups contract together. Exact balance is difficult to achieve. When errors appear as alternate domination of antagonistic pairs, tremor occurs. The absence of these errors is a measure of steadiness.

Steadiness may be required in guided movement, as well as in stationary holding. The dominance of one muscle group, the mover, then exceeds the force of the other, the antagonist—the difference being roughly proportionate to the speed and force of the total movement. Examples of guided movement are writing; repairing a watch; threading

a needle; lifting a very full cup of coffee; and even such skills as dart throwing for accuracy over a short distance. In addition to the guiding, dragging, controlling contraction of antagonists in these movements, a number of other muscles may act in graded contraction, constantly or intermittently, for the sole purpose of preventing deviations of the movement from the desired path. These guiding muscles also probably act sometimes simultaneously in antagonistic pairs, sometimes in alternation. The existence or timing of these contractions is almost impossible to predict, for they result primarily as feedback from error signals.

Dynamic Balance (DB) Movement. Muscle spindles detect deviations from a desired position of balance and initiate a servocontrol system to make corrections. The result is a series of irregular oscillations, precisely mediated by reflex contraction of appropriate muscle groups, in order to maintain the balanced position. Example: erect "stationary" standing. Chapter 5 details the sensorimotor systems involved.

Oscillating (OSC) Movement. The movement is rapidly reversed at the end of each short excursion, with contracting antagonistic muscle groups alternating in dominance. Examples: tapping; shaking an object. The maximum possible speed of such alternating movement is highly subject to motor learning and is also dependent on the weight or inertia of the moving parts and on the strength of the active muscles.

The following "maximum rhythms" have been established for movements of the various segments of the upper extremity:

Shoulder—5 to 6 movements/sec
Elbow—8 to 9 movements/sec
Forearm—3 to 4 movements/sec
Wrist—10 to 11 movements/sec
Fingers—8 to 9 movements/sec

Flexions are faster than extensions. There appears to be little correlation between power and velocity of movement and various anthropometric measurements. The validity of the hypothesis that speed of muscular contraction is conditioned by a general factor has not been clearly demonstrated. The maximum rate of high-speed movement may depend on some intrinsic physiologic property of the reflex circuit. Maximum velocity is presumably limited not by the properties of muscle itself but by the need for the agonists to relax in order to permit the antagonists to halt the movement. The limiting factor may be the speed with which excitation and inhibition can be made to alternate in the central nervous system.

REFERENCES

1. Ruch, T.C., and Patton, H.D.: Physiology and Biophysics. 20th Ed. Philadelphia, W.B. Saunders Co., 1982, p. 125.
2. Peachey, L.D.: Muscle. Ann. Rev. Physiol., *30*:401, 1968.
3. Goldberg, A.L., et al.: Mechanism of work-induced hypertrophy of skeletal muscle. Med. Sci. Sports, *7*:185, 1975.
4. Feinstein, B., et al.: Morphologic studies of motor units in normal muscles. Acta Anat., *23*:127, 1955.
5. Brunnstrom, S.: Comparative strength of muscles with similar functions. Phys. Ther. Rev., *26*:59, 1946.
6. MacConaill, M.A.: Spurt and shunt muscles: Some minimal principles applicable in myomechanics. Biomed. Eng., *1*:498, 1966.

RECOMMENDED READING

Bourne, G.H. (ed): The Structure and Function of Muscle. Vol. I. 2nd Ed. New York, Academic Press, Inc., 1972.

Huxley, A.H., and Simmons, R.M.: Proposed mechanism of force generation in striated muscle. Science, *233*:533, 1971.

Huxley, H.E.: The structural basis of muscular contraction. Proc. R. Soc. Lond., *B178*:131, 1971.

Rasch, P.J.: Some aspects of muscular movement: A review. Am. Correct. Ther. J., *23*:151, 1969.

Rasch, P.J.: The present status of negative (eccentric) exercise: A Review. Am. Correct. Ther. J., *28*:77, 1974.

4 THE PHYSIOLOGY OF MUSCLE CONTRACTION

ROBERT J. GREGOR

The function of nerve fibers is to conduct impulses. Any analysis of this propagation involves both chemical and electrical considerations.

PROPAGATION OF NEURAL IMPULSES

The membranes of all living cells have one characteristic in common: the ability to separate charged ions. Under resting conditions the concentration of sodium (Na) ions in the fluid inside of the living cell is 10 to 20 times greater than in the fluid on the outside. The opposite is true for potassium (K), resulting in negative electrical potential outside the cell with respect to the inside. Nachmansohn[1] hypothesized that acetylcholine (ACh) is stored in the nerve fibers in an inactive form. Release of ACh resulting from an environmental change (stimulus) triggers a transient local change in the ionic permeability of the cellular membrane. Na ions flow inward; K ions slightly later and more slowly flow outward. This process is known as depolarization. For a brief period the interior of the cell becomes positively charged and the exterior of the cell becomes negatively charged. These changes in the ionic concentration gradients generate small bioelectric currents called action potentials (Fig. 4–1). It is thought that the influx of sodium is responsible for the rising action and that the later efflux of potassium takes place during the descending limb of the spike, which lasts approximately 500 msec and attains an amplitude of approximately 130 mv.

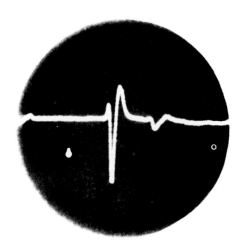

FIG. 4–1. Normal motor unit wave, showing large characteristic negative phase both preceded and followed by smaller positive phases. (Meditron Co.)

The spike is followed by a negative after-potential lasting 12 to 80 msec and by a positive after-potential lasting from 40 to 1000 msec. The origin of these after-potentials is not clear, but they appear to reflect the metabolic process associated with recovery. An action potential stimulates the adjacent area in the neuron to undergo the same depolarizing process. In this way the entire membrane is successively activated and the electrical impulse is propagated along the axon, with its velocity and duration determined by the electrical properties of the neuron involved.

Within 1 msec or less, ACh is inactivated by hydrolysis and the permeability barrier is restored. During rest the initial electrolytic distribution is restored and the nerve becomes ready to respond to the next stimulus.

Neuromuscular Transmission. At rest, miniature end-plate potentials (epp) are continually discharged at the motor nerve ending, probably resulting from a spontaneous, random discharge of quantities (quanta) of ACh from globular bodies called vesicles. Depolarization of chemosensitive areas of the nerve ending by a neural impulse appears to release relatively large quantities (quanta) of ACh and produces a prolonged negative discharge perhaps 100 times the amplitude of the resting epp. This discharge in turn propagates the muscle action potential. The excitatory event is believed to be transferred from the cell membrane to the fibrils by means of the T (transverse tubular) structures found on both sides of the Z lines. The link between depolarization of the membrane by an action potential and the subsequent contraction of the I bands appears to be the release of calcium ions at the level of the Z lines. This release establishes the active state of the muscle by offsetting troponin, an inhibitory protein preventing cross-bridge attachment. The result is the formation of actomyosin, ATPase activation, and contraction.

Admittedly, these phenomena are complex and somewhat confusing. Neuromuscular transmission and the spread of electrical charge to the myofibrils proceeds in a number of discrete stages and may be summarized as follows:

1. Reduction of the resting potential of the nerve terminal.
2. Release of quanta of ACh.
3. Diffusion of ACh across the synaptic gap.
4. Combination of ACh with receptor molecules in the end-plate membrane.
5. Increased permeability and entrance of sodium and other ions.
6. Propagation of an all-or-none action potential along the muscle fiber.
7. Inward spread of membrane potential via the T system to release calcium from the lateral vesicles (terminal cisternae) of the triads.
8. Inhibition of the troponin molecule, cross-bridge formation, and subsequent contraction.

Muscle Fiber Action Potential. Activity in a nerve fiber may set off an action potential in a muscle fiber. Starting at the neuromuscular junction, this activity passes over and depolarizes a muscle fiber, causing it to contract. In mammalian muscle, conduction velocity is approximately 5 msec. The duration of action potentials shows no significant difference among individuals of both sexes 20 to 40 years of age, but it becomes prolonged with age or low muscle temperature, leading to a longer reflex response time.

Contraction passes down the muscle fiber like a wave emanating from the point of stimulation. Between the arrival of the electrical stimulation at the muscle and the beginning of tension development in the fibers is a latency period of about 3 msec. During this time the muscle actually relaxes. This delay between stimulus and contraction may be due to the molecular rearrangements required for the release of the chemical energy necessary for contraction, although the chemical reactions may be well advanced before any detectable shortening begins. The loss of tension at higher speeds of shortening may be related to the rate at which chemical energy is made available, because the viscous resistance of the muscle appears insignificant.

MECHANICS OF MUSCLE CONTRACTION

The physical rearrangements that take place during muscle contraction are as controversial as are the chemical processes involved. Current theory, the sliding filament theory, holds that changes in muscle length are a result of the actin filaments in the I band sliding past the myosin filaments in the A band. This theory accounts for the active length-tension curve commonly mentioned in the literature. Tension decreases at very short lengths and very long lengths because the filaments and consequently the cross-bridges are not in the ideal or optimal zone of overlap. At long muscle lengths, however, total tension increases, because while the number of overlapping cross-bridges decreases and the active length-tension curve goes down, the tension from stretching passive connective tissue dramatically increases. Total tension is the summation of both active and passive components. Therefore, at longer muscle lengths, total tension goes up primarily because of an increase in the passive connective tissue contribution (Fig. 4–2).

Another well-defined property of skeletal muscle that governs its force production capability is its force-velocity property (Fig. 4–3). While the exact shape of the force-velocity curve will differ for different muscles, in general, as load increases, the speed of the shortening contraction decreases. Fast muscles (predominantly fast-twitch motor units) will produce higher forces than slow muscles at the same velocity of shortening. Because power is the product of force and velocity, fast muscles are usually more powerful, though only at the same muscle activation level (see the section on EMG). Additionally, for all muscle, enhanced or higher forces will be produced at a given velocity of shortening if the shortening contraction is preceded by active stretch on the muscle. As mentioned in the previous chapter, this stretch-shorten cycle is common in many daily activities.[4]

Twitch. When studying muscular contraction, physiologists use what is known as a muscle-nerve preparation. This usually consists of a freshly excised muscle, e.g., the gastrocnemius of a frog or the gastrocnemius or soleus of a dog, cat, or rabbit, together with the muscle's motor nerve. When an electrical stimulus of sufficient size is applied to the motor nerve, the muscle responds with a single contraction known as a muscle twitch (Fig. 4–4).

When recorded under standardized conditions, the shape of the twitch curve is similar for all striated muscle, but the time factors involved show great variations in different muscles, in different species, and at different temperatures.

The action potential contains an absolute refractory period. During this period a stimulus in the area cannot initiate a fresh potential, nor can an impulse generated elsewhere pass through the area. The next few milliseconds comprise a relative refractory period. A very strong stimulus can excite the fiber, but the spike evoked is submaximal and conduction velocity is below normal. These changes reflect alterations in the inward flow of sodium ions and the outward flow of potassium ions as a result of depolarization of the membrane during the impulse.

Treppe. When a muscle is stimulated in such a way that complete single twitches rapidly follow each other, the first few contractions progressively increase in height. This effect is known as treppe, or the staircase ef-

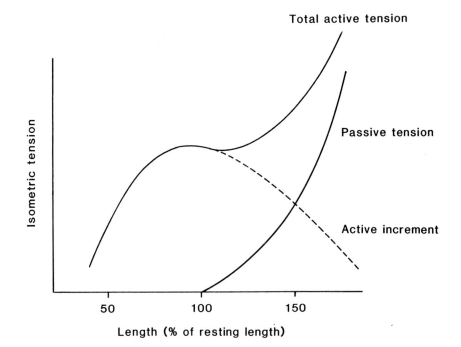

FIG. 4–2.   The length-tension relation in skeletal muscle.

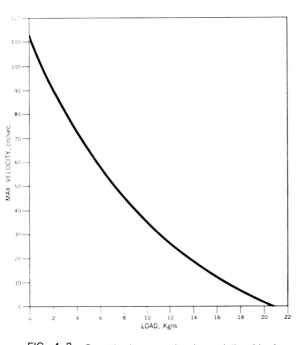

FIG. 4–3. Smoothed curve showing relationship between load and maximal velocity of contraction in human pectoralis major muscle. (Based on data of Ralston, et al.[3])

second the first time the muscle is used, whereas the asserted warm-up benefits presumably require a prolonged preliminary activity.

Wave Summation. An adequate stimulus produces a muscle contraction that lasts for a definite period. If a second stimulus is received while the muscle is still contracted, its shortening and tension are increased. The force finally exerted may be four times as great as that afforded by a series of single twitches. The phenomenon of summation has been demonstrated with single fibers as well as with whole muscles.

Tetanus. If successive stimuli are administered very rapidly, no time is allowed for the muscle to relax. This fusion of superimposed twitches is known as tetanus or tetanic contraction. It is the normal type of voluntary muscular contraction and may be maintained until fatigue sets in. Tetanic contraction in voluntary muscle is maintained by a series of 10 to 50 or more nerve impulses/sec in each nerve fiber. Slow motor units and consequently slow muscles reach tetanus at a lower discharge rate than do fast motor units or fast muscles, partly because of the differences in latency periods.

The refractory period of cardiac muscle, on the other hand, is so long that the muscle becomes almost completely relaxed before a second stimulus can become effective. For this reason, tetanus cannot develop in normal cardiac muscle and the heart does not display

fect (Fig. 4–5). This successive increase in the extent of the contraction has led some authors to cite it as the mechanism responsible for the benefits of warm-up in sports. The fallacy in this reasoning is that treppe occurs only in well-rested muscle and only as the result of spaced, single-nerve impulses. In the intact muscle, even the briefest stimulation consists of a volley of closely spaced nerve impulses. Treppe would take place in a fraction of a

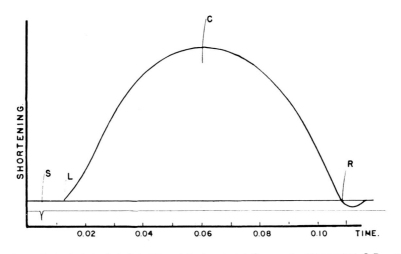

FIG. 4–4. Curve form of a typical single twitch. S-L = latent period; L-C = contraction period; C-R = relaxation period.

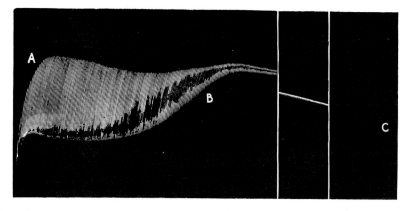

FIG. 4–5.   Effects of repeated stimulation of frog muscle. *A*, Treppe; *B*, Contracture; *C*, Fatigue. (From Francis, Knowlton, and Tuttle: Textbook of Anatomy and Physiology, courtesy The C.V. Mosby Co.)

fatigue in the same manner that skeletal muscle does.

All-or-None Law. In the past, the all-or-none law has been stated as follows: If a muscle fiber contracts at all, it contracts to the maximum extent to which it is capable. Although it is much more accurate to say that the amount of contraction of a muscle fiber is independent of the strength of the stimulus, even this concept is subject to severe, if not disqualifying, limitations. Under laboratory conditions, in which it is possible to stimulate a muscle fiber by special direct methods (rather than through the usual action potential), the amount of contraction is shown to be proportionate to the strength of the stimulus over a wide range of stimulus intensities. Even under normal conditions of stimulation through an action potential in the innervating neuron, the law is at best an oversimplification.

It is helpful to distinguish between the conductile mechanism and the contractile mechanism of a muscle fiber. The conductile processes, like those of nerve fibers, do indeed follow the all-or-none law; that is, the magnitude of the response is independent of the magnitude of the stimulus, provided that the stimulus achieves at least a certain threshold level. This level in turn depends on many factors, such as temperature, chemical state, and elapsed time from a previous stimulus (whether adequate or subthreshold). The contractile processes, on the other hand, do not follow strictly the all-or-none law. For example, summation may occur if successive stimuli are sufficiently rapid.

GRADATION OF CONTRACTION

Obviously, whole muscles do not follow the all-or-none law. Whole muscles have the ability to contract very weakly or very strongly, or at any of a large number of finely graded intermediate levels. The strength of contraction or gradation results mainly from the interaction of three factors—the number of motor units stimulated (recruitment), the frequency of the stimulation (rate of firing), and the timing of stimulation of various motor units (synchronization).

The major mechanism of gradation is the ability of the central nervous system to send stimuli to a greater or lesser number of motor units. When greater tension is needed, more motor units are stimulated. This factor is known as recruitment. According to the "size principle" as it relates to the size of motor neurons innervating a number of fibers, the slow motor units are recruited first.[5] These slow motor units typically have smaller fibers, produce lower maximum tensions, and are fatigue resistant (possess abundant mitochondria). Next in order of recruitment are the fast motor units, which can be either oxidative or fast glycolytic units. Although all fast motor units have high contraction speeds, the oxidative units (which can be a result of high-endurance training) can have slightly smaller fibers and lower maximum tensions than the fast glycolytic units. The fast glycolytic units are recruited later, when a great deal of force and power are needed to perform a given movement. Once a motor unit is recruited, whether it is fast or slow, it can increase its tension only by increasing its firing rate. It is believed that motor units in small muscles have a broad range of firing rates (9 to 50 pulses/sec) and use this range to better control tension than can larger muscles, which have a smaller range of firing rates (13 to 30 pulses/sec) but recruit more units to increase tension.[5]

Differences in muscle fiber composition, i.e., the percentage of fast and slow fibers, appear to be genetically determined, but certain forms of training might affect the oxidative capacity of both fast and slow motor units, as well as affect the size of the fibers in each type of motor unit. For example, long-distance runners may have large slow-twitch fibers and high oxidative capacity in both slow- and fast-twitch fibers, whereas power lifters may have large fast-twitch fibers and lower oxidative capacity in both types of motor units. Aerobic training as compared to power training will have different specific effects on the muscles, which must be kept in mind when athletes prepare for different types of sporting activities.

Summation is a function of the frequency of stimulation. Impulses spaced at intervals greater than the time required for a single twitch will result in minimal muscle contractions and may produce only one fourth the tension that would be produced in tetanus. A somewhat smaller interval between stimuli will result in partial summation, or incomplete tetanus. Even when successive stimuli are equal in strength, very rapid volleys of impulses to the whole muscle will cause maximum response (tetanus).

Ordinarily, the impulses reaching different motor units are out of phase (asynchronous). When a sudden great effort is required, impulses to many or all of the motor units may occur simultaneously (synchronization). In this situation the muscle cannot wait to follow some orderly recruitment process. It needs a great deal of tension very quickly and therefore calls in all the motor units at approximately the same time. The extra strength resulting from synchronization cannot be

employed for a sustained period; it is used most often in short explosive efforts. The firing rate of each motor unit increases quite evenly with gradually increasing effort, whereas the addition of each new motor unit represents a discrete step. It appears that the change in firing rate is the more delicate method of grading the strength of a contraction, whereas the accession of motor units is probably a quicker and more potent factor. Under experimental conditions the strongest voluntary effort does not drive motor units at frequencies much above 50 pulses/sec. It is possible that under the stimulus of an emergency or athletic competition this rate can be increased.

To complicate matters further, there are two separate nerve-muscle systems, innervated by the large neurons and the gamma neurons, respectively (see Chapter 5). Reflex contractions and inhibitions initiated by proprioceptors and the gamma neurons are responsible for feedback, which exerts critical control over the activity of the larger motor neurons; indeed, this is the basis for the mechanisms of posture regulation and of other delicate reflexive controls.

Although a single neuron cannot activate more than the total number of muscle fibers it innervates, it need not activate all the muscle fibers it innervates. A stimulus may be inadequate to activate some of the least irritable muscle fibers in a motor unit (that is, those whose thresholds are at the moment relatively high), because the various fibers may differ from each other in temperature, accumulation of fatigue products, or adequacy of circulation. One of the benefits of training with near-maximal weights in progressive resistance exercise may be that such training brings some of the high-threshold neurons within the orbit of voluntary activity. Such factors as those mentioned in this and the preceding paragraph may modify the three major gradation mechanisms considerably.

RHYTHMIC AND ARRHYTHMIC CONTRACTIONS

Normally the contraction of a muscle as a whole is smooth because the individual responses of the motor units are out of phase with each other, continuously alternating. If the activity of the units becomes synchronous and the contractions appear alternately and rhythmically in muscle groups and their antagonists, tremor results. If the contractions appear simultaneously in both an agonist and antagonist muscle group, rigidity is seen. Coordinated grouping of the discharge of muscle units results in the gross tremor of shivering.

Training produces a reduction in the electrical activity required for a muscle to produce a given degree of tension, indicating that the process of muscle stimulation by the central nervous system becomes more economical.

CONTRACTURE

Any state of prolonged resistance to passive stretch in a muscle may be called contracture. Physiologic contracture results from mechanical, chemical, or other agents acting directly on the contractile mechanism without involving an action potential. Figure 4–5 shows the result of one kind of physiologic contracture in which complete relaxation fails to occur between stimuli. This sort of physiologic contracture occurs when a working muscle becomes fatigued (e.g., in a runner who "ties up"), but its mechanisms are not well understood. Myostatic contracture is a fibrotic condition of the supporting connective tissues of a muscle or joint, resulting from immobilization of the muscle in the short position while the nerve-muscle unit remains intact. Myostatic contracture occurs after a limb has been immobilized in a cast, after a tendon has been severed or detached, or after antagonistic muscles have been paralyzed.

CRAMPS

During vigorous exercise or during sleep, healthy persons may experience involuntary, sustained, painful contraction of skeletal muscle termed cramp. For experimental purposes cramps can be induced by a maximum voluntary effort while the muscle is in a shortened position. The pattern of the action potentials indicates that cramps are due to excitation of most of the muscle fibers in a given motor unit, suggesting that the cramp can be

explained in terms of motor unit activity originating in the central nervous system. The pain seems to be proportionate to the total number of active units. Hypertrophied muscles appear more liable to cramp than normal muscles, but, physiologically, hypertrophy is not associated with any known change in excitability.

The cause of cramps may be centered in the muscle, in peripheral nerves, or in the central nervous system. These causes are poorly understood and in many instances are impossible to identify. It is known that cramps in healthy persons and athletes may be caused by local fatigue; rapid changes in deep-muscle temperature, as when exertion is not preceded by adequate warm-up; extreme effort at sustained muscular contraction, especially when the muscle is in a shortened position; restricted circulation caused by tight clothing or prolonged static contraction; and imbalance of ions caused by excessive perspiring. The obvious antidotes may be tried, such as rest, warm-up, massage, fluid intake to compensate for fluid loss, and salt supplementation to maintain ion concentrations. Administration of salt does no good, however, unless salt was previously depleted. Often, acute cramps can be relieved by passive stretching of the muscle group involved.

MUSCLE SPASM

Muscle spasm resembles cramps but tends to be less severe and more persistent. Postexercise soreness and the pain of idiopathic low-back syndrome often result from muscle spasm. Low-back syndrome may be complicated by arthritic pressure on spinal nerves or by abnormality of intervertebral disks and should be evaluated by an orthopedist before any remedy is sought.

SPASTICITY

The central nervous system receives information about changes in the length of muscles by means of proprioceptive impulses arising from the muscle spindles (see Chapter 5) and other end organs. Normally, when the muscle surrounding a spindle contracts, the discharge from the spindle ceases. A disturbance in the gamma efferent control over the spindle can result in its continued discharge, producing in the muscles an exaggerated stretch reflex (hypertonus). Motor unit activity in the affected limb at rest does not differ from that in the normal limb. However, if exaggerated motor unit activity is observed when an attempt is made to move the limb, the limb is said to be spastic. In humans, such hypertonus occurs only in the antigravity muscles. Efforts to flex the hip, knee, or ankle, which result in a stretch of spastic extensor muscles at each joint, encounter marked resistance. The same joints can be extended freely, however. In the arm, the flexors normally counteract the force of gravity, and a spastic arm resists attempts at extension.

RECIPROCAL INNERVATION AND CO-CONTRACTION

Sherrington observed that in decerebrate or anesthetized animals, in whom voluntary control is abolished, afferent neural impulses that stimulate the motor neurons of a given muscle reflexively inhibit the motor neurons of the antagonistic muscles. This effect is known as reciprocal innervation, and the mechanism by which it functions is reciprocal inhibition of antagonistic muscles. Uncoordinated movement can result if the excitation of the agonist is not accompanied by this corresponding reflex inhibition of the antagonist. Sherrington also noted that antagonistic muscles can contract simultaneously with the agonists, which he attributed to double reciprocal innervation.[6] Studies on the role of the muscle spindles in the production of a stretch reflex suggest that this theory is no longer tenable.[7]

Sherrigton further observed that after being subjected to reflex inhibition, the neural drive to a skeletal muscle tends to increase (rebound discharge). As a result, application of a stimulus that causes flexion (or extension) of a limb tends to be followed by active extension (or flexion) of the same limb (successive induction) when the inhibitory effect is withdrawn. Theoretically, then, when the discus thrower swings his arm backward, the horizontal extensors of the shoulder joint are activated and the horizontal flexors are inhib-

ited. The resulting rebound and successive induction of the horizontal flexors reflexively give greater force to the subsequent swing forward. An additional consideration is the use of elastic strain energy in the horizontal flexion that was stored when the arm swung backward.

As early as 1925, Tilney and Pike found that under normal conditions they were unable to observe Sherrington's phenomena and concluded that "muscular coordination depends primarily on the synchronous co-contractive relationship in the antagonist muscle groups."[8] They suggested that one possible result of the disturbance of this co-contractive relationship is overextension by the agonists, followed by overcorrection by the antagonists. An irregular series of oscillations would result, which might explain the clinical symptoms of ataxia.

Only muscles acting on a single joint are assumed to be true antagonists. Muscles acting on more than one joint can act at times as antagonists and at other times as synergists. The rectus femoris normally acts as an antagonist to the hamstrings, but if the hip and knee are flexed simultaneously, the rectus femoris acts synergistically with them. In some multipennate muscles one part may act as an antagonist and another part as a synergist.

As an agonist goes into the final range of contraction, it begins to cause proprioceptive stimulation of the antagonist muscle. The resulting contraction of the antagonist then offers resistance to the final phase of movement of the agonist. The position in the movement where this resistance occurs varies with the joint and muscles involved.

It is possible to demonstrate reciprocal innervation in the human in unresisted voluntary movement, reflex movements such as the knee jerk, and, in cases of spasticity, a condition that leads to structural shortening of the muscles involved. Electrical stimulation of muscles antagonistic to those in spasm has been found to result in relaxation of the spastic muscles. Some investigators[9] believe that, in normal voluntary movement, co-contraction is the rule rather than the exception, and satisfactory evidence that reciprocal innervation plays the part usually assigned to it by kinesiologists is lacking; others contend that during movement the antagonist relaxes completely, with a single exception—the finish of a whip-like motion of a hinge joint.

The evidence suggests that antagonistic muscles behave in at least three distinct ways:

1. When external resistance is so great that the joint cannot move, the antagonists relax.
2. When the muscles are acting against moderate resistance, the antagonists become active to decelerate the movement.
3. When there is no external resistance to be overcome and the limb must move with great precision, tension tends to be maintained in both the agonist group and the antagonist group, with the agonist group predominating.

ISOMETRIC TENSION

When force is exerted by a muscle against an object that it cannot move, the muscle-tendon unit remains at the same length and technically accomplishes no external work. The energy that would normally be displayed as external mechanical work is used in the structural rearrangement of muscle fibers and tendon, i.e., fibers shorten and tendon stretches, and some is dissipated as heat. In such a case, the muscle is said to develop isometric tension, and the contractile elements may shorten about 3% of their length by stretching the elastic components (e.g., tendon). Evidence suggests that the muscle fibers are not of uniform strength; some of the heat produced may result from the stronger fibers extending the weaker fibers. Posture is maintained largely by relatively isometric contractions of certain muscles of the back and legs, in which muscle tension is required to offset the pull of gravity on the body. Isometric exercise is also employed for "muscle setting" exercises in physical medicine.

ISOTONIC CONTRACTION

When a muscle is able to move a load, work is accomplished and the muscle is said to have performed an isotonic contraction. At a constant velocity of shortening, the motor unit activity has been found to be directly pro-portionate to the tension. At a constant velocity of lengthening, such as occurs when a weight is slowly lowered to the ground, motor unit electrical activity is again proportionate to tension; however, less electrical activity is required in lengthening because the elastic structures of the muscle help lower the weight.

The A bands remain at a constant length during normal muscle shortening, the I bands shorten, and the H bands close up, creating a dark line in place of the H zone. This line may be interpreted as a crumpling of the ends of the actin filaments and may constitute the M band.

Muscle, tendon, and bone have different strengths and are affected differently by situations that place different rates of strain on these tissues. As a rule, slow strains create avulsion fractures, in which the rupturing tendon actually pulls a section of bone with it. Fast strains, produced, for example, by unexpectedly dropping your heel into a hole in the ground during running, would cause the tendon to rupture and not necessarily affect the bone. (For information on the effects of age, exercise, and immobilization on the connective tissue in the body, additional reading is necessary.[10])

CONTRALATERAL EXERCISE (CROSS EDUCATION)

Under certain conditions, training of one limb has been shown to produce an increase in strength, endurance, or skill of the opposite (contralateral) limb. This effect probably has little importance for the normal individual but may be of value in maintaining muscle tone and preventing atrophy in an immobilized limb during convalescence. The explanation is not entirely clear. It appears that in situations in which a muscle is overloaded, there may be an overflow from neurons in the motor cortex to those that supply the contralateral limb.

STRETCHING

When a muscle is stretched, the A bands remain at a constant length, the I bands increase in length, the actin filaments are pulled out of the A bands, and the H bands become longer by an amount equal to the increase in the length of the I bands. A muscle can resist a stretch with a force greater than it can develop in either an isometric contraction or a shortening contraction. Muscle stretching is very common in normal movements, and these lengthening contractions are used to control limb movement. For example, in walking, as the nonsupporting limb swings through and prepares for heel strike, the knee is extending. To control this extension, the hamstrings are active. Knee flexors, then, not knee extensors, are needed to control and slow down knee extension and prepare the limb for contact with the ground again.

The three types of muscular contraction and the characteristics of each are summarized in Table 4–1.

WORK DONE BY MUSCLE CONTRACTION

The amount of work done by a contracting muscle is a combination of two elements of equal importance: the amount of force used and the distance of the movement. Stated mathematically, the amount of work done is the product of the force and the distance ($W = Fd$). One unit of work is the amount involved in exerting one unit of force through one unit of distance, regardless of what these units are, so that work may be expressed in gram-centimeters, foot-pounds, kilogram-meters, or any other appropriate combinations, according to the units of force and distance employed.

The force that a muscle can exert depends on the physiologic cross-sectional area of its fibers; the distance through which it can contract depends on the length of its fibers. Absolute muscle force varies with the length of the muscle at the time of the test and the velocity of shortening during the test. When muscle strength is being measured, allowances must also be made for the angle of insertion of the fibers. Unless each of these factors is equated, data from different studies may not be compared, and in fact the literature contains widely varying estimates of muscle strength. Muscle force varies from muscle to muscle, but approximately 3.3 kg of isometric force per cm² of cross section is generally accepted.[11] Normal muscle can shorten up to 25% of its relaxed state. On the average, the dynamic strength of women is 68.6% that of men, ranging from 59% to 84%, depending on the area of the body tested.[12]

Negative Work. In the case of an eccentric (lengthening) contraction, as occurs when lowering a heavy weight slowly or when walking down stairs, no external work is being done, according to the preceding definition. In such cases, work is done by the weight on the muscles, which is referred to as negative work, instead of being done by the muscles on the weight. Its numeric value is calculated exactly as in the aforementioned formula; if a 50-kg weight is lowered slowly through 25 cm, the work done is 1250 kg-cm.

Two-Joint Muscles. The fact that some muscles affect two or more joints of the skeleton affects their work efficiency. For example, when the leg is moved forward, tension developed in the rectus femoris contributes, simultaneously, to flexing the hip and extending the knee. When the leg is moved backward, tension in the hamstrings contributes, simultaneously, to extension of the hip and flexion of the knee. There are many examples of two-joint muscles in the human body, and the advantages of using them rather than the single-joint muscles are obvious. For example, hip flexion and knee extension occur together very often in normal movement. The effect on the rectus femoris is shortening at the hip and lengthening at the knee. Positive work is done at the hip and

Table 4–1.   Types of Muscle Contraction

Type of Tension	Type of Contraction	Function	External Force Opposing Muscle	External Work by Muscle	Energy Supply
Isotonic	Concentric	Acceleration	Less	Positive	Increases
Isometric	Static	Fixation	Equal	None	
Lengthening	Eccentric	Deceleration	Greater	Negative	Decreases

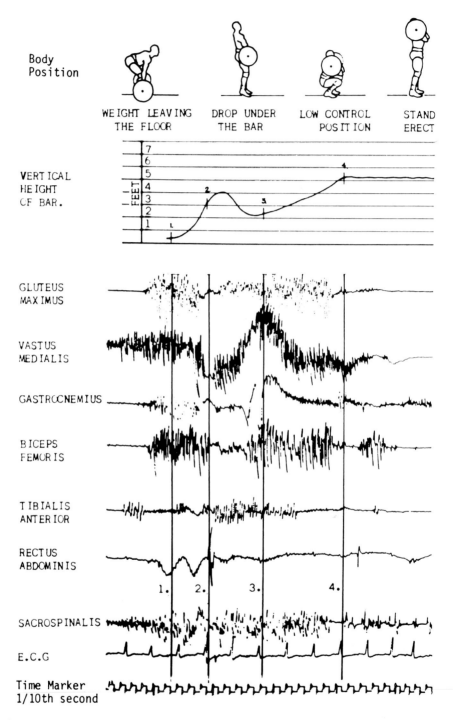

Body Position

WEIGHT LEAVING THE FLOOR

DROP UNDER THE BAR

LOW CONTROL POSITION

STAND ERECT

VERTICAL HEIGHT OF BAR.

GLUTEUS MAXIMUS

VASTUS MEDIALIS

GASTROCNEMIUS

BICEPS FEMORIS

TIBIALIS ANTERIOR

RECTUS ABDOMINIS

SACROSPINALIS

E.C.G

Time Marker 1/10th second

FIG. 4–6. Legend on facing page.

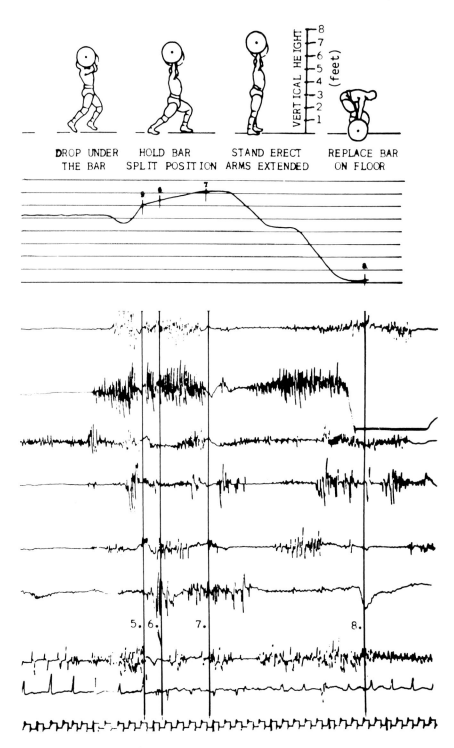

FIG. 4–6.   Recording of electromyograms and other data during a two-hands clean and jerk. (Courtesy V. Thomas: Sportsmen Under Stress. New Scientist, 1969. Copyright Corser, Saville & Thomas.)

negative work is done at the knee, with the net mechanical result being a saving in energy cost. Additionally, the total length of the muscle may change very little, thus keeping it in a more ideal position to generate tension according to its length-tension curve. (See Chapter 16.)

METHODS OF STUDYING MUSCULAR ACTION

There are at least five ways of studying a muscle to determine its action.

1. Study the conditions under which a muscle acts by the use of a mounted skeleton, noticing the muscle's points of attachment, direction of pull, leverage, and any other points pertaining to the problem.
2. Pull on the partly dissected muscles of a cadaver and notice the resulting movements.

Both of these methods have their uses, but it does not necessarily follow that muscle action in vivo can be deduced from either one of them. Synergistic actions cannot be determined by such methods. Normal movements usually involve groups of muscles, and the same muscle may work in different movements.

3. Stimulate individual muscles by electric current and observe the resulting movements. This was the classic methodology of Duchenne. Though it increased our knowledge, it can be applied only to the superficial muscles and is subject to the objections made in the use of the first and second methods.
4. Study subjects who have lost the use of certain muscles to determine what loss of power and movement has resulted and whether any abnormal postures have been produced. Studies of this kind have added materially to our knowledge of muscular action, but it is difficult to obtain a sufficient variety of subjects to study the muscles in a systematic way.
5. Study the normal living body to find what muscles contract in certain exercises and what movements call certain muscles into action. This is perhaps the

most practical approach to kinesiologic problems. Neither observations made on a cadaver or skeleton, nor data provided by electrical stimulation experiments can tell what a muscle will do. They may, however, tell what a muscle *can* do. We need to learn not only what action a muscle is able to perform because of its position and opportunity, but also what, in an actual case, the nervous system requires of it and when the nervous system permits it to lie idle. Some of Duchenne's most brilliant discoveries by means of electrical stimulation have been found to be misleading, because observation of the living body shows that certain muscles that might help greatly in a movement are actually never called on. An example is the gluteus maximus, which could participate in leg extension in walking but does not.

Observations on normal subjects may be made by two quite different techniques. The first technique, best suited to beginners, is to determine the action of muscles in a given exercise by seeing or actual feeling the muscle contract. This method does not always produce dependable results, however, because many muscles are so situated that they cannot be observed directly.

The student with some technical background can make use of an electromyogram (EMG), which is a record of the muscular excitation resulting from stimulation by the nervous system. The electrical activity in a contracting muscle is roughly proportionate to the isometric tension in the muscle. In isotonic contractions, however, the EMG output is affected by the load, velocity, acceleration, and length of the muscle. The EMG is lower for an eccentric contraction than for a concentric one when the same tension is produced in each contraction. The action of a number of muscles may be observed simultaneously when EMG is used in conjunction with some visual records (film or video), and the student can tell exactly at which point each muscle comes into play and when its action ceases (Fig. 4–6). Surface electrodes are used most commonly in kinesiologic studies, whereas indwelling electrodes are used more clinically for disease diagnosis and for recording activity of deep muscles, e.g., iliopsoas.[6]

The electromyogram is affected by the degree of training of the muscle as well as by the age of the individual. With progressive training of a muscle, the average duration of its electrical potentials gradually increases and the average frequency decreases, and antagonists are progressively inhibited.[6] Studies of older persons show a decreased amplitude for motor unit potentials, believed to result from a decrease in muscle fibers' size and number; a high incidence of polyphasic motor unit potentials, suggesting a delay in endplate transmission or muscle fiber response; and a decay in amplitude on sustained contractions, which presumably reflects an inability of the fibers to maintain sustained tension.

REFERENCES

1. Nachmansohn, D.: Chemical and Molecular Basis of Nerve Activity. 2nd Ed. New York, Academic Press, Inc., 1975.
2. Aidley, D.J.: The Physiology of Excitable Cells. New York, Cambridge University Press, 1978.
3. Ralston, H.J., et al.: Dynamic features of human isolated voluntary muscle in isometric and free contractions. J. Appl. Physiol., *1*:526, 1949.
4. Komi, P.V.: Physiological and biomechanical correlates of muscle function: effects of muscle structure and stretch-shortening cycle on force and speed. *In* Exercise and Sport Sciences Reviews. Edited by R.L. Terjung. Lexington, Mass., Collamore Press, 1984, p. 81.
5. Basmajian, J.V., and DeLuca, C.J.: Muscles Alive: Their Functions Revealed by Electromyography. Baltimore, Williams and Wilkins, 1985, p. 157.
6. Denny-Brown, D. (ed): Selected Writings of Sir Charles Sherrington. New York, Paul N. Hoeber Inc., 1940, pp. 237.
7. Herman, R.: The physiologic basis of tone, spasticity and rigidity. Arch. Phys. Med., *43*:108, 1962.
8. Tilney, F., and Pike, F.H.: Muscular coordination experimentally studied in its relation to the cerebellum. Arch. Neurol. Psychiat., *13*:289, 1925.
9. Levine, M.G., and Kabat, H.: Cocontraction and reciprocal innervation in volunary movement in man. Science, *116*:115, 1952.
10. Frankel, V.H., and Norden, M.: Basic Biomechanics of the Skeletal System. Philadelphia, Lea & Febiger, 1980, p. 55.
11. Elftman, H.: Biomechanics of muscle. J. Bone Joint Surg., *48-A*:363, 1966.
12. Laubach, L.L.: Comparative muscular strength of men and women: Review of the literature. Aviat. Space Environ. Med., *47*:534, 1976.

RECOMMENDED READING

Carlson, F.D., and Wilkie, D.R.: Muscle Physiology. Englewood Cliffs, N.J., Prentice-Hall, 1974.
Cavanagh, P.R.: Electromyography: Its use and misuse in physical education. JOHPER, *45*:61, 1974.
Hall, E.A.: Electromyographic techniques: A review. Phys. Ther., *50*:651, 1970.
Rasch, P.J.: Isometric exercise and gains of muscle strength. *In* Frontiers of Fitness. Edited by R.J. Shephard. Springfield, Illinois, Charles C Thomas, 1971, p. 98.

5 NEUROLOGY, KINESTHESIA, AND SERVOMOTOR CONTROL

ROBERT J. GREGOR

Neurons transmit electric pulses, whose sizes are constant but whose frequency may be varied; the greater the stimulus, the greater the frequency. Consequently, muscle action potentials and neural action potentials are identical; the discharge of a motor neuron can hardly be distinguished from the discharge of a sensory organ, and reflex response to electrical stimulation gives an electromyogram (EMG) similar to those EMGs obtained by mechanical percussion of a tendon. The only way the brain can distinguish among the inputs from the various sensory organs is for it to be aware of which nerves have been stimulated. It follows that for the brain to be really sure of what is happening to the body, several sources of sensory input are desirable. Most of this chapter will be devoted to considering the brain's sources of sensory information.

THE NEURON AND ITS FUNCTIONS

The structural and functional unit of the nervous system is the single nerve cell, or neuron (Fig. 5–1). It consists of a nucleated cell body and two or more processes called nerve fibers. The processes may be divided into axons (axis cylinders) and dendrites. Usually there are several dendrites, which may traverse either a very long or a very short distance between the cell body and the many branches at their terminal arborizations. Dendrites are receivers and normally conduct impulses toward the cell body. Generally, a neuron has only one axon, which may be up to

3 ft long, which carries impulses away from the cell body and passes them along to the dendrites of the next neuron. The cell bodies are located in the gray matter of the spinal cord and brain or in ganglia (collections or bunches of cell bodies) located outside of, but relatively close to, the spinal cord. Nerve fibers may be found intermingled with the cell bodies of the gray matter, or they may be arranged longitudinally in white bundles. White bundles within the spinal cord and brain are known as tracts, columns, or commissures, while those outside the spinal cord and brain are known as nerves. Neurons are generally considered to be the individual nerve cells, whereas nerves are typically bundles of fibers (e.g., median nerve).

The nerve fiber is essentially a protoplasmic extension (axis cylinder) of the body of the cell. This axis cylinder is sometimes clothed with a fatty myelin or medullary sheath. In some areas, a thinner nucleated membrane, the neurilemma, invests the axis cylinder, and if a myelin sheath is present, it lies between the neurilemma and the axis cylinder. Both of these coverings, when present, insulate to prevent irradiation of impulses. The neurilemma is an essential factor in the regeneration of nerve fibers.

Axons and dendrites may or may not have specialized end organs. Motor axons have motor end-plates (Fig. 5–2) that lie on individual muscle fibers and are necessary for transmission of an impulse across the myoneural junction. Sensory fibers sometimes have specialized receptor end organs, such as

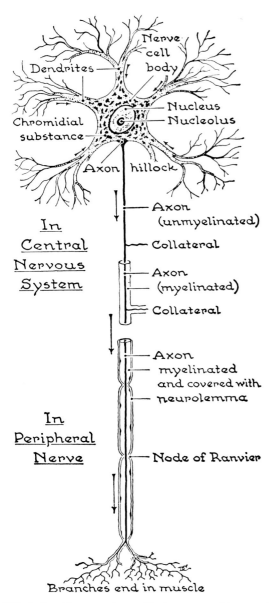

FIG. 5–1.   Diagram of a multipolar neuron. (Ham and Lesson: Histology. 4th Ed. Courtesy J.B. Lippincott Co.)

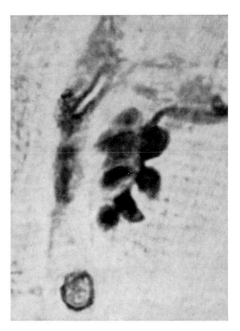

FIG. 5–2.   The terminal arborization of the motor end plate in man. (Coërs.)

the proprioceptor end organs discussed later in this chapter.

If a cell body is sufficiently damaged, the entire neuron will degenerate irreversibly; if a process is only severed or damaged, usually only the portion peripheral to the cell body will degenerate. If the cell body and the neurilemma of the degenerated portion remain intact, the central end of the process may grow out (regenerate) along its former course by following the path provided by the neu-

rilemma. In the case of a cut nerve, the suturing together of the severed nerve ends may enhance the possibility of regeneration by approximately restoring the continuity of the neurilemma pathway. Unfortunately, no regeneration is possible if the cell bodies of motor nerves lying in the spinal cord are destroyed, as is the case in poliomyelitis. When a muscle atrophies, both the muscle fibers and the motor endings diminish in size (Fig. 5–3).

Peripheral neurons (those extending outside the brain and spinal cord) may be divided into afferent (sensory) neurons and efferent (motor) neurons. Most nerves are mixed nerves—that is, they contain both afferent and efferent fibers. Neurons within the spinal cord and brain are known as internuncial or intercalary neurons, serving as connectors, collators, integrators, analyzers, and organizers of sensory and motor impulses.

NEURAL CONDUCTION

A neuron is potentially capable of responding to electrical, mechanical, chemical, or thermal stimuli, although a receptor end organ may make it especially susceptible to a certain kind of stimulation. In any event, an

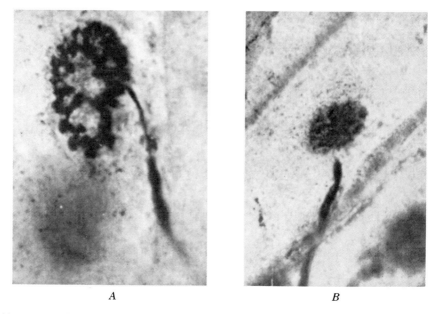

A   *B*

FIG. 5–3.   Motor ending (myoneural junction) in gastrocnemius of rat. (Cole.) *A,* Normal male rat. (×450.) *B,* Male rat whose femur has been immobilized for 14 days. (×450.)

adequate stimulus causes a physiochemical change known as a local excitatory state (les). If the stimulus has sufficient strength, duration, and rate of change of intensity, the les triggers the propagation of a wave of excitation (nerve impulse) along the fiber—this process is known as conduction. The nerve impulse is self-propagating, like a spark traveling along a string of gunpowder. It is carried from the point of stimulation to all parts of the neuron, at speeds up to 120 m/sec, depending on the diameter of the fiber and its physiologic state at that moment. A neuron obeys the all-or-none law—that is, conduction depends on a stimulus whose intensity reaches a certain threshold value. A stimulus of greater than threshold value has no extra effect on the quality of the impulse, although it may irradiate at its point of application and cause conduction in adjacent neurons as well.

After conduction, there is an absolute refractory period (about 0.0004 sec in mammals) during which no stimulus will arouse a response from the neuron. This period is followed by a relative refractory period (about 0.01 to 0.02 sec) during which excitability gradually returns to normal, and only an intense stimulus will arouse a response from the neuron.

The Synapse. The junction between two nerve fibers is called a synapse. Here the ends of the axons are in very close contact with the brush-like endings of the dendrites and other neurons. Because each neuron is a discrete anatomic unit, the synapse becomes the point of communication between one neuron and another. The nervous impulse travels along an axon and across the synapse to the dendrites of the other neuron, never in the reverse direction. The synapse offers varying resistance, depending on the synapse, to the passage of the nervous impulse. The synapse also causes a slight delay, about 0.002 sec, in the transmission of the nervous impulse.

The synapse acts as a one-way valve or gate that permits the passage of the nervous impulse from one neuron to another. Because of their variable resistance, synapses tend to be selective and direct the pathway of the nervous impulse, both that result from the conduction of feeble stimuli across only the synapses with low resistance, and nervous impulses that result from the conduction of powerful stimuli across those synapses with high resistance.

Inhibition. The foregoing material on synaptic transmission pertains to neurons whose function is excitatory. In the brain and spinal cord, however, there are many presynaptic neurons whose function is inhibitory rather than excitatory. Inhibitory neurons have only one major difference from excitatory neurons: instead of depolarizing the postsynaptic neuron, they increase the resting potential. Like local excitatory states, local inhibitory states are additive when several occur simultaneously. The postsynaptic neuron will "fire" only when the algebraic sum of inhibitory and excitatory states balances out on the excitatory side, at or above threshold level. An inhibitory neuron receives its neural stimulation by a preponderance of excitatory influence, just like any other neuron, even though its influence across its terminal synapse is inhibitory.

Some of the reason for the complexity of neural functioning should now be clear. Although we can define two-neuron reflex arcs and even isolate them functionally under sophisticated laboratory circumstances, in vivo a nerve cell body is subject to the modulating influence of several, or even hundreds, of impinging excitatory and inhibitory neurons. Thus, the net effect on the motor neuron is determined by a myriad of modulations, feedbacks, and filtering from both peripheral and central sources, including some from higher brain centers.

Examples of graded inhibition are seen in most voluntary movements. The concept of co-contraction (Chap. 4) specifies that movement usually involves the simultaneous contraction of antagonistic muscle groups, although there may be a distinct difference in the forces exerted by the members of the pair. When the external resistance to the agonists is great, the co-contraction of the antagonists is minimal. Apparently a central inhibitory effect acts on the antagonists to reduce the resistance to the movement. This inhibition occurs in involuntary, though perhaps learned, reflexes. It is controlled in the spinal cord and lower levels of the brain and is roughly proportionate to the amount of force required for the agonists to perform the movement.

A therapist, first-aid administrator, or athlete can sometimes make use of the phenomenon of inhibition of antagonists. Muscle cramps and spasms, especially when acute, can sometimes be relieved by a strong voluntary or electrical stimulation of the muscle's antagonist.

As with other reflexes, the inhibition of antagonists may be overridden or modified under certain conditions. For example, at the extreme range of motion the inhibited antagonist may be stretched sufficiently to initiate a myotatic contraction.

Excessive general tension associated with emotional stress can also modify the reflex inhibition of antagonists. In the early stages of motor learning, such factors as fear, embarrassment, and intense motivation can result in indiscriminate contractions of muscle groups, thus interfering with smooth and effective performance. Expert performers have learned coordinated patterns of contraction and inhibition; these have been so strongly conditioned that only intense stresses are capable of interfering. In any performer, the removal of excess general tension minimizes the output of irrelevant motor impulses, allowing the conditioned reflexes for contraction and inhibition to occur. Coaches, teachers, and therapists who stress general relaxation, minimize fear, and use care in applying motivational stresses during the learning process are acting on sound physiologic and psychologic principles.

ORGANIZATION OF THE NERVOUS SYSTEM

The nervous system may be divided into the central nervous system, consisting of the brain and spinal cord, and the peripheral nervous system, consisting of all ganglia and nerves outside of the brain and spinal cord (Fig. 5–4). From another aspect, the nervous system may be divided into the autonomic nervous system, which involves responses of the heart, intestines, urogenital tract, blood vessels, and endocrine glands receiving a nervous supply, and the somatic system, which deals with sensory impulses and motor responses of the skeletal musculature.

Cranial Nerves. The peripheral nerves arising from the brain innervate skeletal muscles, such as the muscles of the eyeball, face, and tongue, but they are concerned mainly with olfaction, vision, taste, balance, audition, and other sensory functions, and with involuntary control of the heart, lungs, stomach, and other viscera. The spinal part of the accessory

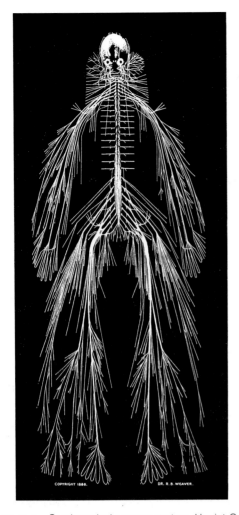

FIG. 5–4. Cerebrospinal nervous system. Harriet Cole, a scrubwoman at Hahnemann Medical College, willed her body to Anatomy Professor Rufus B. Weaver. The doctor used it for what is probably the only preserved dissection of the human nervous system. The brain was removed, but the spinal cord and the peripheral nervous system are shown. (Hahnemann Medical College and Hospital.)

nerve (CN XI) is the only cranial nerve that innervates important postural muscles—the sternocleidomastoid and trapezius muscles.

Spinal Nerves. There are 31 pairs of spinal nerves arising from the spinal cord and leaving the vertebral canal through the intervertebral foramina. Each of the 8 pairs of cervical nerves is named for the vertebra just below it (except the eighth, which arises between the seventh cervical and the first thoracic vertebrae), and each of the 12 thoracic, 5 lumbar, 5 sacral, and 1 coccygeal pairs is named for the vertebra just above it. Spinal nerves are

called mixed nerves because they are made up of both sensory and motor fibers along most of their length. They are mixed in another sense, too, for most of them carry fibers of both the autonomic and somatic nervous systems (Fig. 5–5).

Pathways of the Spinal Nerves. As the spinal nerve root approaches the spine, it bifurcates into an efferent root and an afferent root that carries impulses of proprioception, touch, pain, heat, cold, etc. The afferent root enters the spinal cord in the region of the posterior horn of the gray matter and hence is termed the dorsal or posterior root; the efferent root enters the spinal cord in the region of the ventral horn of the gray matter and is termed the ventral or anterior root (Fig. 5–5). After entering the cord, the afferent fibers take various courses, some ending in the gray matter at the same level, some taking a vertical course in the white columns and sending terminal endings into the gray matter at higher or lower levels, and some traversing the white columns as far as the base of the brain. They make synaptic contact in an exceptionally versatile manner, either joining dendrites of motor neurons directly or joining dendrites of internuncial neurons. The internuncial neurons serve as middlemen in transferring impulses to motor neurons at the same or different spinal levels or to higher centers in the brain.

The dendrites and cell bodies of efferent (motor) neurons are located in the gray matter of the spinal cord. They collect impulses from fibers descending from the brain, from internuncial neurons, or directly from afferent spinal neurons at the same or different levels of the cord.

The basic plan of distribution of spinal nerves is clearly an evolutionary holdover from that seen in limbless segmented lower forms. At the cervical and upper thoracic spinal regions and in the lumbar and sacral spinal regions, the adjacent spinal regions, the adjacent spinal nerves interconnect with each other in complex patterns. These five plexuses are the cervical plexus, the brachial plexus, the lumbar plexus, the sacral plexus, and the coccygeal plexus. The acroparesthesia sometimes seen in women engaged in manual work results when the supporting muscula-

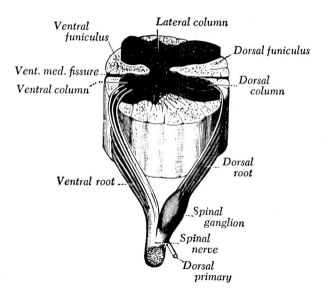

FIG. 5–5. A spinal nerve with its anterior and posterior roots. (Gray's Anatomy. 30th Ed. Philadelphia, Lea & Febiger, 1985.)

ture becomes atonic and permits the shoulder girdle to sag. Pressure by the first rib and traction and compression of the lower components of the brachial plexus follows. Elevating the arms overhead is restful, because it relieves the pull on the brachial plexus.

SPINAL REFLEXES

A reflex is an involuntary muscular contraction or glandular secretion resulting from a sensory stimulation. Reflexes can be very complex and can involve the higher brain centers. The simplest reflex is the spinal reflex, requiring a minimum of two neurons. An afferent neuron receives a stimulus at its peripheral end and carries the resulting impulse along a spinal nerve to the gray matter of the spinal cord by way of the dorsal root. The impulse crosses a synapse in the spinal cord to a motor neuron that transmits the impulse along the ventral horn, along a spinal nerve, and to a muscle or gland. More frequently, a third neuron (an internuncial neuron) lying in the gray matter of the spinal cord mediates the impulse between the sensory and the motor neurons.

Simple spinal reflex arcs involving only two or three neurons exist but are hardly typical even of the most elemental reflex activity. At the synapse in the spinal cord, the impulse

from the sensory neuron is likely to trigger not only the motor neuron that completes the reflex arc, but also a number of others that carry sensory or motor impulses along parallel pathways to the contralateral side of the body, to higher or lower spinal levels, to the lower brain center, and even to the higher levels of consciousness. The original sensory neuron itself can send branches to adjacent spinal levels. Internuncial neurons generally connect with not one but numerous motor neurons at several spinal levels (Fig. 5–6).

Each involved neuron has a threshold of sensitivity governed at any given moment by the algebraic sum of various inhibitory and excitatory influences supplied through many other existing synaptic connections. Some of these additionally impinging influences arise locally; others originate from distant sources, perhaps including voluntary cortical emanations. The most elementary activity usually involves thousands of neural elements, giving a picture of reverberating circuits and a multitude of continuous modulations from positive and negative feedback mechanisms.

A great proportion of our actions are reflexive. Even a simple pinprick on the hand, which can cause a sleeping person to withdraw a limb without waking, irradiates to the lower brain centers. It is difficult to conceive

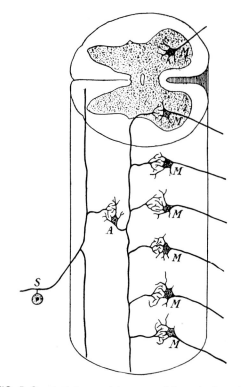

FIG. 5–6.   An internuncial neuron of the spinal cord. *S*, Sensory neuron. *A*, Internuncial neuron. *M*, Motor neurons. This diagram has been simplified to show only one sensory neuron being stimulated to initiate a reflex.

such reflex actions as being either simple or spinal in any limiting sense of the words.

Corrective and physical therapists make use of some of the more complex reflexes in the treatment of certain types of patients. Thus, the spastic hand may be "unlocked" by placing it palm up over the buttocks of the prone patient and turning his head away from the involved side. The evolutionary mechanisms underlying such phenomena and the ways in which reflexes of this type may be utilized have been summarized by Fay.[1]

KINESTHETIC AND SERVOMOTOR CONTROL

Kinesthesis or kinesthesia is the perception of the position and movement of one's body parts in space. It also includes perception of the internal and external forces tending to move or stabilize the body parts. Various kinds of receptors contribute to kinesthesis, including (1) free, unencapsulated nerve endings sensitive to pain, (2) Meissner's corpus-

cles, sensitive to touch, (3) joint receptors resembling flower-spray endings and giving a steady discharge proportionate to changes in joint capsule tension resulting from changes in the joint's position (Fig. 5–7A), (4) joint receptors resembling elongated pacinian corpuscles, giving a discharge proportionate to changes in capsule tension during movement (Fig. 5–7B), (5) pacinian corpuscles sensitive to deep pressure resulting from deformation of body tissues (Fig. 5–8), (6) labyrinthine receptors, (7) visual receptors, (8) auditory receptors, (9) Golgi tendon organs, and (10) muscle spindles.

Kinesthetic perceptions generally are relayed to cortical centers of consciousness, although the process of motor learning may allow them to exert their influence automatically or subconsciously. However, two of the above-listed receptors operate essentially at a peripheral level, although they are markedly susceptible to central control. The Golgi tendon organs and the muscle spindle, in association with skeletal muscle fibers, form a basic servomotor system, knowledge of which is essential to an understanding of terminal muscle function. Consequently, the structure and function of these organs must be considered in some detail.

Golgi Tendon Organs. The Golgi tendon organs (Fig. 5–9) consist of fusiform fibrous capsules enclosing myelinated nerve fibers. Because most of them are located at the junction of muscle fibers and their tendinous attachments at both ends of the muscle, the Golgi tendon organs are said to be "in series" with the muscle. They are sensitive to both muscle stretch and muscle contraction but cannot distinguish between the two. In other words, they discharge as the result of tension in the tendon. Their discharge causes inhibition of their own muscle and facilitation of its antagonist. This safety valve action prevents damage from excessive contraction by the muscle in which they occur.

Muscle Spindles. A muscle spindle (Fig. 5–10) consists of a connective tissue capsule about 1 mm long, six or more intrafusal ("within the spindle") muscle fibers, and some specialized motor and sensory nerve endings. Spindles are located between and parallel to the extrafusal muscle fibers of the

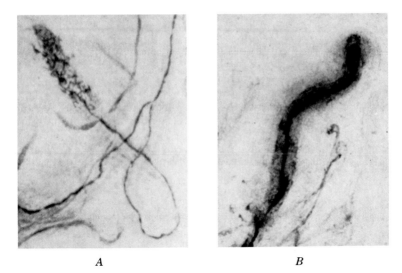

A   *B*

FIG. 5–7. Sensory endings in human synovial joint capsule. *A*, Flower-spray ending, slowly adapting and believed to signal joint position in the steady state. *B*, Lamellated or paciniform ending, rapidly adapting and believed to respond to movement and pressure. (McCarry, with permission. J. Physiol., November, 1965.)

whole muscle. The ends of the capsule extend into and merge with the connective tissue of the whole muscle. The important point is that the spindles lie parallel with the muscle, in contrast to the "in series" arrangement of the Golgi tendon organs. Like the Golgi tendon organs, the receptors of the muscle spindles are sensitive to stretch (Fig. 5–11). Stretching the muscle will accelerate the discharge of both Golgi receptors and spindle receptors, but contraction of the muscle will stimulate only the Golgi receptors, because as the muscle shortens it tends to slacken the tension on the muscle spindles, with a consequent decrease in the discharge rate of its receptors. Combinations of sensory information received from the various receptors render an accurate report of the situation in the muscle to the spinal level, and hence to higher centers. It is the superior recognition of and response to clues of this nature that enable the skilled performer to accomplish movements

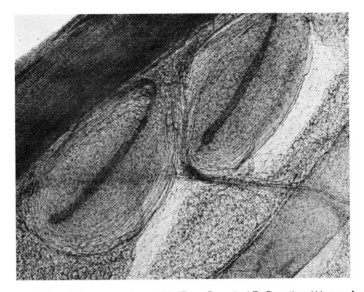

FIG. 5–8. Photomicrograph of pacinian corpuscles, × 30. (From Crouch, J.E.: Functional Human Anatomy, Philadelphia, Lea & Febiger, 1985, p. 366.)

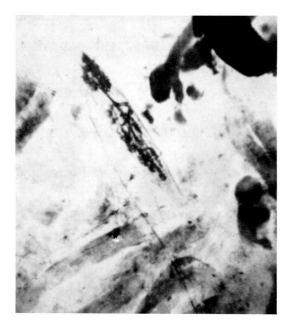

FIG. 5–9.   Golgi organ of a rat. (×100.) (Cole.)

Nuclear chain or intracapsular fibers terminate within the capsule, are smaller in diameter, and have their nuclei dispersed along their length in a nuclear chain. Muscle spindles have two kinds of sensory receptors. Primary (annulospiral, A2, or nuclear bag) endings wrap around the larger intrafusal nuclear bag muscle fibers at the equatorial regions (Fig. 5–12). The afferent nerve fibers leading from them are relatively large Group I fibers (8 to 12 μ in diameter), indicating fast conduction rates. Some but not all muscle spindles have secondary (flower-spray, A1, or nuclear chain) endings on the smaller intrafusal nuclear chain muscle fibers or on the larger intrafusal nuclear bag muscle fibers at the polar regions (Fig. 5–13). The afferent nerve fibers in this case are relatively small Group II fibers (6 to 9 μ in diameter), indicating slower conduction rates. These secondary endings are believed to be responsible for a flexor reflex, with inhibition of the extensors.

The primary endings have a lower threshold than do the secondary endings. They are sensitive to stretch, and their discharge produces a reflex contraction known as the stretch reflex. This reflex causes the muscle to contract to a degree roughly proportionate to the amount of the applied stretch, thus restoring the muscle to its original length. The increased tension and the rate of develop-

requiring a remarkable degree of neuromuscular coordination.

The types of intrafusal fibers occur within the same spindle. Nuclear bag or percapsular fibers perforate the capsule at both ends and extend beyond them. These large fibers are striated at their polar ends but have a nonstriated, noncontractile central equatorial region with cell nuclei clusters in a nuclear bag.

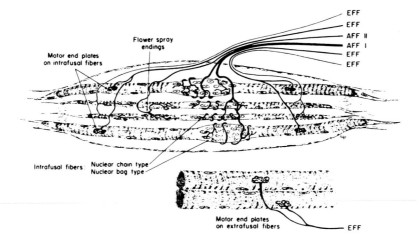

FIG. 5–10.   Diagrammatic illustration of elements comprising a muscle spindle. Within a capsule of perineural epithelium, there are nuclear bag and nuclear chain intrafusal muscle fibers (vs extrafusal muscle fibers that comprise the bulk of the muscle). Annulospinal endings around the nuclear regions constitute the primary ending of a large myelinated axon (AFF I). Flower spray or secondary endings are also shown. Intrafusal muscle fibers are innervated by fusimotor or gamma efferent axons (EFF) that terminate as end-plates or else trail along the fiber surface. (From Ham, A.W.: Histology. 7th Ed. Philadelphia, J.B. Lippincott Co., 1974, Fig. 28–2, with permission.)

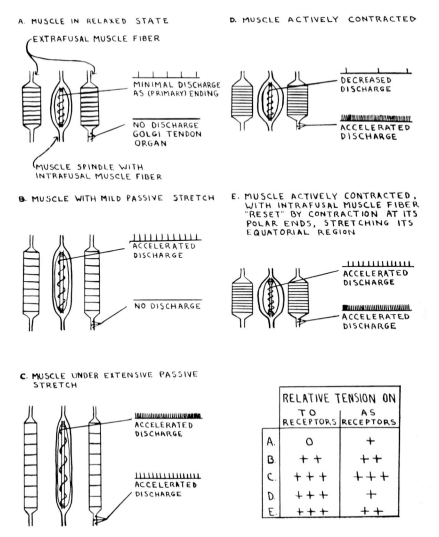

FIG. 5–11.   Simplified scheme of possible variations in afferent discharge from Golgi tendon organs (TO) and from muscle spindle primary or annulospiral receptors (AS), under various conditions of extrafusal relaxation, stretch, and contraction. Both TO and AS receptors are sensitive to passive stretching, although TO receptors have a higher threshold (A, B, and C). The TO receptors respond indiscriminately to extensive stretch *(C)* and to active extrafusal contraction *(D* and *E)*. Active contraction relieves the tension on AS receptors *(D)*, unless gamma efferent activity "resets" the tension within the intrafusal fiber *(E)*. Intrafusal secondary or flower-spray receptors have been omitted here, although in actuality they add still another variable factor to the array of afferent information.

ment of tension in stretched muscle fibers have been attributed to an increase in the calcium ions released for the activation of contractile proteins.[2] The familiar knee jerk or patellar tendon reflex is an example of the stretch reflex. The athlete attempts to take advantage of this phenomenon by a quick stretch during the preparatory back swing in overarm throwing and other similar movements. The afferent impulse from the primary endings also connects, through inhibitory internuncial neurons in the spinal cord, with the antagonist of a particular muscle. Output from these primary endings is responsible for reciprocal innervation, which reduces the "drag" of the antagonist on the agonist. If the stretch reflex is too extensive, however, it will stretch the antagonist as well, stimulating the antagonist's primary endings, thereby initiating a stretch reflex in the opposite direction and causing double reciprocal inhibition.

Not as much is known about the effects of discharge from the secondary endings. Eldred[3] presents evidence that the discharge

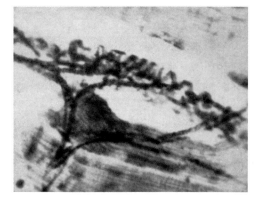

FIG. 5–12. Primary (annulospiral) endings around the intrafusal fibers in the mouse. (×450.) (Cole.)

of secondary endings in flexor muscles facilitates the flexors and inhibits the extensors (like a stretch reflex), but discharge of secondary endings in extensor muscles also facilitates the flexors and inhibits the extensors (unlike a stretch reflex). Therefore, the arrangement is not doubly reciprocal (Fig. 5–14). Recent work suggests that the stretch reflex depends on the excitation of both the primary and secondary endings of the spindle.

While these findings have cast doubt on Sherrington's explanation of some of his observations, the fact remains that, through their interplay, these reflexes serve to correct each other, and the interplay provides a means of fine adjustment and control over body position and movement. However, attempts to exploit these phenomena to augment the development of muscular strength have proved disappointing.[4]

The Fusimotor or Gamma System. The muscle spindle has been the subject of a comprehensive review by Matthews.[5] A number of the body's sensory systems are subject to central control by which their sensitivity can be set at various levels, somewhat like a thermostat. These sensitivity settings can be predictive—that is, the sensitivity level can be set at one moment in order to serve an anticipated sensory need that will occur several moments later. Were it not for such settings, body reactions would always be a little bit late because of the inevitable delay in the working of any system employing negative feedback controls.

In the muscle spindle, the mechanism for selective sensitivity settings depends on its gamma motor neurons, which are functionally independent from the alpha motor neurons that initiate contraction in the extrafusal fibers of the whole muscle (Fig. 5–11). The gamma neurons end on the intrafusal fibers, and their impulses result in contractile shortening of the spindle without any detectable influence on the strength or shortening of the whole muscle. When a whole muscle contracts under the influence of the alpha motor neurons, the muscle spindles are slackened (Fig. 5–11D). The result is a cessation of discharges from the primary and secondary endings within the spindles, and abolition of the stretch reflex. As the spindles become slack, however, gamma motor discharge can be increased, restoring tension within the spindles and resetting the sensitivity of the sensory mechanism (Fig. 5–11E). The same thing may happen when the whole muscle slackens as the result of muscular relaxation. The gamma neurons and the intrafusal muscle fibers appear to be a servomechanism for controlling afferent discharge. In the spinal cord, the gamma motor neurons are under the integrated control of several efferent tracts originating in both the subconscious and the volitional centers of the brain. These higher centers can "decide" in advance what level of reflex sensitivity will be required and set the tension within the "follow-up length servo."

CONDITIONED REFLEXES

Although some reflexes are developed prenatally, most are learned; it is a mistake to

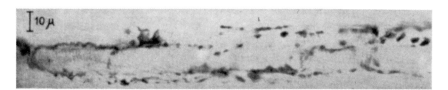

FIG. 5–13. Secondary (flower-spray) ending of the cat's muscle spindle. (Coërs.)

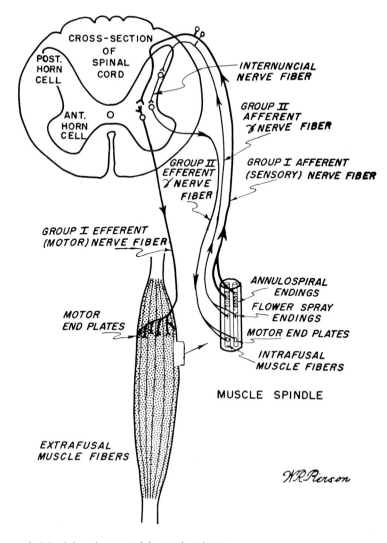

FIG. 5–14. Schema of alpha (α) and gamma (γ) neural systems.

think of all reflexes as inherited reactions, or as a limited number of very primitive reactions. The usual goal in motor learning is to reduce the new movement patterns to subconscious automaticity, dependent merely on a push-button sort of stimulus at either the conscious or subconscious level. Although highly complex motor activities, such as those involved in sports situations, may at first seem to be predominantly under conscious modification according to the changing environmental situation, if the performer is an expert the activity is likely to be a complex learned reflexive response, although attention must be paid to cues. The many redirections occurring during the performance are also reflexive, arising directly in response to the stimuli of the changing situation, rather than being deliberately and rationally inaugurated by the highest levels of the brain. The conscious mind of a star shortstop while he is making a sensational pick-up of a hard-driven bounding ball is likely to be concerned more with the possible wisdom of starting a double play than with specific direction of his bodily actions.

These concepts have implications for understanding and treating certain neurologic disfunctions. Harris[6] suggests that the fluctuating muscle tone seen in athetosis (constant slow writhing movements of the fingers and hands) in cerebral palsy may result from a malfunctioning proprioceptive system. The muscle stretch receptors continually vary in their sensitivity and feed faulty signals regarding the position of the body parts into the central nervous system. This interferes with postural stability and phasic movement control. In spastic cerebral palsy, the stretch receptors in the spastic muscles may be so highly sensitized from constant excessive gamma efferent activation that they generate afferent impulses even under the minimal passive muscle stretch caused by gravity. This results in elevated tone, or at least in increased resistance to stretch, in the affected muscles. The outcome is the condition called spasticity. This neurophysiologic model provides a rationale for special therapeutic regimens, with which Harris claims to have had considerable success.

PSYCHOMOTOR BEHAVIOR

Psychomotor behavior has emerged as an important specialized field of study. Its scope and principles are presented in texts such as those by Schmidt,[7] Singer,[8] and Cratty.[9]

Maturation and Motor Learning. Maturation means growth accompanied by changes in functional ability. The emphasis is on ripening rather than on changes in size, shape, and volume. Every teacher of motor skills should be familiar with the crucial relationship between physical or physiologic maturation and motor learning. For example, motor learning during the first 2 years of life is limited by the degree of myelination of nerve fibers, which is incomplete during this period. Certain coordinations such as creeping and walking must await the development of myelin sheaths in the appropriate nerves and spinal tracts, perhaps to prevent a chaotic short-circuiting of the necessary impulses. Because maturation is highly correlated with age, parents and teachers should become familiar with descriptions of average ability at various age levels to adjust teaching processes to the known periods of readiness of the child. However, because maturation is not *perfectly* correlated with age, an intelligent person should guard against a blind application of such norms. Norms are guides and should never substitute for observation and testing of the individual child.

The development of motor skills follows a progressive sequence, partly dependent on maturation. Although a particular kind of skill cannot be mastered prior to the necessary physical maturation, the opportunity to attain the skill can be lost, perhaps irretrievably, if the environment does not allow the skill to be mastered in the normal sequence, soon after maturation produces the potential. It is well known among physical education teachers that basic sports and aquatic skills are most easily achieved before or during adolescence, although the proportionate influence of physical factors and social or psychologic factors remains obscure.

Progression. It is a matter of common observation that a child stands before he walks and walks before he runs. Complex motor learning requires an order of prerequisites, a background of specific attainments. Complex coordinations cannot be mastered until certain basic movement patterns have been reduced to the automaticity of conditioned reflexes. In general, fine movements are distilled out of gross movements; new skills are based on recombinations of the elements of old skills. It is a principle of physical education based on neuromuscular principles that early motor training should be broad, varied, and general to provide a basis for later learning that is more refined, specialized, and complex.

This concept has implications for therapy as well. Rood emphasizes that general functional activities, muscle groups, and patterns of movement pass through developmental sequences. In her system the therapeutic approach is designed essentially to reproduce the normal developmental sequences that are missing from the abnormal sequences of the patient.[10]

Individual Differences in Structure. The properties of bone and muscle and the way in which these tissues are constructed may account for many psychomotor abilities, because structure influences performance. The relationship may be either permissive or restrictive and varies according to the nature of each separate activity. Each of several factors, many of which are discussed extensively elsewhere in this text, contributes to the individual differences affecting motor performance. The factors are somatotype or body type;

height of the body and length of bony levers; proportions of bone, muscle, and fat; specific gravity or buoyancy of the body; acuity of vision, audition, proprioception, and other sensations; mobility of various joints; hereditary or congenital structural abnormalities; and residual defects from disease or trauma. The trained kinesiologist views a performer or a would-be performer with an analytic eye, assessing his individual abilities and capabilities for particular activities.

Standard Form. Much of kinesiology has implications for determining the mechanical technique or form to be employed by the learner. Class teaching methods often imply that there is a best way to perform a given activity, whether it be postural adjustment, crutch-walking, or participation in a sport, but teachers should not insist on too rigid a form. In the first place, better forms are still being discovered for most activities, as the history of championship performance clearly demonstrates. In the second place, individual differences can never be completely understood. There is a wisdom of the body that supersedes academic knowledge or analysis, and a little trial-and-error learning frequently produces a more effective performance technique than could rigid direction.

The seemingly authoritative descriptions of technique by champion athletes are sometimes at variance with the form they actually employ as indicated by motion picture analysis and EMG studies. The expert performer functions so largely on the reflex level that he does not find it necessary to analyze routine movements and is therefore often unconscious of precisely how he executes them. For this reason experts are sometimes poor teachers, whereas less accomplished individuals may be forced to develop the ability to analyze performance effectively. Additionally, techniques used by champion performers do not necessarily apply to all performers. Individual variation must be considered.

Practicing for Speed and Accuracy. If a finished skill requires both high speed and great accuracy, as does serving a tennis ball, practice should emphasize both of these qualities from the start. If accuracy is emphasized to the neglect of speed, much relearning must take place in the final stages of practice when

a faster speed is employed. A target-directed skill like pitching a baseball involves one kinesiologic pattern when performed slowly and an entirely different pattern when performed rapidly. The difference consists largely of variation in the degree of contraction of muscles antagonistic to the prime movers. This difference between slow controlled movements, rapid controlled movements, and ballistic movements has been discussed in Chap. 3.

Speed of movement should not be confused with haste in performance. In most gross skills, speed implies the application of great force, and the performer might well be advised to perform "harder" or "more forcefully" rather than "faster." General haste is likely to cause a central irradiation of neural impulses to muscles whose contraction would be unnecessary or disadvantageous. This is one reason why a performer "ties up."

SUMMARY

Though the varieties and qualities of human motion are infinite, at the level of terminal action the effector mechanism is basic. The operational structure is the motor unit—a group of skeletal muscle fibers innervated by a motor neuron arising in the spinal cord. This motor unit either will act by contraction of its muscle fibers, or it will not act. There are no other possibilities. All the versatility of human motion depends on the selective activation of individual motor units in various combinations.

The functioning of motor units, however, is only superficially simple. Variety, versatility, and complexity are inherent in the very nature of this effector system. The first variable is the great number of individual motor units and their independence of action. None, some, or many motor units may be activated, in all sorts of combinations, at any given moment. The second variable is the possibility of graded contraction of the motor units, dependent largely on the frequency with which motor impulses arrive at the muscle fibers. The third variable is the organization of groups of muscle fibers into separate muscles, with tendons arranged variously to produce different joint actions. The fourth variable is the variety of combinations in which different muscles can be activated synergistically; for example, a flexor and an abductor can work together to produce an intermediate diagonal movement, or a flexor and an extensor can cooperate to attain rigid stability. The fifth variable is the physiologic condition of the tissues, involving relative states of nutrition, fatigue, training, oxygen availability, and other factors.

Spinal reflexes are the basis for control of human movement. Certain sensory and motor neurons are structurally located to provide for reflex action. Some of these reflexes appear to be functionally innate; others are acquired or learned through complex processes, after which they become relatively simple and peripherally automatic. Some reflexes are opposite or antagonistic to each other, for example, an extensor thrust and a flexor withdrawal. Obviously, control mechanisms must account for the selecting, in terms of activation or inhibition, of reflexes in various combinations or patterns at different times.

An interesting example of the functioning of the proprioceptors is seen in the knockdown in boxing. The blow causes a violent rotational movement of the head. The subsequent synchronous discharge of the proprioceptors results in an intense reflex counter-rotation, with the result that the boxer falls in the direction from which the blow came.[11]

One major determinant for the selection of reflex patterns is sensory input. Here, variety is evident with respect not only to kinds of inputs, but to numbers of individual units available and the intensity of their stimulations. Light pressure might elicit a mild extensor thrust reflex; obnoxious pressure might result in a more vigorous thrust; a pinprick might generate a withdrawal reflex.

Numerous as they are, the different kinds of sensations are inadequate to provide effective versatility of response; however, the possible responses are tremendously increased by combinations of sensations. For example, three of the more important sensory detectors are Golgi tendon organs, spindle primary endings, and spindle secondary endings. These can act separately or in various combinations and permutations, multiplying the

possible effects. Further, there are built-in-feedback circuits, some complex and indirect, others simple and direct. In the interneuron (Renshaw) loop, a motor neuron gives off side branches before leaving the spinal cord, so that whenever it activates a muscle it simultaneously activates an internuncial inhibitory neuron that is functionally connected to the cell body of the original motor neuron. This connection results in a self-inhibiting or "start-stop" circuit. An example of a more indirect servomechanism is double reciprocal inhibition, whereby two similar stretch reflexes in antagonistic muscles limit and modulate each other, producing a postural position that is stable except for minute oscillations.

Although the foregoing discussion of peripheral neuromotor mechanisms is schematic and simplified, it does indicate the complexity and versatility of this system. Obviously, the peripheral neuromotor pathways must be capable of producing all possible human movement. Supraspinal mechanisms do not increase the repertoire of possible responses; rather, they provide control and coordination by facilitating or inhibiting the peripheral neurons. The descending nerve tracts from the various brain centers may be classified as part of the voluntary system, from the cerebral cortex; part of the antigravity system, from the vestibular nucleus; or part of the suppressor system, from the red nucleus and the reticular formation.[12] Each of these systems can have both excitatory and inhibitory elements, and each transmits the selected and filtered output of various processing stations of the brain. One of the more important centers of motor coordination is the cerebellum, which has no direct communication with the spinal motor neurons but directs its output to other centers of integration. (Man's nervous system is not capable of detailed rational understanding of its own complexity.)

Plasticity—the ability of the nervous system to fashion and modify itself functionally through functioning—constitutes the highest level of neural complexity. Conditioning, learning, remembering, forgetting, relearning, and other sophisticated psychophysical aspects of man's behavior give evidence of the plasticity of his nervous system. At the limits of human understanding are the qualities of personality, motivation, body image, consciousness, meaning, and significance. All of these are crucial considerations in even the least complex human body motions, including simple spinal reflexes.

REFERENCES

1. Fay, T.: The origin of human movement. Am. J. Psychiatry, *111*:644, 1952.
2. Gonzales-Serratos, H., et al.: Effect of muscle stretching on tension development and mechanical threshold during contraction. Nature (New Biol.), *246*:221, 1973.
3. Eldred, E.: The dual sensory role of muscle spindles. J. Am. Phys. Ther. Assoc., *45*:290, 1965.
4. Awad, E.A., and Kottke, F.J.: Effectiveness of myostatic reflex facilitation in augmenting rate of increase of muscular strength due to brief maximal exercise. Arch. Phys. Med., *45*:23, 1964.
5. Matthews, P.B.C.: Muscles spindles and their motor control. Physiol. Rev., *44*:219, 1964.
6. Harris, F.A.: Muscle stretch receptor hypersensitation in spasticity. Am. J. Phys. Med., *57*:16, 1978.
7. Schmidt, R.A.: Motor Skills. New York, Harper & Row, 1975.
8. Singer, R.N.: Motor learning and human performance: an application to physical education skills. 3rd Ed. New York, Macmillan Publishing Co., 1980.
9. Cratty, B.J.: Movement behavior and motor learning. 3rd Ed. Philadelphia, Lea & Febiger, 1973.
10. Stockmeyer, S.A.: An interpretation of the approach of Rood to the treatment of neuromuscular dysfunction. Am. J. Phys. Med., *46*:900, 1967.
11. Govons, S.R.: Brain concussion and posture: the knockdown blow of the boxing ring. Confin. Psychiatr., *30*:77, 1968.
12. Ritchie, A.E.: Physiological control of muscle. Physiotherapy, *49*:16, 1963.

RECOMMENDED READING

Granit, R.: The Basis of Motor Control. New York, Academic Press, 1970.

6 BIOMECHANICS I

JOHN GARHAMMER

Mechanics is an area of physics and engineering that deals with the evaluation of forces responsible for maintaining an object or structure in a fixed position, as well as with the description, prediction, and causes of motion of an object or structure. The kinesiologist is concerned with the human body when both stable and moving. Thus, the kinesiologist must be able to apply basic laws and principles of mechanics in order to evaluate human activities. Such an application of mechanics falls in the domain of biomechanics, which can be defined as the application of mechanics to living organisms and biologic tissues.

This chapter introduces basic concepts, principles, and laws of mechanics and illustrates their application to kinesiologic problems. Much of this information is of immediate value in understanding the kinesiology of the body's joints in the following chapters. Chapter 7 covers additional topics about mechanics that are useful in analyzing more complex movements of the body, as well as the motion of objects interacting with or propelled by the body.

CENTER OF GRAVITY

The concept of center of gravity (CG) is useful in describing and analyzing mechanically the motion of the human body and other objects. CG is the point associated with an object at which all its mass—that is, all the material making up the object—may be considered to be concentrated. A meter stick, for example,

may be balanced on one's finger at the 50-cm point. This is its CG in the length dimension, while its CG in the width dimension is halfway across the relatively narrow stick. Gravity pulls downward on every mass point (atom or molecule) making up the stick, but because the stick is of uniform density the total pull on each side of the CG point is equal; hence, support under the CG will prevent the stick from turning and falling. Determining the CG of the human body, which is not rigid, of uniform density, nor symmetric, is very difficult. Some methods to estimate the CG of the human body and its segments will be presented at the end of this chapter.

LINE OF GRAVITY AND BASE OF SUPPORT

The location of the CG of the body as a whole varies greatly depending on body position. In a standing person it can be approximated as lying on a line formed by the intersection of a plane cutting the body into right and left halves with a plane cutting the body into front and back halves (see anatomic reference planes). The position of the CG point along this imaginary line can be estimated, as is shown later in this chapter. Gravity can be considered to act on this single CG point of the body by pulling straight downward toward the center of the earth. This line or direction of pull is known as the line of gravity.

The base of support for the body is the area formed under the body by connecting with one continuous line all points in contact with the ground. In normal standing, for example, the base of support is approximately a rectangle formed by straight lines across the toes and heels and along the sides of each foot. When the body is in a fixed position with the line of gravity passing through the base of support it is said to be balanced, stable, or in static equilibrium. If the gravity line passes outside of the base of support, balance and stability are lost and the supporting limbs must move to avoid a fall. This situation occurs continuously as we walk, run, and change direction. Balance and stability are easier to maintain when the base of support is increased or CG is lowered. Both actions are commonly seen in wrestling, when the low CG and wide base of support make it difficult for one opponent to shift the line of gravity outside the other's support base. During certain types of movement, particularly as seen in many sport activities, the line of gravity falls far outside the base of support (Fig. 6–1). These are highly dynamic situations during which other considerations, such as centrifugal force (see Chapter 7), tend to offset the pull of gravity. If a person carries a load, the body's position is shifted so that the line of gravity acting on the combined CG of the body and the load passes through the base of support. If the load is on one side of the body, as when a person carries a suitcase, the body leans toward the opposite side. If the load is on the back, as when a person carries a backpack for hiking, the body leans forward.

Much practical work in kinesiology has been sponsored by the armies of the world in order to determine the effect of various types and positions of army packs on the line of gravity, and many studies have been undertaken in efforts to determine where this line should fall ideally, but differences in human physique have made it difficult to generalize from the findings.

When an external force is applied to the body, the resulting movement depends on the direction of the force with reference to the center of gravity. An unopposed force from any direction that is directed through the center of gravity causes the whole body to move in the direction of the force, with no rotational effect. An external force directed anywhere except at the CG tends to cause both movement of the whole body in that direction and rotation of the body around its CG. The "secret" of judo is simply that it is a highly developed technique of applying the above laws. The judoka applies force, or utilizes the force developed by an opponent, to cause the latter first to move and then to fall in a desired direction (Fig. 6–14). More familiar examples may be found in football, in which it will be observed that a horizontal charge aimed at the level of the center of gravity of an opponent tends to move him to another place; a higher charge tends to tip him over while moving him, and a lower charge tends to topple him forward over the charge while moving him.

MECHANICS

The field of mechanics can be divided into statics, which considers particles and rigid bodies that are in a state of static equilibrium, and dynamics, which studies objects that are in accelerated motion. Dynamics may be further subdivided into kinematics and kinetics. Kinematics is the geometry of motion, which includes displacement, velocity, and acceleration without regard for the forces acting on a body. Kinetics considers forces, the causes of motion.

DYNAMICS

There are three general types of motion: rectilinear (translatory), angular (rotary), and curvilinear. In rectilinear motion, every particle of a body moves the same distance along a straight line parallel to the path of every other particle. Motion of the whole human body seldom fulfills these conditions. Even when a person jumps feet first off a diving board with the body perpendicular and rigid, there is some slight rotation of the body around its CG, and the path of the CG follows a slight curve. Perhaps some point on the fist of a boxer executing a straight left jab exhibits rectilinear motion, but most parts of his arm will move neither in a straight line nor parallel to the first point. In practical problems, small discrepancies from strictly rectilinear motion are ignored; thus, the approximate horizontal

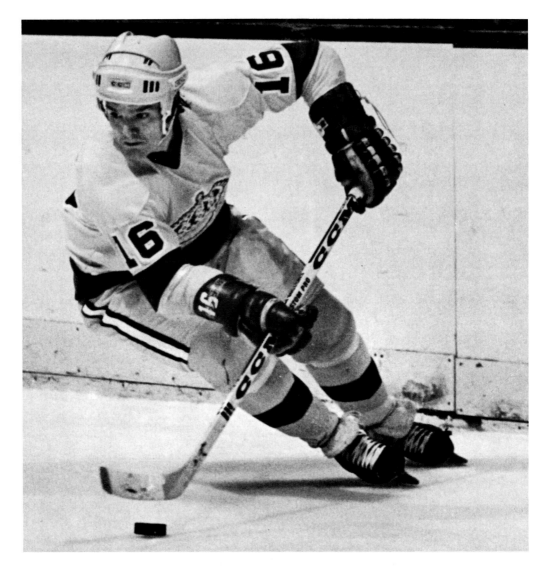

FIG. 6–1. Marcel Dionne, formerly of the Los Angeles Kings ice hockey team, displays the unstable position that may be assumed by an ice skater making an abrupt change of direction. Why does he not fall when his line of gravity is so far outside the base of support? (Los Angeles *Times* photo.)

distance traversed by the CG of a walking person is sometimes referred to as the translatory motion of the person, even though the CG actually oscillates laterally, forward and backward, and up and down slightly during the "straight" walking, and that other body points deviate even more radically from a rectilinear path (Fig. 6–2).

In angular motion, the paths of various particles of a rigid body are described with reference to a center of rotation or "axis." This center of rotation may be either within the volume of the body, as in the case of a pir-

ouetting dancer, or outside of the body, as in the case of a gymnast on the rings or high bar. If the body and its connection to the center of rotation is rigid, then all mass-points move along arcs of concentric circles and result in circular motion, a special case of angular motion. The human body more commonly changes shape as it moves around the center of rotation, and the resulting motion is angular (if the center of rotation may be considered as fixed), but not purely circular.

In curvilinear motion, the center of rotation itself may be continuously moving, causing

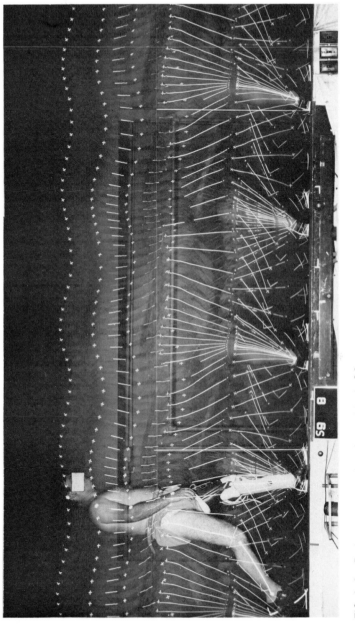

FIG. 6–2.   During normal walking, the total body CG oscillates in a cyclic up-and-down manner similar to the pattern shown here for the shoulder. In this cyclogram of an amputee walking, the sequence of the swing and support phases of the artificial limb as compared to the normal limb is evident. (R. Drillis, courtesy Prosthetic Devices Studies, New York University.)

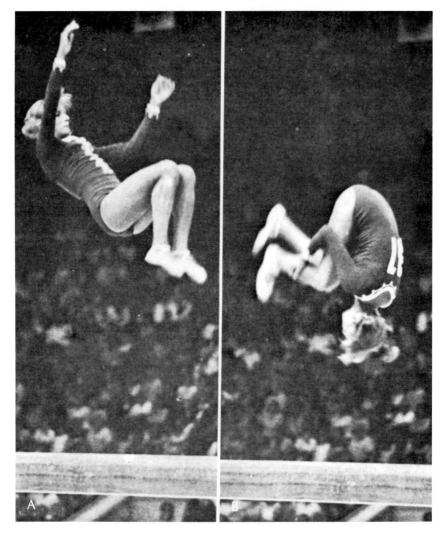

FIG. 6–3.   Olga Korbut, of the U.S.S.R., Olympic gymnast and winner of two gold medals and one silver medal at Munich in 1972, performs a back somersault on the balance beam. In *A*, shortly after takeoff, the center of gravity of the body is well along its parabolic path determined by the directional angle and velocity at takeoff, as modified continuously by the acceleration of gravity. A slow backward rotation, also established at takeoff, is beginning to be accelerated by the transition of body parts from layout to tuck position. In *B*, the rotation has been nearly completed. Proper timing of the emergence from the tuck decelerates the rotation and places the body in a position for landing. The separation of the feet is not a departure from good form, but is preparation for balanced landing on the 4-inch beam. Korbut is 4 ft 10 in. tall, when competing weighed 83 lb., and had only 1.5% body fat. This may be compared with 36% for a noted distance swimmer, who is 5 ft 6 in. tall and weighs 200 lb. Korbut was the 1972 Female Athlete of the Year. (Photo by Glenn Sundby, publisher of *Gymnast* magazine.)

the individual mass-points to follow irregular paths that are neither rectilinear nor circular. Such a path may be complex and irregular, or it may take the form of one of the defined curves, such as a parabola. Consider the example of a gymnast performing a back somersault with a tuck (Fig. 6–3). Some randomly selected point of the body, such as the tip of the right big toe, traverses an extremely irregular path of motion with respect to the ground. Such a curvilinear path would be difficult to describe mathematically or by name. Even if the path were described, the meaning would be limited, since every other point of the body traverses an essentially different curve. Mechanical analysis of a back somersault is more feasible, and much more useful, if the mass-point selected for study is the overall CG of the body.

In mechanical analysis, all of the mass of the body may be considered to be concentrated at the CG. Furthermore, the CG of any projectile under the influence of gravity follows a perfect parabola (neglecting air resistance and assuming that no other outside force acts on the body during its flight). The particular shape of the parabolic curve depends entirely on takeoff velocity and takeoff angle, so that simple equations can be written to predict or describe the maximum height, distance traversed, time in flight, and other descriptive characteristics. The effects of changing takeoff velocity and angle also can be predicted. In sports performance and teaching, such analytic information is often valuable.

Although velocities and directions can be measured accurately by simple engineering analysis derived from force platforms, sequential motion picture frames, and other devices, a practiced observer can gain considerable insight by estimating the location of the CG and other variables, as well as their relative changes during flight or from trial to trial. Thus, a modern coach closely observes performance and makes estimated comparisons of various angles, velocities, and trajectories, based on knowledge of the underlying equations of motion.

In addition to analysis of the overall trajectory of the body's CG, other mechanical aspects of the performance can be determined. For the back somersault, it is useful to consider the body's CG as a point of reference, just as if it were stationary. The motion of all other body points can be considered as angular around the CG, simplifying the analysis greatly. (If the body were kept rigid, further simplification would be possible by treating the rotation as truly circular around the CG. The moving human body is seldom rigid, however, except for assumed momentary periods. In the back somersault example, the body enters a tuck position soon after takeoff and then emerges to an open position shortly before landing.)

A further analysis, of intermediate complexity, results from measuring or estimating the location of the CG of each segment of the body and considering the movement of segments around the overall CG of the body. Because most body segments are essentially rigid, this method compromises accuracy only a little or not at all.

The joints of the body permit only angular or curvilinear motion. The gliding motions of some joints are slight and usually occur along a curved surface. Any translatory movement of a part of the body must be produced by multiple angular movements at two or more joints or by some force originating outside the body.

NEWTON'S LAWS OF MOTION

The above paragraphs defined and discussed various terms associated with the study of dynamics. To actually apply dynamics to movement situations, some basic principles must be introduced. The most important of these are Newton's laws of motion, first published in 1686, which are fundamental to the solution of engineering problems.

Newton's first law states that a body at rest tends to remain at rest, and a body in motion tends to remain in motion with constant velocity (no change in speed or direction) unless acted on by unbalanced forces. This tendency to resist change is evident to athletes who are moving rapidly when they try to change direction.

Newton's second law states that the sum of forces acting on a body in a given direction is equal to the acceleration of the body in that direction multiplied by the mass of the body. Because acceleration is defined as rate of change of velocity (speed, direction of motion, or both), this law also states that the sum of forces acting on a body in a given direction is proportionate to the rate of change of its state of motion (with mass being the proportionality constant). In equation form the second law can be written

$$\Sigma F = ma = m \, \Delta v / \Delta t$$

where Δv is change in velocity and Δt is change in time. Note that if the sum of forces acting on a body is zero ($\Sigma F = 0$), such as 10 lb pulling to both the left and right, the acceleration and change in velocity will be zero ($a = \Delta v = 0$). Thus, the first law of Newton is really a special case of the second law.

To further discuss and apply Newton's second law, an additional concept must be explained. This is the concept of vector versus scalar quantities. In the statement of the second law above, forces in a given direction must be added and velocity is associated with speed and direction of motion. Both force and velocity are vector quantities, meaning they contain information about magnitude and direction. Clearly, when a wrestler pushes an opponent, the direction as well as the magnitude of the push is important; when a football player runs, both his direction and his speed must be controlled. Scalar quantities, by contrast, contain only information about magnitude, such as mass of an object or temperature of pool water.

Newton's third law of motion is sometimes called the action-reaction principle. It states that the force one body exerts on a second is equal in magnitude and opposite in direction to the force the second body exerts on the first. When a collision occurs between two rugby players, each experiences the same level of force but in opposite directions; the more massive player (with the greatest body weight) recoils the least, assuming that running velocities at impact are equal (see impulse-momentum and conservation of momentum, Chapter 7). An example in which the initial velocities of the interacting bodies are zero is that of a bullet being released and the gun recoiling after firing. The forces exerted on the bullet and the gun are equal and opposite, but the greater weight of the firearm causes it to move relatively little compared with the projectile. Another example is the "takeoff" of a jumper. The push that the athlete makes against the earth causes an equal and opposite reaction force from the ground. Because of the difference in size, the earth is not moved, but its reaction pushes the jumper up into the air.

VECTOR QUANTITIES

Vector quantities have both magnitude and direction as definitive attributes and must be added vectorially, as opposed to arithmeti-

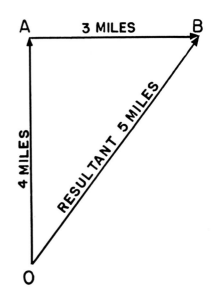

FIG. 6–4.   Determining the actual track of a swimmer by the addition of vector quantities.

cally (as scalar quantities are added), if correct information is to result. Displacement, velocity, acceleration, momentum, and force are common examples of vector quantities.

A vector quantity can be expressed graphically by an arrow whose length indicates its magnitude according to some convenient scale and whose head indicates its direction. Suppose that a channel swimmer swims 4 mi north in a calm sea. His displacement can be represented by drawing an arrow 4 in. long in a direction representing north. Suppose this same swimmer is affected by a tidal current sufficient to displace him 3 mi to the east. This displacement could be represented by drawing another arrow 3 in. long in a direction representing east, starting at the terminal point of the first arrow. If these two quantities are added arithmetically, the total distance is indicated as 7 mi. But will the man be found at a point 7 mi from his starting point? As indicated in Figure 6–4, if arrow OB is drawn and measured, his actual displacement is found to be 5 mi from the starting point. OB is the vectorial sum of vectors OA and AB. Since OB is a vector, it is appropriate to apply a protractor and determine its direction, which is found to be about 37° east of north.

If an analytic solution to such problems is

preferred, the Pythagorean theorem may be utilized. This states that the square of the hypotenuse of a right triangle is equal to the sum of the squares of the other two sides. Hence

$$\overline{OB}^2 = \overline{OA}^2 + \overline{AB}^2$$

$$\overline{OB}^2 = 4^2 + 3^2 = 16 + 9 = 25$$

$$OB = \sqrt{25} = 5 \text{ mi}$$

The direction may be determined from the sine function. The sine of an acute angle of a right triangle is the ratio of the side opposite the angle to the hypotenuse. This ratio is constant for any given angle:

$$\text{Sin AOB} = \frac{3}{5} = 0.6$$

By consulting the table of sines in Appendix A and interpolating, a sine of 0.6 is found to correspond to an angle of 36.9°, and the diagram shows that angle to be east of north.

A typical example of the use of such computations in kinesiologic problems is found in a study by Pugh et al.,[1] in which it was necessary to determine the distances actually swum by participants in the 1955 race across the English Channel. One of the first contestants to finish was found to have actually covered 25.8 mi, although the displacement through the water was only 21.5 mi. Slower swimmers suffered more from tidal effects and were forced to swim greater distances, the result being that most of them failed to finish.

Composition of Vectors. Such problems as that of the swimmer affected by the cross-current, in which two displacements are known and the resultant must be calculated, are solved by the methods of composition (or combination) of vectors. In such problems it is customary to use the parallelogram method instead of the triangle method employed above.

Suppose two muscles with a common insertion but with different angles of pull contract simultaneously (Fig. 6–5). Point O represents the common insertion of the lateral and medial heads of the quadriceps on the

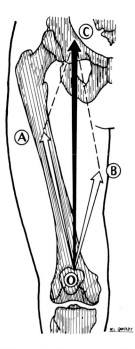

FIG. 6–5. Diagrammatic illustration of the composition of forces by the parallelogram method.

patella. OA is a vector depicting the magnitude and direction of the pull of the lateral head, OB of the medial head. From point A, the line AC is drawn parallel to OB; from point B, the line BC is drawn parallel to OA. The resultant, OC, represents the combination of the forces developed by the two muscles and might be regarded as a hypothetical muscle pull that could replace the pull of the original muscles without changing the effect of their action on the bone to which they are attached.

If there were three muscles pulling on a common point of insertion (as in the case of the three parts of the deltoid muscle), the composition of all could be found by determining the resultant from any two and then combining it with the pull of the third muscle in order to get the final resultant. Any number of forces acting at a given point can thus be combined by taking two at a time.

Resolution of Vectors. In dealing with the composition of vectors, the problem is to find the resultant of two or more component vectors. Sometimes the opposite problem must be solved—a single vector is known, and its components in perpendicular directions must be found. This is a problem in resolution of vectors.

The kinesiologist is often interested in the

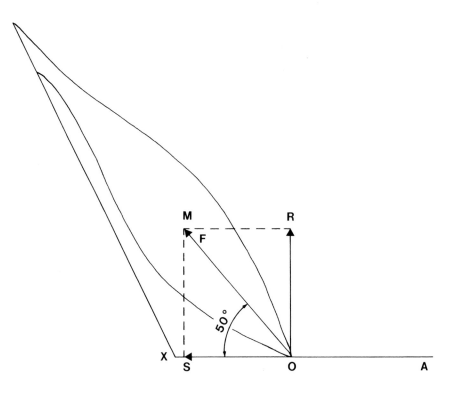

FIG. 6–6. Resolution of a vector representing muscular force. X is the center of the joint, around which bone XA turns. OM is a vector representing a muscle pulling with a force of 100 lb at an angle of 50° to the bone. OR is the rotary component; OS is the stabilizing component.

resolution of muscle forces. For example, suppose that a muscle is pulling with a force of 100 lb at an angle of 50° to the long axis of the bone on which it inserts. In Figure 6–6, OM is the vector representing the pull of the muscle on bone XA. This force OM can be analyzed into two components, OR or OS. OR is the rotary component, acting at right angles to the bone and representing the force that tends to turn the bone around the fulcrum X. OS is the stabilizing component, acting along the long axis of the bone and tending to pull it tightly into the socket at X. The point R is located by erecting a line from O perpendicular to XO, and by then drawing a line parallel to XO from M to R. The point S is located by dropping a line from M perpendicular to XO and parallel to OR. Knowing the magnitude of OM to be 100 lb and the angle MOS to be 50°, one can compute the magnitude of OR and OS as follows:

$$OR = OM \times \sin 50° \text{ or } OR = OM \times \cos 40°$$
$$= 100 \times 0.766 \qquad = 100 \times 0.766$$
$$= 76.6 \text{ lb.} \qquad = 76.6 \text{ lb.}$$

$$OS = OM \times \sin 40° \text{ or } OS = OM \times \cos 50°$$
$$= 100 \times 0.643 \qquad = 100 \times 0.643$$
$$= 64.3 \text{ lb.} \qquad = 64.3 \text{ lb.}$$

Note that the arithmetic total of the force vector components is greater than 100 lb.

The components of the various forces acting within the body are also often given other names to further clarify their effects. Some components of muscle forces tend to compress bone and are called compression force components. Others tend to cause bones (e.g., vertebrae) or regions of bone to slide over each other and are called shear force components. Similarly, components of muscle force that tend to rotate a bone about a joint also tend to bend it and are said to create

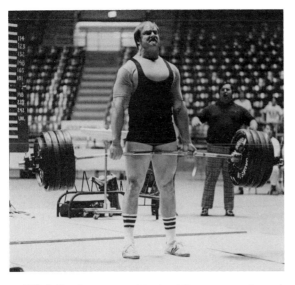

FIG. 6–7. Completion of the dead lift event as performed in competitive powerlifting by John Kuc. (Photo by B. Klemens.)

bending torques. Muscle contractions tending to elongate tendons are said to cause tensile forces in the tendons. Such considerations indicate the usefulness of composition and resolution of vectors.

APPLICATION OF NEWTON'S SECOND LAW

As a simple application showing the importance of vector analysis, consider the dead lift exercise (Fig. 6–7. See also Chapter 7). In this exercise the lifter stands and lifts a barbell from the floor and holds it at thigh level. If one knows the maximum upward force the lifter can exert in the starting position (e.g., 325 lb) and the weight of the barbell (e.g., 300 lb), the upward acceleration can be determined. Newton's second law is a vector relationship between the sum of forces acting on an object in a given direction and the resulting acceleration in that direction. In the current example, the forces acting on the barbell are the pull of gravity (the weight, W) straight downward and the (ideally) straight upward force (F) exerted by the lifter. To complete the determination of the barbell's initial acceleration (A) upward, the mass (M) of the barbell must be known. The mass is simply the weight divided by the constant 32, which gives the proper value in units consistent with pounds. Thus,

$$\Sigma F = ma$$
$$F - W = MA$$
$$A = \frac{F - W}{M} = \frac{325 - 300}{(300/32)} = \frac{25}{9.375}$$
$$A = 2.67 \ ft/sec^2$$

This means that as long as the lifter exerts an upward force of 325 lb on the barbell, it will increase its upward velocity 2.67 ft/sec every second. In actuality, because the lifter's force would be constantly changing during the lift as a result of many factors (e.g., leverage and muscle length changes), the acceleration would also vary.

Two important points are evident from this simple example. First, even if the lifter's pull of 325 lb were not straight upward, only the upward component would tend to lift the barbell; the sideward component would tend to move the barbell toward the lifter. The upward component would then be less than 325 lbs and result in less movement (acceleration), whereas the sideward component could cause movement detrimental to balance. Second, note that to lift a barbell, the force applied must be greater than the weight of the barbell, and because applied force can vary during the lift, so can acceleration. Lifting free weights (barbells and dumbbells) is often referred to as isotonic (constant tension) exercise. However, biomechanical analysis of various lifts shows that barbell acceleration varies greatly during movement and indicates that applied forces must also vary.[2] Thus, free-weight lifting exercises are more accurately described as dynamic rather than isotonic.

Additional examples of vector methods and applications of Newton's laws are given in Chapter 7. For an understanding of how muscle forces produce movement of body segments, the topic of rotary or angular motion must be discussed in more detail, along with the concept of torque—the rotational effect caused by forces.

TORQUE AND ROTARY MOTION

If a force is exerted on a body that can rotate about some pivot or fulcrum point, the force is said to generate a torque.* In the human body a standard example of a muscle force creating a torque is found at the elbow joint. The pull of the biceps and other muscles causes the forearm to rotate about the pivot point, the elbow joint. Usually the contraction force of a muscle cannot be measured directly. Because the human body moves by a series of rotations of its segments, the amount of torque that a muscle can develop is a very useful measure of its effect.

To apply the very valuable concept of torque, factors related to its magnitude and techniques for its calculation must be understood. The magnitude of a torque is clearly related to the magnitude of the force generating it, but an additional factor is the direction of that force relative to the position of the pivot point. The perpendicular distance from the pivot (fulcrum) to the line of action (direction) of the force is known as the lever arm of the force. One method to calculate the magnitude of torque (Γ) is to multiply the magnitude of the force (F) creating it by the length of the lever arm (d), $\Gamma = F \times d$. The concept of perpendicular distance used to determine lever arm length is sometimes confusing to beginning students. Consider the situation illustrated by Figure 6–6, which has been discussed previously. Assume that XO is 3 in. or 0.25 ft. Although the actual force developed in the muscle is 100 lb, the torque is not 100×0.25, because XO is not perpendicular to the line of the force. There are two alternative methods of determining the torque. The first, which was indicated previously, requires the resolution of the actual muscle force into components, one of which was OR, the rotary component, which was calculated to be 76.6 lb. Since this rotary component is perpendicular to the lever arm XO, the torque is given by

$$\text{Torque} = \text{Rotary component} \times \text{perpendicular distance}$$

$$\Gamma = 76.6 \times 0.25$$
$$= 19.15 \text{ ft-lb}$$

In the method just described, torque was computed by taking the component of force

---

*The term "torque" is equivalent to the older terminology "moment of force."

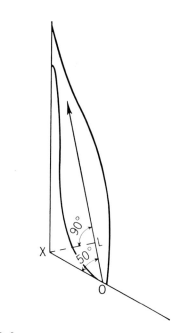

FIG. 6–8. Torque is equal to the force exerted by the muscle in direction OL, multiplied by the perpendicular distance from the center of rotation (X) to the line of the force (OL).

that is perpendicular to the lever arm. The second method requires that the lever arm perpendicular to the original force be computed. Figure 6–8 illustrates the method. From center of rotation X, draw XL perpendicular to OL. The length of XL may be determined as follows:

$$XL = XO \times \sin 50°$$
$$= 0.25 \times 0.766$$
$$= 0.1915 \text{ ft}$$

Then, torque is given by

$$\Gamma = 100 \times 0.1915$$
$$= 19.15 \text{ ft-lb}$$

which agrees with the result obtained by the first method.

When a torque is applied to an object with a pivot, the object will begin to rotate if the magnitude of the torque is sufficient to overcome the object's rotational inertia. Rotational inertia is analogous to mass in rectilinear motion. Newton's second law showed that an object subjected to a given force will accelerate; the greater the mass of the object, the smaller the acceleration. Likewise, an object will begin to rotate about its pivot when subjected to a torque. Because the rate of rotation or angular velocity changes when sufficient torque is applied, it is said that torque causes angular acceleration. The greater the rotational inertia (also called "moment of inertia") of an object, the smaller its angular acceleration for a given torque. (This topic will be covered in more detail in Chapter 7.)

LEVER SYSTEMS—APPLICATION OF TORQUE PRINCIPLES

In Chapter 2 the skeleton was presented as a supportive structure composed of articulated bones. This is the classic anatomic approach. Scientists involved with problems of human engineering often speak of links and pivots rather than of bones and joints. Links are defined as straight lines extending through a body segment between adjacent pivot points. These are functional rather than structural entities. Although links cannot be accurately measured from surface landmarks, using this concept the body can be represented using stick figures for mechanical analysis (Fig. 6–9). The joints are the pivots, and the contraction of the muscles results in the movement of the links around their centers of rotation. Movement can take place only in the direction or directions and to the extent permitted by the configuration of the joints and their supporting structures. Almost all joint movements are rotational and can be measured in degrees or radians (see Chapter 7).

The various possible combinations of links and pivots give the body a wide variety of movements. An understanding of leverage and the various kinds of levers is essential in comprehending the movements of the body.

A lever is a rigid bar revolving about a fixed point called the pivot, axis, or fulcrum. The length of the lever between the fulcrum and the weight or resistance is termed the resistance arm; the length between the fulcrum and the applied force is termed the force arm. The mechanical advantage of a lever is the ratio of the length of the force arm to that of the resistance arm. The usual function of a lever is to gain a mechanical advantage whereby a small force applied at one end of a lever over a large distance produces a greater force operating over a lesser distance at the other. In the human body, the action of contracting muscles normally constitutes the force, the resistance is furnished by the center of gravity of the segment moved plus any additional weight that may be in contact with that segment, and the axis is the joint at which the movement takes place. In most cases the force arm in the human body is shorter than is the resistance arm, resulting in a mechanical disadvantage.

When a lever turns on its pivot, all points on the lever move in arcs of a circle, and the distance through which any given point moves is proportion to its distance from the axis. Because these different distances are traversed in the same time, it follows that the points more distant from the pivot move faster than do those closer to it. Thus, a gain in distance is also a gain in speed. The biceps muscle in Figure 6–11 is at a mechanical disadvantage to lift a weight in the hand, but a small shortening of the bicep will cause the hand to move a large distance.

The arrangement and structure of muscles can give a comparatively large amount of force, and the arrangement of the bony levers gives distance of movement and speed. Because force is usually applied with a short force arm and a long resistance arm, the muscles lie close to the bones, and a compact structure is achieved. Baseball bats, hockey sticks, tennis rackets, and similar instruments represent artificial extensions of the resistance arms of body levers, thus increasing the speed at the striking point but requiring an increase in muscular force. On the other hand, wheelbarrows, pliers, and crowbars are designed to decrease the resistance arms and increase the force arms, thus increasing the mechanical advantage and allowing a greater application of force with a small muscular effort, but with a necessary decrease in range of motion.

Levers are divided into three classes, depending on the relative positions of the force, the axis, and the resistance (Fig. 6–10). In all three classes, balance or equilibrium exists when the product of the force times the length

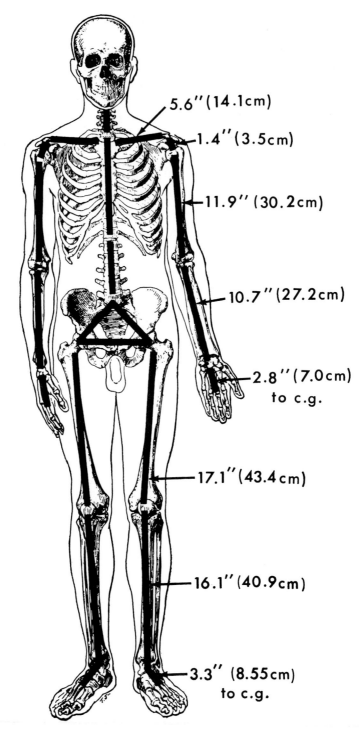

FIG. 6–9. The link system of the human body. The straight black lines indicate the effective levers for rotatory actions between one joint center and the next in sequence. Length dimensions are means for 50 percentile of Air Force flying personnel. (After Dempster.)

of the force arm is equal to the product of the resistance times the length of the resistance arm (f × fa = r × ra). It should be emphasized that f and r in the formula refer only to rotary components of the actual forces. These components are directed at 90° to the lever arms. Each side of this formula represents a torque:

$$f \times fa = \text{force torque}$$

$$r \times ra = \text{resistance torque}$$

Graphic and computational techniques for determining such torques were discussed previously. The application of an unbalanced torque will cause the lever to move, and the effects of changes in any of the components of the lever can be easily determined by substitution in the above formula.

First-Class Levers. Levers of the first class have the fulcrum located between the force and the resistance. As a consequence, the two arms of the lever move in opposite directions, as in a crowbar, a pair of scissors, or a teeter-totter. First-class levers can favor either force or range of motion, at the expense of the other. A typical example is the triceps (Muscle I, in Fig. 6–11). Assume the elbow is at the side, flexed at an angle of 90° and the palm is exerting a force of 10 lb against a table top. The palm is 12 in. from the elbow joint (fulcrum), and the triceps has a force arm of 1 in. What is the rotary force of contraction of the triceps?

$$f \times fa = r \times ra$$

$$f \times 1 = 10 \times 12$$

$$f = 120 \text{ lb}$$

Second-Class Levers. In levers of the sec-

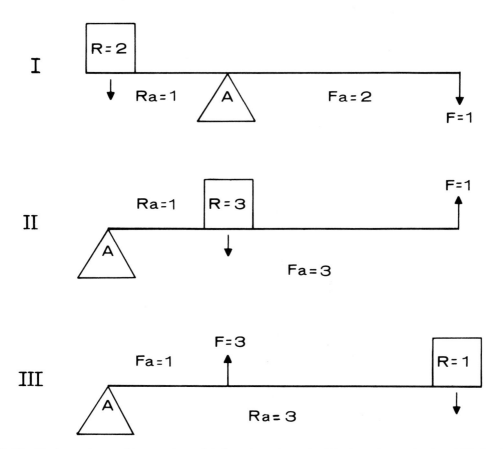

FIG. 6–10. The three classes of lever systems. A is the axis or pivot point, R is the resistance load, and F is the effort force. Fa is the lever arm distance from the force to the axis (or force arm), and Ra is the lever arm distance from the resistance to the axis (or resistance arm). The product of force and force lever arm balances the product of the resistance and resistance lever arm in this example, since the resulting torques (or turning effects) are equal.

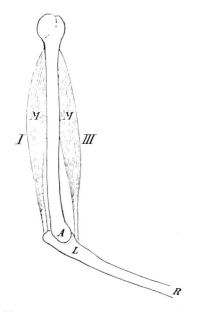

FIG. 6–11. Illustration of first-class and third-class levers by muscles acting on the elbow joint. The bone *LR* is the lever, with the axis at *A*, the weight or resistance at the hand, which is beyond *R*. *M and M* are the muscles, and *L* is the insertion of muscle *III*. See discussion in text.

ond class, the resistance is between the fulcrum and the force. Here, range of motion is sacrificed to gain force. Examples are found in the wheelbarrow and the nutcracker. Almost no levers of this type are found in the body, but opening the mouth against resistance is an example.

Third-Class Levers. In third-class levers, the force is applied between the fulcrum and the resistance. A common example is found in the spring that closes a screen door. This class of lever is the one most common in the body, since it permits the muscle to be inserted near the joint and to produce distance and speed of movement, with minimal muscle shortening, although at a sacrifice of force.

A typical example is found in the biceps when the forearm is flexed against resistance (Fig. 6–11). Assume that the elbow is flexed at 90° and that a 16-lb shot is held in the hand. The fulcrum is at the elbow joint. If the biceps is assumed to have a 2-in. force arm and the distance from the fulcrum to the center of the shot is 14 in., the rotary force exerted by the

biceps in supporting the shot can be calculated by the previous formula:

$$f \times fa = r \times ra$$

$$f \times 2 = 16 \times 14$$

$$f \times 2 = 224$$

$$f = 112 \text{ lb}$$

In this example, however, the weight of the forearm has been neglected. If we wish to include it, we must know its weight and the location of its center of gravity. If we assume the weight of the forearm and hand to be 4 lb and the center of gravity to be 6 in. from the fulcrum, the torque (i.e., force times perpendicular distance) about the elbow from this source is equal to $4 \times 6 = 24$ lb. Since the torque of the shot equals 224 lb, a total torque of 248 lb results. In order to keep the forearm and the shot in equilibrium, the rotary force exerted by the contraction of the biceps must also equal 248 lb. Since

$$\text{force} = \frac{\text{Resistance torque}}{\text{Force arm}}$$

$$f = \frac{248}{2} = 124 \text{ lb force exerted by biceps}$$

A more complicated example of a third-class lever is seen in the Monteggia (nightstick) fracture (Fig. 6–12).

Effect of the Angle of Pull. Figure 6–13 shows how the angle of pull changes as the muscle contracts. When the bony lever is in position BC, the angle of pull (DEB) is 12°; in the position BC_1, it is 20°; at BC_2, 25° degrees. The smaller the angle of pull, the farther and faster a given amount of muscular contraction (shortening) moves the bone. In Figure 6–13, the muscle DE is represented as making four successive contractions, each one equivalent to one eighth of the muscle's length. Starting at position BE, where the angle of pull is only 12°, the first contraction moves the bone BE through an angular distance of 32° as the angle of pull increases, the same amount of contraction turns it 25°, 21°, and 19°, respectively. When the angle of pull is 10° to 12°, movements are about the same.

From the standpoint of force alone, the optimal angle of pull for any muscle is 90°, because at this angle the entire force of the mus-

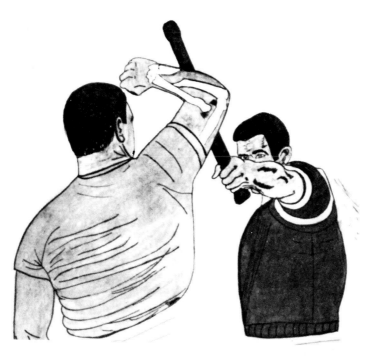

FIG. 6–12. Simultaneous fracture of the ulna and anterior or posterior dislocation of the head of the radius while the forearm is in a pronated position is known as a Monteggia fracture. One form of this fracture may occur while defending one's head from a blow from a nightstick. The direct trauma fractures the ulna. The fulcrum formed by the fractured ulna causes the head of the radius to dislocate posteriorly. A more common form results when a falling person catches his weight on an extended arm, with the forearm pronated and with the body and upper arm twisting, creating more pronational force, in which case the radial head dislocates anteriorly.

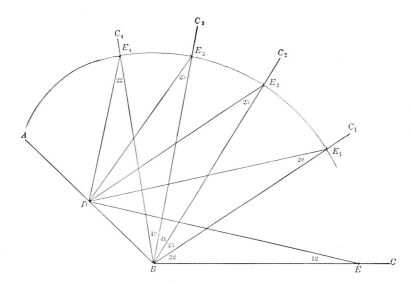

FIG. 6–13. Diagram to show how the angle of pull changes as the bony lever is moved by the muscle: AB is a stationary bone with axis at B; DE is the muscle and BC the moving bone, coming to positions BC_1, BC_2, etc.; as the muscle shortens, the muscle comes to positions DE_1, DE_2, etc.; DEB is the angle of pull.

cle is acting to rotate the bony lever around its axis. This is the only case in which the force arm is equal to the perpendicular distance along the bone. At angles of less than 90°, part of the muscular pull acts to pull the bone lengthwise into the joint, thereby stabilizing but increasing the friction of the joint and reducing the amount of pull available to perform external work. At angles greater than 90°, part of the pull can tend to pull the bone out of the joint, again reducing the amount for external work. As a result, the increased distance and speed of movement at small angles of pull is achieved only at the sacrifice of efficiency, and the actual movement at angles other than 90° is the result of two-force components.

Stabilization is of particular importance in the case of the shoulder, where the head of the humerus is only loosely held in place. In the absence of a relatively large stabilizing force, certain strenuous efforts might cause the joint to dislocate (luxation). In the upper range of movement where this is a definite possibility, the supraspinatus muscle aids greatly by providing a relatively large force for stabilization. In the case of the hip, the stabilizing component need not be large because the socket is deep and the head of the femur is held firmly in place by strong, taut ligaments. In many positions the weight of the body also tends to push the head of the femur into the socket.

Because the stabilizing component of force cannot contribute to useful work, it represents wasted energy insofar as mechanical efficiency of the machine is concerned. In any movement in which the stabilizing force is relatively large compared to the rotary force, the efficiency of movement must be low. As will be discussed later in this chapter, in some cases the body has endeavored to overcome this situation by the introduction of pulleys into the mechanical system.

Effect of the Angle of Resistance. When an object is moved, the resistance that is overcome is usually the force of gravity. Gravity is always effective vertically downward from the center of gravity of the object. As a muscle contracts and moves an object through space, the angle of the resistance to the force continually changes, just as has been shown to be true for the angle of pull of a muscle. As a result, two calculations are necessary before the force required at any given stage in a movement can be calculated.

Assume a weight lifter curls a 100-lb barbell. The distance between the axis at the elbow and the insertion of the biceps is 2 in.; the angle of pull of the elbow flexors is 75°, the distance from the axis to the weight is 14 in., and the angle between the forearm and the line of gravity of the barbell is 82°. The torque developed by this weight is equal to the amount of weight (100 lb) times the sine of the angle of the weight (sin 82° = 0.99027) times the length of the resistance arm (14 in.), or 1386.38 in.-lb. To this must be added the torque developed by the weight of the forearm itself—say 25 in.-lb—for a total resistance torque of 1411.38 in.-lb. By use of the formula

$$f = \frac{\text{Resistance torque}}{\text{Force arm}}$$

we find that the rotary force component of the muscular contraction necessary to offset this torque is 705.5 in.-lb. This is the *rotary force*, which must be produced by the muscle's pulling at an angle of 75°. The *entire force* of contraction that will be needed must now be found. Substituting known quantities in the formula

$$f = F \times \text{sine angle of pull}$$
$$705.5 = F \times 0.966$$
$$F = \frac{705.5}{0.966}$$
$$= 730.33 \text{ lb}$$

Ordinarily, several muscles act on a joint at once, necessitating very complex computations. Usually the distances from the axis, the angle of muscle pulls, and the weights of the body segments cannot be determined with any degree of accuracy. Even allowing for these inherent inaccuracies, however, such studies clearly show the extent to which the third-class lever system of the body sacrifices force for range of motion, and, conversely, the great amount of force required to lift relatively light weights. When a 170-lb man performs a straight-legged dead lift of 200 lb, the forces of the weight lifted, the weight of the upper body, and the contraction of the deep muscles of the spine generate a theoretical reaction of 2071 lb at the lumbosacral disk, although certain compensating mechanisms in the torso reduce this to 1483 lb.[3] Examples of this type clarify why such movements occasionally result in serious trauma and they emphasize the need for proper body mechanics (see also Chapter 15).

WHEEL AND AXLE ACTION

A modification of the lever is found in the wheel and axle principle, which is used in the body to effect or prevent rotation of a segment. In trunk twisting exercises, for example, the oblique abdominal muscles pull on the trunk as though it were the rim of a wheel, and the trunk is turned in the direction of the pull. This action actually constitutes a lever of the second class.

Usually rotation is the result of the synergic action of many muscles, whose pull is oblique rather than direct. Frequently a muscle inserts on a tuberosity, or bony process. This increases the torque by increasing the length of the lever arm.

PULLEY ACTION

The pulley provides a means of changing the direction of a force, thereby applying it at a different angle and perhaps resulting in a line of movement quite different from that which would otherwise have occurred. The tendon of insertion of the peroneus longus muscle offers a good example. This tendon goes directly down the lateral aspect of the leg, passes around the external malleolus, goes to a notch in the cuboid bone, turns under the foot, and inserts in the medial cuneiform and the first metatarsal. The pulley action of the external malleolus and the cuboid bone thus accomplishes two changes of direction that would otherwise be impossible. The result is that contraction of this muscle causes plantar flexion of the foot; without the pulleys the muscle would insert in front of the ankle and on top of the foot, so that it would cause dorsiflexion of that segment.

By changing the direction of the application of force, a pulley may provide a greater angle of insertion than would otherwise be possible. An example is found in the patella. By passing over this sesamoid bone, the patellar ligament inserts at a greater angle, which increases the rotary component of force of the quadriceps muscle of the thigh and decreases the stabilizing component. In this case a change of direction of force achieves an increased effective force in the movement.

Figure 6–14 shows a typical example of human movement in athletics. It describes how mechanical analysis can be applied to such an activity, the results of such analysis may be used to produce improved performance by showing the athlete exactly what he is trying to do, why he is trying to do it, and how he can accomplish his end most efficiently, and may point the way to more effective performance.

REHABILITATION OF THE KNEE

As an additional example of the application of torque concepts, consider the common knee extension exercise often used for quadriceps conditioning and strengthening of the knee joint after injury. One method used to perform knee extensions is to attach a weighted boot to the foot while seated on a padded table. In the starting position, with the knee flexed about 90° and the shank, foot, and boot hanging off the table perpendicular to the floor, the line of the pull of gravity on the boot passes vertically through the knee joint. Thus, there is zero lever arm distance from the rotational axis of the knee to the pull of gravity and the boot provides almost no resistance (other than inertia) to initial extension of the knee joint. As the knee extends, the line of pull of gravity moves away from the knee joint so that the weight of the boot continuously acts through a larger and larger lever arm until full knee extension is reached. This type of knee extension exercise, therefore, subjects the knee joint musculature to increasing loads to overcome the torque created by gravity on the boot as the knee extends.

A cable and pulley type leg extension bench produces a different overload pattern on the knee joint. The pulley and cable system directs the pull of gravity on an adjustable weight stack so that it is perpendicular to the

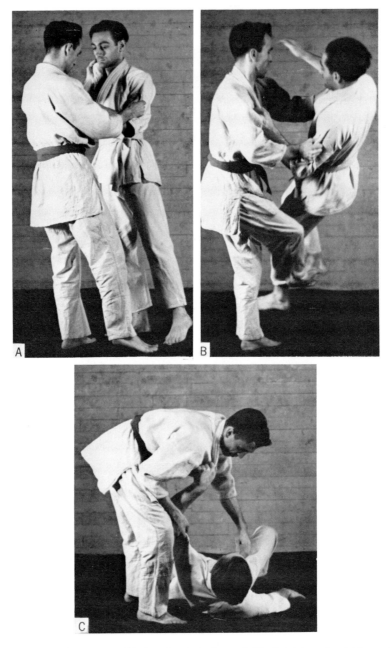

FIG. 6–14. Okuri-ashi-harai (sweeping ankle throw), a judo throw. *A,* The judoist on the right may be thought of as essentially a second-class lever, with the fulcrum at his feet, his weight at his center of gravity, and a force couple applied at feet and chest. *B,* The mv with which the right foot of the opponent sweeps against his left ankle as he steps sideward develops an F that moves his foot against the right ankle (Newton's first law), thus narrowing his base of support to his right foot alone. Simultaneously the combined Fs of the lift-push of the opponent's left arm and the pull of the right arm rotate him on his narrowed base (Newton's second law) and cause his line of gravity to fall outside of his base. If the F of the opponent's foot is great enough, it overcomes the friction between the man's supporting foot and the mat and sweeps his base out from under him. *C,* The torque created by the force couple (Fd center of gravity to ankle + Fd center of gravity to chest) developed by the combined leg and arm maneuvers causes him to rotate around his center of gravity and crash to the mat on his back. By landing on his back (and by the preliminary slap of his right arm on the mat) the thrown judoka receives the landing shock on the padded parts of the body and minimizes the impact per square inch by dissipating it over as large an area as possible. Expressed as a formula, Pressure = $\frac{force}{area}$. A similar analysis of aikido throws will show that this art depends to a much greater extent on the use of centrifugal force. (Photos reproduced from *Modern Judo,* Volume I, by Charles Yerkow, with permission of the publishers. The Stackpole Company, Harrisburg, Pa.)

shank and applied to the ankle joint area via a padded bar. Thus, the load acts through a maximal lever arm distance at the start of knee extension (from approximately 90° of flexion) and through slightly smaller lever arms as knee extension occurs and the pulley cable moves closer to the knee joint. This type of knee extension exercise, therefore, subjects the knee joint musculature to maximal overload at the start of extension and gradually decreasing overload as the knee extends. Which of the above two types of knee conditioning exercise is better depends on the type of injury or deficiency experienced by the individual. An understanding of torque and lever arm concepts can help the therapist or physical educator evaluate the overload produced by the ever-increasing variety of exercise devices available.

BALANCE BOARDS AND CENTER OF GRAVITY

As a final example of the application of torque principles in kinesiology, the balance board method to estimate the position of the center of gravity (CG) in the body is presented.

Consider the simple apparatus illustrated in Figure 6–15, which consists of a rigid board (approximately 3 ft by 7 ft), a scale for weighing, and two pointed-edge pivots. The height of the subject's CG above the ground is to be determined. The subject lies on the board with his feet at the point of the first pivot (considered to be the rotation point for the calculations). The scale reading (S1) is noted before the subject is positioned on the board and again (S2) in the lying position (Fig. 6–15). The pull of gravity on the CG of the board creates a torque about the first pivot that tends to rotate the board clockwise. Rotation is prevented by a counterclockwise torque created by the upward force (S1) applied toward the other end of the board by the second pivot resting on the scale. When the subject is in position, gravity also pulls on the CG of the body, with a force equal to body weight (W), and creates an additional torque tending to rotate the board clockwise about the first pivot. This torque is counteracted by an increased upward force (S2 − S1) on the board by the second pivot. Note that the lever arm (X) of the pull of gravity on the body's CG is just the parameter needed and that it is shorter than the lever arm (L) for the increased force (S2 − S1) applied by the second pivot. L can be measured directly with a measuring tape or ruler. The equation for this balanced or equilibrium situation is

$$\text{Torque 1} = \text{Torque 2}$$
$$W X = (S2 - S1) L$$
$$X = (S2 - S1) (L/W)$$

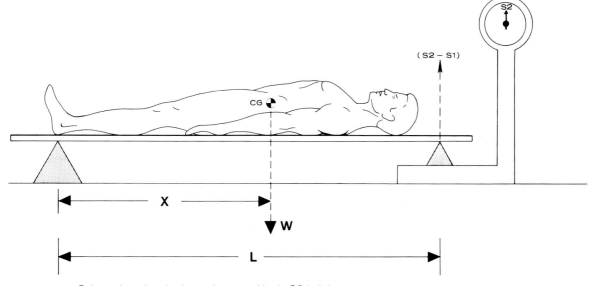

FIG. 6–15.   Balance board method to estimate total body CG height.

If W = 150 lb, L = 7 ft and (S2 − S1) = 75 lb, then

$$X = 75 \ (7/150)$$

$$X = 3.5 \ \text{ft}$$

The CG of the subject's body is approximately 3.5 ft above the ground when he is standing with the arms in the same position they were in while he was lying on the board for the measurement. Because blood distribution and internal organs may shift slightly toward the feet when standing as opposed to lying horizontally, the CG is actually a little lower than calculated.

The above method is useful to estimate CG position in the vertical dimension. For more complex body positions the CG can be estimated in two dimensions (Fig. 6–16). Balance board techniques for determining segment CG's are discussed elsewhere.[4]

CALCULATION OF MULTISEGMENT CENTER OF GRAVITY

If an object is composed of several parts, each of which has a known CG location, the CG of the object as a whole can be calculated. Similarly, the CG of any part of the body composed of two or more segments can be computed if the CG location for each segment is known. The procedure can be illustrated by

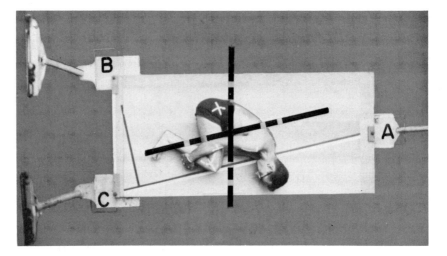

FIG. 6–16. Apparatus for locating the center of gravity in two planes simultaneously, photographed from directly overhead. The rectangular balance board rests on three weighing scales by means of pointed bolts (A,B,C). Theoretically, only two scales are needed; the third permits an accuracy check. The center of gravity of the subject will be located (as shown by the intersecting broken lines on the photograph) directly above a point that is G_A distant from line BC and G_B distant from line AC, as calculated by the formulas

$$G_A = \frac{(a_2 - a_1) \ (D_A)}{W} \quad \text{and} \quad G_B = \frac{(b_2 - b_1) \ (D_B)}{W}$$

where

   G_A = perpendicular distance of center of gravity from line BC.
   G_B = perpendicular distance of center of gravity from line AC.
   a_1 = scale reading for board alone at Scale A.
   a_2 = scale reading for board and subject at Scale A.
   b_1 = scale reading for board alone at Scale B.
   b_2 = scale reading for board and subject at Scale B.
   D_A = perpendicular distance from line BC to point A.
   D_B = perpendicular distance from line AC to point B.
   W = weight of the subject.

using the arm as an example. If the arm is held out to the side parallel to the ground, the arm's CG is located an unknown distance between the shoulder and the hand. Information about the weight of the upper arm, forearm, and hand as a percentage of body weight, as well as the distance from the proximal end of each of these segments to its CG location as a percentage of segment length, can be found in numerous biomechanics textbooks. From this information the location of the entire arm's CG relative to a reference point, for instance the shoulder joint, is calculated by making the product of the entire arm's weight and its lever arm distance to the shoulder (L_{cg}, the desired unknown location of the arm's CG) equal to the sum of the products of each segment's weight and its lever arm distance to the shoulder (Fig. 6–17). Hence,

$$(W_a + W_f + W_h)L_{cg} = W_a(C_a \times L_a)$$

$$+ W_f([C_f \times L_f] + L_a) + W_h([C_h \times L_h] + L_a + L_f)$$

where C_a is the fraction of the upper arm's length (L_a) from its proximal end to its CG position, W_a is its weight, and similarly for the other segments.

Using the parameters of body weight = 140 lb, L_a = 12 in., L_f = 10 in., and L_h = 7 in., and if available data indicates that C_a = 0.43, C_f = 0.43, C_h = 0.5, W_a = 4 lb., W_f = 2.4 lb, and W_h = 0.8 lb, then the above equation yields

$$(4 + 2.4 + 0.8)L_{cg} = \begin{array}{l} 4(.43 \times 12) + 2.4([.43 \times 10] + 12) \\ + .8([.5 \times 7] + 12 + 10) \end{array}$$

$$7.2 \times L_{cg} = 20.64 + 39.12 + 20.4$$

$$L_{cg} = 80.16/7.2 = 11.1 \text{ in.}$$

Thus, the total arm's CG is located 11.1 in. from the shoulder.

FORCE AND STRENGTH

The term force has been used frequently in previous sections in connection with dynamics and Newton's laws of motion. In addition to having a precise meaning in mechanics, it has an almost intuitive connection to how hard one pulls or pushes to lift or move an object.

Strength is more difficult to define because the force or tension muscles create is not directly measurable or applicable in everyday activities—muscle tension acts via the skeletal leverage system. Strength is not a standard term in mechanics. It may be used to designate an ability to produce or resist a force, but because it can be measured only in terms of the force, torque, or work produced, it tends to be ambiguous in the context of quantitative physics. Muscular strength, for example, may be measured in terms of the ability to overcome a resistance (concentric, isometric, or dynamic strength), to resist forces (eccentric strength), or to support a load (isometric or static strength). The correlation between strengths measured in any of these ways is high, but the scores and positions of maximal force are not identical (Fig. 6–18).[5]

WORK AND POWER

In mechanics, work is defined as the product of force and displacement (W = F × D, where F is the force component in the direction of the displacement D). Thus, isometric force results in the performance of no mechanical work because, by definition, there is

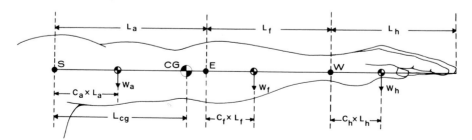

FIG. 6–17. Model of the arm as used to determine its CG location from segment CG locations and anthropometric measures.

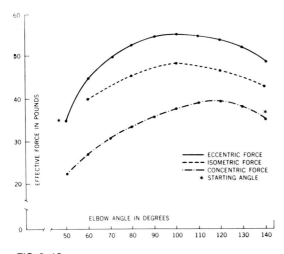

FIG. 6–18. Curves of maximum eccentric, isometric, and concentric forces of forearm flexors. (Singh and Karpovich,[5] by permission J. Appl. Physiol.)

no movement. Physiologic work, however, is performed, because energy must be used to generate muscle tension. Power is defined as the rate of doing work or work done per unit time ($P = W/t$). During a workout, average power output is related to the intensity of the exercise, which is very important in obtaining a training effect (see Chapter 16).

An estimation of the maximum power output capacity of an individual can be obtained by several methods. Two of the most popular are the Lewis formula,[6] using the standing vertical jump test, and the Margaria-Kalaman test, in which the subject is timed while running up a standardized flight of stairs.[6] Other methods involve use of cycle ergometers and isokinetic testing machines.

A good example to illustrate the differences between force, strength, work, and power comes from the sports of weightlifting and powerlifting. One of the lifts in powerlifting is the dead lift. If an athlete completes a 600-lb dead lift in 2 sec by elevating the weight to mid-thigh level 2 ft above its starting height (see Figs. 6–7, 15–6), the following mechanical factors were required:

(1) max force = slightly more than 600 lb because acceleration is minimal in heavy dead lifts
(2) work done = (600+ lb) × (2 ft) = 1200+ ft-lb

(3) power = (1200+ ft-lb)/(2 sec) = 600+ ft-lb/sec

NOTE: Power is often given in horsepower (hp). 1 hp = 550 ft-lb/sec, so the above dead lift required 1.1 hp (600/550).

One of the lifts in Olympic-style weightlifting is the snatch lift, in which the barbell must be lifted from the floor to arms' length overhead in one motion. If an athlete completes a 300-lb snatch in 1 sec and elevates the barbell 5 ft, the required mechanical factors were

(1) max force = approximately 450 lb based on published acceleration data for this lift[7]
(2) work done = (400 lb) × (5 ft) = 2000 ft-lb (average force of 400 lb based on published data[7])
(3) power = (2000 ft-lb)/(1 sec) = 2000 ft-lb/sec or 3.6 hp (2000/550)

Thus, mechanical analysis shows that the Olympic weightlifter is the more powerful athlete, while the powerlifter is the stronger athlete.[8] In 1960, Wilkie[9] reviewed the literature dealing with the mechanical power output of champion athletes under various conditions and concluded the output is limited:

1. To less than 6 hp in single movements having a duration of less than 1 sec, owing to the intrinsic power production of muscle and the difficulty of coupling a large mass of muscle to a suitably matched load.

2. To 0.5 to 2 hp in bouts of exercise lasting 1 to 5 min owing to the restricted availability in the muscles of stores of energy-yielding substances.

3. To 0.4 to 0.5 hp in steady state work of 5 to 150 min or more, owing to the restricted ability of the body to absorb and transport oxygen.

4. To perhaps 0.2 hp in long-term work, owing to wear and tear of muscles, the need to eat, etc.

In the past two decades, athletic performance has increased greatly in all sports, and the above maximal estimates have been surpassed.[7,10,11]

REFERENCES

1. Pugh, L.G.C.E., et al.: A physiological study of channel swimmers. Clin. Sci., *19*:257, 1960.

2. Garhammer, J.: Longitudinal analysis of highly skilled Olympic weightlifters. *In* Science in Weightlifting. Edited by J. Terauds. Del Mar, California, Academic Publishers, 1979, pp. 79–88.

3. Morris, J.M., et al.: Role of the trunk in stability of the spine. J. Bone Joint Surg., *43A*:327, 1961.

4. LeVeau, B.: Biomechanics of Human Motion. Philadelphia, W.B. Saunders Co., 1977, pp. 205–215.

5. Singh, M., and Karpovich, P.V.: Isotonic and isometric forces of forearm flexors and extensors. J. Appl. Physiol., *21*:1435, 1966.

6. Stone, M., and O'Bryant, H.: Weight Training—A Scientific Approach. Minneapolis, Burgess Publishing Co., 1987, pp. 166–171.

7. Garhammer, J.: Power production by Olympic weightlifters. Med. Sci. Sports Exerc. *12*(1):54, 1980.

8. Garhammer, J., and McLaughlin, T.: Power output as a function of load variation in Olympic and powerlifting. J. Biomech., *13*(2):198, 1980.

9. Wilkie, D.R.: Man as a source of mechanical power. Ergonomics, *3*:1, 1960.

10. Garhammer, J.: Evaluation of human power capacity through Olympic weightlifting analyses. Doctoral dissertation, University of California at Los Angeles, 1980.

11. Garhammer, J.: Biomechanical profiles of Olympic weightlifters. Int. J. Sport Biomech., *1*(2):122, 1985.

RECOMMENDED READING

Hay, J.G.: The Biomechanics of Sports Techniques. Englewood Cliffs, Prentice-Hall, Inc., 1985.

Laws, K.: The Physics of Dance. New York, Schrimer Books, 1984.

Nave, C.R., and Nave, B.C.: Physics for the Health Sciences. Philadelphia, W.B. Saunders Co., 1975.

Winter, D.A.: Biomechanics of Human Movement. New York, John Wiley & Sons, 1979.

Wiktorin, C.V.H., and Nordin, M.: Introduction to Problem Solving in Biomechanics (Physical Therapy). Philadelphia, Lea & Febiger, 1986.

7 BIOMECHANICS II

JOHN GARHAMMER

In Chapter 6, the area of study called dynamics was introduced as a subdiscipline of mechanics. Kinematics was mentioned as the subdivision of dynamics that concentrates on describing the pattern of motion. Such a description of motion is often very useful for studying the motion of the human body and its segments, as well as the motion of objects interacting with it, and thus requires that both linear and rotary kinematics be considered in more detail. This discussion is followed by additional topics from kinetics and topics related to the motion of projectiles, such as baseballs and tennis balls.

KINEMATICS

Kinematics is essentially the descriptive geometry of motion with respect to time, ignoring the causes of motion and the concepts of mass, force, momentum, and energy. In pure form, kinematics refers to the motion of an infinitesimally small massless particle. However, the kinematics of a rigid body of finite mass may be analyzed if its mass is considered to be concentrated at one point. Even a deformable mass, like the human body, under some circumstances can be treated as a particle by analyzing the motion of its center of gravity. In studying the motion of a runner, for example, we ordinarily are interested in the motion of his center of gravity and not in the irrelevant flapping of a lock of his hair, his shoelace, or his wrist. Nevertheless, if there is some reason to be interested in the motion of his wrist, there is no reason why

we cannot follow its motion as a point, so long as the analysis is not interpreted as describing the overall motion of his body.

Kinematic analyses can be important in understanding the mechanisms of athletes' injuries. For instance, if the axis of a blow to the head runs through the center of gravity of the skull, as occurs when a boxer falls backwards and strikes his occiput on the mat, translatory motion results, and the injury is usually found opposite to the point of impact. In the case of an uppercut, however, the axis of the blow traverses the skull obliquely. Translation of the center of mass of the head and a rotation about this center occur. The farther a given point is from the center of mass, the greater its acceleration and hence the greater the possibility of injury. It follows that in such cases the spinal cord, as well as the brain, may suffer lesions.[1]

Displacement. Displacement (d) is the change in position of a particle with reference to some set of coordinate axes; d is a vector, since it has a positive or negative direction. Distance is a scalar quantity describing the length of path traversed, including actual changes in direction; thus, it is always positive. With reference to some arbitrary x axis, d is the difference between the terminal and initial coordinate of the particle on the scale:

$$d = x_t - x_i$$

Velocity. Average velocity (v_{avg}) is the displacement divided by the elapsed time

$$V_{avg} = \frac{x_t - x_i}{t_t - t_i} = \frac{d}{t}$$

If the coordinate x_i is numerically greater than x_t on the scale being used, both displacement and velocity will be negative. When the elapsed time is very short (as between frames of a slow motion movie), average velocity may be treated as though it were instantaneous velocity without introducing serious error for most purposes in human motion analysis. Of course, if velocity is constant (or uniform), average velocity and instantaneous velocity have the same value.

Note that average speed is the total distance traversed divided by the elapsed time and is different from average velocity. If a sprinter runs the 100-m race in 9.9 sec, the average velocity is $d/t = 100/9.9 = 10.1$ m/sec. Here we are interested in the average linear velocity and not in the average speed of the runner's center of gravity as it wandered from side to side and up and down, nor are we interested in the response time between the go signal and his first movement, although these are important factors from the point of view of the athlete and his coach.

Acceleration. The rate of change in velocity is acceleration. When motion is characterized by fluctuating velocity, analysis is complex unless the motion is broken down into its component parts. Motion characterized by constant acceleration is subject to analysis by relatively simple equations, however. The remainder of this discussion will pertain only to conditions of constant or uniform acceleration, of which there are two subconditions. When acceleration is zero, velocity is constant and a graph of displacement plotted against time is a straight line with a slope proportionate to the constant velocity. When acceleration is constant but not zero, the graph of velocity against time is a straight line with a slope proportionate to the constant acceleration. In this instance, the acceleration may be positive or negative, with the former indicating an increase of velocity with time, and the latter indicating a decrease of velocity with time. Negative acceleration is also called, non-technically, deceleration. For constant acceleration, the plot of acceleration against time is a horizontal straight line, with its magnitude proportionate to the degree of slope of the plot of velocity against time.

The motion of a particle under constant ac-

celeration may be described by the following equations, in which v_o = initial velocity at time $t_o = 0$, v = terminal velocity, t = elapsed time from time t_o, and d = displacement. When $v_o = 0$, the simpler equations in the right-hand column are valid.

$$a = \frac{v - v_o}{t} \quad \text{or} \quad a = \frac{v}{t}$$

$$d = v_o t + \tfrac{1}{2}at^2 \quad \text{or} \quad d = (at^2)/2$$

$$d = \tfrac{1}{2}(v_o + v)t \quad \text{or} \quad d = \tfrac{1}{2}vt$$

$$v = v_o + at \quad \text{or} \quad v = at$$

$$v^2 = v_o^2 + 2ad \quad \text{or} \quad v^2 = 2\,ad$$

The above equations contain a total of four variables, v, d, a, and t. Each of the equations lacks one of these but contains the other three. Therefore, if v_o and any two of the other four variables are known, the remaining two unknown factors may be determined by selecting and solving two equations, each of which contains only one of the two unknowns. For example, if a distance runner accelerates uniformly from 60 ft/sec to 85 ft/sec in 10 sec, his acceleration is

$$a = \frac{v - v_o}{t}$$

$$= \frac{85 \text{ ft/sec} - 60 \text{ ft/sec}}{10 \text{ sec}}$$

$$= 2.5 \text{ ft/sec/sec, or } 2.5 \text{ ft/sec}^2$$

The result is read as "2.5 feet per second per second" or "2.5 feet per second squared." This indicates that the velocity increases by 2.5 ft/sec each second.

Consider a gymnast who loses his handgrip and falls from a stationary position ($v_o = 0$) to the ground in 0.75 sec. We know that g, the acceleration of gravity, is equal to 32.2 ft/sec.[2] His velocity on impact is

$$v = at = (32.2 \text{ ft/sec}^2)(0.75 \text{ sec})$$

$$= 24.15 \text{ ft sec}$$

From another equation, we can find the distance he fell, as follows:

$$d = \tfrac{1}{2}vt = \frac{(24.15 \text{ ft/sec})(0.75 \text{ sec})}{2}$$

$$= 9.05 \text{ ft}$$

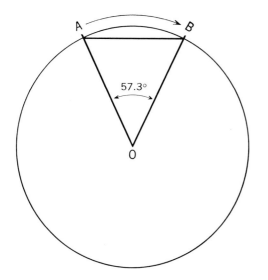

FIG. 7–1. Diagrammatic illustration of a radian. Arc AB is equal in length to the radius of the circle. A radian is defined as "the angle subtended by an arc on a circle equal in length to the radius of the circle," and is equivalent to 57.3 degrees. 2π radians = one revolution, or 360°. This seemingly arbitrary measurement is used because it relates linear velocity to angular velocity and linear displacement to angular displacement. Consequently, equations such as those for linear and angular acceleration can be expressed identically except for the distinguishing symbols.

Rotary Motion. The concepts employed to describe rotary motion are analogous to those that have been set forth for linear motion. Assume that in a given time (t) a point advances from A to B on a circle (Fig. 7–1). The angle AOB, which subtends arc AB, is termed angular displacement and may be measured in radians, degrees, or revolutions. Because 1 radian is defined as the angle that subtends an arc equal in length to the radius (r) of the circle (Fig. 7–1), linear and angular displacement (θ) are related by the equation $d = \theta r$. Average angular velocity (ω) is defined as angular displacement divided by elapsed time, or $\omega = \theta/t$. Using the above equation connecting linear and angular displacement, and dividing by t, $d/t = r\theta/t$ or $v = r\omega$, the equation relating average linear and angular velocity during motion along the arc of a circle. Angular acceleration (α) is defined analogously to linear acceleration $\alpha = (\omega - \omega_o)/t$. If angular acceleration is constant, kinematic equations for rotational motion can be derived

that are completely analogous to those for linear motion.

$$\theta = \omega_o t + (\alpha t^2)/2 \quad \text{or} \quad \theta = \alpha t^2/2$$

$$\theta = (\omega_o + \omega)\, t/2 \quad \text{or} \quad \theta = \omega t/2$$

$$\omega = \omega_o + \alpha t \qquad \text{or} \quad \omega = \alpha t$$

$$\omega = \omega_o^2 + 2\alpha\theta \qquad \text{or} \quad \omega = 2\alpha\theta$$

Rotary motion problems are solved in the same manner as linear motion problems except that the units are radians, radians/sec, or radians/sec². Radians are easily converted to degrees, 1 radian equalling 57.3°. Note that, because of the definition of a radian, the above equations connecting linear and angular displacement and velocity are valid only when using radian units. As an example, consider a figure skater who begins a spin ($\omega_o = 0$) with uniform angular acceleration and reaches $\omega = 5$ rev/sec in 3 sec. What was the magnitude of α and how many revolutions were completed in the 3-sec period of constant angular acceleration? Also, what is the linear velocity of the skater's hands when $\omega = 5$ rev/sec if they are 20 cm from the vertical axis of rotation through the body?

$$\alpha = (\omega - \omega_o)/t$$

$$= (5 \text{ rev/sec} - 0)/3 \text{ sec}$$

$$= 1.67 \text{ rev/sec}^2$$

$$\text{or} = (1.67 \text{ rev/sec}^2) \times (2\,\pi \text{ rad/rev})$$

$$= 10.49 \text{ rad/sec}^2$$

$$\text{or} = (10.49 \text{ rad/sec}^2) \times (57.3°/\text{rad})$$

$$= 600.9°/\text{sec}^2$$

Angular displacement in revolutions is found from

$$\theta = \alpha t^2/2$$

$$\theta = 1.67 \text{ rev/sec} \times (3 \text{ sec})^2/2$$

$$\theta = 7.5 \text{ rev}$$

or

$$\theta = (\omega\, t)/2$$

$$\theta = (5 \text{ rev/sec} \times 3 \text{ sec})/2$$

$$\theta = 7.5 \text{ rev}$$

To determine linear velocity of the hands, remember that rotary values must be in radian units.

$$v = r \, \omega$$

$$v = (20 \text{ cm}) \times (5 \text{ rev/sec}) \times (2 \, \pi \text{ rad/rev})$$

$$v = 628 \text{ cm/sec}$$

KINETICS

Kinetics is the second major area of study in the field of dynamics. It is concerned with the causes of motion and changes in motion. Kinetics is based largely on applications of Newton's second law of motion, which was discussed in Chapter 6. Additional topics in kinetics will be presented here, starting with another look at Newton's second law, which states that the vector sum of forces acting on an object equals the mass of the object times its acceleration ($F = ma$). Since $a = (v - v_o)/t$, the second law can be expressed as

$$F = (mv - mv_o)/t$$

The product of mass times velocity is known as momentum; hence, the second law states that the net force acting on an object equals the change in its momentum per unit time. Multiplying this equation by t yields

$$Ft = mv - mv_o$$

which expresses the "impulse–change in momentum" relationship, where force (F) acting on an object multiplied by the time during which it acts is known as the impulse given to the object.

Note when using this and other relationships involving mass that weight and mass are not equivalent. Weight equals the mass of an object multiplied by gravitational acceleration ($W = mg$). The value of "g" varies slightly at different places on earth but can generally be taken as 32.2 ft/sec² or 9.81 m/sec.² Weight is measured in units of pounds or Newtons, and mass in slugs or kilograms, depending on whether the British engineering or metric system units are being used (see Appendix B). Weight, being a force, is a vector quantity. Mass is a scalar quantity.

The impulse-momentum relationship is useful in the solution of problems in which force is applied to an object for a given period of time and produces a change in the momentum of the object. Typical examples are those in which balls are struck with various sports implements. Simplifying assumptions are made for these types of calculations, for example, regarding deformation of the ball.

Assume that a standard 1.6 oz golf ball is struck with a club and given a velocity of 200 ft/sec. If it is known that the club head is in contact with the ball for 0.0005 sec, by using the impulse-momentum equation it is possible to calculate the force in pounds with which the ball is struck.

$$Ft = \frac{W}{g} v - \frac{W}{g} v_o$$

$$F = \frac{\dfrac{W}{g} v - \dfrac{W}{g} v_o}{t}$$

The second term in the numerator disappears because the ball starts from rest and its initial velocity is zero.

Converting ounces to pounds,

$$F = \frac{\dfrac{0.1}{32.2} \times 200}{0.0005} = 1242 \text{ lb}$$

It is also possible to calculate the distance through which the club head is in contact with the ball.

$$\text{Average velocity} = \frac{v - v_o}{2} = \bar{v}$$

$$= \frac{200 - 0}{2}$$

$$= 100 \text{ ft/sec}$$

$$\text{Distance} = \bar{v}t = 100 \times 0.0005$$

$$= 0.05 \text{ ft}$$

Curiously enough, since it takes 0.0006 sec for the shock of the impact to reach the grip, and a further period before the brain receives the signal from the hands, the ball will have flown about 2 ft before the player becomes conscious of the impact. Consequently, it is impossible for him to correct a faulty shot.²

From the foregoing equations it is apparent that the racket of a tennis player strikes the ball with a momentum proportionate to the racket's mass and the velocity with which it is moving. The player can hit the ball harder by "getting his body" into the serve, and thus increasing the mass, or by increasing the velocity with which the racket moves, and hence the velocity that it imparts to the ball. In either case, in order to produce a larger mv in the object, a larger Ft must be applied to the object.

In physical contact sports these relationshps are especially important. If a relatively small halfback must block a big lineman, his principal hope lies in moving fast enough so that he develops an mv great enough to overcome his adversary's advantage in mass.

CONSERVATION OF MOMENTUM

Note from the impulse-momentum equation that if no net force acts on an object (i.e., Ft = 0), then mv = mv$_o$. Newton's third law states that when two objects interact, such as during a collision, they experience equal forces but in opposite directions. Thus, because in a collision there is no net force acting on the objects involved, the total momentum of the objects must remain the same. The principle of conservation of momentum states that in the absence of any net external force, the sum of the momentums of two interacting particles remains constant. That is,

$$m_1v_a + m_2v_b = m_1v_{a'} + m_2v_{b'}$$

where v$_a$ and v$_b$ are the velocities of two particles, a and b, at time 1, respectively, and v$_{a'}$ and v$_{b'}$ are the velocities at time 2.

When one moving body strikes another, the momentum involved is said to be "conserved," that is, the total mv after the collision of two bodies is exactly equal to the total of the two momentums before the impact. If a heavy man is tackled by a light man, he may be slowed down but keep moving. In such cases his loss of velocity is offset by the fact that he has gained in mass by the addition of the tackler. When a runner is tackled head-on by a man possessing equal momentum, both come to a halt because the momentums were in opposite directions.

KINETICS AND ROTARY MOTION

Basic kinematic considerations for rotary motion were presented earlier in this chapter and analogies with the linear kinematic equations were pointed out. The concept of torque is fundamental to rotary kinetics, and basic considerations related to torque and lever systems were presented in Chapter 6. A few additional concepts from rotary kinetics that have frequent application in kinesiology will now be presented.

A fundamental equation in linear kinetics is F = ma. The analogous equation in rotary kinetics is $\gamma = I\alpha$. Torque (Γ) was explained in Chapter 6, and angular acceleration (α) was introduced there and further discussed in this chapter. The moment of inertia or rotational inertia (I) was also introduced in Chapter 6 but requires more discussion.

Rotational Inertia. Rotational inertia (I) in angular motion is comparable to the mass in linear motion. For relatively small objects centered at a relatively great distance from the center of rotation (like a stone being swung at the end of a string, or a gymnast swinging on the rings), rotational inertia is approximately equal to the mass of the object multiplied by the square of its distance from the center of rotation (I = mr^2). In most kinesiologic and athletic problems, this special situation does not hold, because the mass of the body or segment is distributed over a large volume and is close to (or contains) the center of rotation. In such cases, it is necessary to take the mass of each elementary particle and multiply by the square of its distance from the center of rotation, and then to add all such products, in order to calculate rotational inertia (I = $m_1r_1^2 + m_2r + \ldots 1\, m_nr^2_n$). Such a task is impractical; therefore, shortcut approximations are employed. For example, the body is divided into segments, each of which is typified by a standard geometric shape. The head is considered to be a sphere, the upper arm a cylinder, the forearm a truncated cone, etc. Physics books give formulas for computing rotational inertia for each idealized segment, and these are added to determine roughly the rotational inertia. Whenever the human body moves, its mass is redistributed, and rotational inertia changes, requiring a recalculation. Because of these complexities, rotational inertia of the human body is difficult to compute accurately.

Rotational inertia is mentioned here primarily because of its relation to the phenomenon of conservation of angular momentum. In this regard, understanding of the concept of rotational inertia is important, even though rotational inertia is difficult to quantify.

Angular Momentum. Angular momentum is analogous to linear momentum (mv). Angular momentum is rotational inertia (I) multiplied by the angular velocity (ω).

$$\text{Angular momentum} = I\omega$$

Conservation of Angular Momentum. The principle of conservation of angular momentum is comparable to the principle of conservation of momentum in linear motion. It is sufficient here to point out that $I\omega$, once established, will remain constant until outside forces act to change it. If a weight on the end of a string is swung around one's head, a certain angular momentum is established. If the string is drawn in so that it is shortened by one half, the angular velocity is increased to four times its original value. Shortening the radius by one half diminishes the rotational inertia (I) by one quarter; therefore, angular velocity (ω) must be increased four times so that the angular momentum ($I\omega$) remains constant.

This principle is a common and an important consideration in a great variety of sports skills. Chapter 16 presents a detailed explanation illustrated by practical examples.

Tangential Velocity. When a weight on the end of a string is swung in a circle, each mass particle has, at any instant, a tendency to fly off in a direction tangent to the circle. If the string breaks (cf. the release of a discus or a thrown ball), the weight flies away tangentially at a velocity termed the tangential velocity. In Figure 7–2, the vector for tangential velocity is labeled v_t. The magnitude of v_t is equal to the radius of the circle multiplied by the angular velocity in radians/sec.

$$v_t = R\omega$$

The equation indicates clearly why a discus thrower emphasizes speed of rotation, and

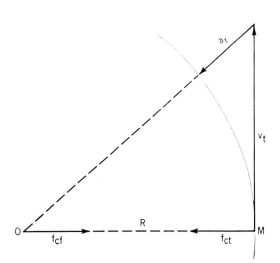

FIG. 7–2.   Diagram showing vectors for tangential velocity (v_t), radial acceleration (a_r), centripetal force (f_{ct}), and centrifugal force (f_{cf}) resulting from constant circular motion of mass-particle M in the counterclockwise direction. O is the center of rotation. The line OM = R is a constraining thread with infinitely small mass. If the thread has mass, then each of its own mass-particles will generate vector quantities like those of mass-particle M.

why he moves the discus through an arc having the largest possible radius.

Radial Acceleration. Newton's first law indicates that an object in motion will tend to remain in motion in a straight line, unless some other force acts on it. In Figure 7–2, the "straight line" is represented by the vector for tangential velocity, v_t, but because the object actually moves in a circle before its release, it is obvious that some force is constantly accelerating it toward the center of the circle. This is called radial acceleration, represented in Figure 7–2 by the vector labeled a_r. The magnitude of a_r at any moment is expressed by

$$a_r = \frac{v_t^2}{R}$$

which shows that radial acceleration is directly proportionate to the square of the instantaneous tangential velocity and inversely proportionate to the radius of the circle.

Centripetal and Centrifugal Force. The force that produces radial acceleration is called centripetal force, expressed by the formula

$$F = m \frac{v_t^2}{R} = \frac{W v_t^2}{g R}$$

Centripetal force appears as tension in the structure connecting the object with the center of rotation, pulling the object toward the center of rotation. It is matched by a reactive force equal in magnitude and opposite in direction, the centrifugal force, which is caused by the object's tendency to travel in a straight line. The formula for centrifugal force is the same as that for centripetal force.

In the common problems of kinesiology and sports analysis, it is not ordinarily necessary to compute centrifugal and centripetal force, but the student should understand that these forces are directly proportionate to the mass (or weight) of the object and the square of the tangential velocity.

In sports performance, centrifugal forces often reach tremendous magnitudes. The maximum momentary centrifugal force generated during a giant swing on the horizontal bar, at the bottom of the swing, has been calculated to be 438 lb for an expert performer weighing about 160 lb, making the total force directed away from the bar about 600 lb.[3]

ACTION OF MECHANICAL FORCES ON PROJECTILES

If we ignore for the moment the effect of air resistance, the horizontal distance a missile will be propelled from the ground can be computed by the formula

$$R = \frac{V^2 \sin 2\theta}{g}$$

where R = horizontal range, V = initial velocity of object, θ = angle of projection, and g = acceleration of gravity.* If it is assumed that a shot is released at a height of 8 ft, the above horizontal range will be the distance to the point at which the shot returns to a height of 8 ft above the ground. To determine the additional distance gained from this point to the place where the shot strikes the ground

---

*A summary of simple trigonometric relationships, together with a table of sines, is located in Appendix A.

requires the use of another formula. In Figure 7–3 the greatest range is achieved when the angle of projection is 45°. This results because sin 2θ is at a maximum when θ = 45°. Modifications of this same formula will give the maximum height attained by the object and the time the projectile is in the air. Height may be computed by the equation

$$Height = \frac{(V \sin \theta)^2}{2g}$$

Since θ reaches its maximum at 90°, the maximum height will also be reached at this angle. The time the projectile is in the air can be calculated by use of the formula

$$Time = \frac{2V \sin \theta}{g}$$

Although the uses of such formulas are largely theoretical, the physical laws they describe may have definite practical applications. In football, for instance, it may be more important to gain height and time on a punt to enable the players to cover the receiver than it is to achieve maximum distance on the kick. The kicker must vary the θ of the ball accordingly. For an "onside" kick an appropriate reduction of V is essential. Again, if a baseball player desires to "pick off" a base runner, the time during which the ball is in the air becomes more important than the maximum distance that it can be thrown. Using the above formula it can be demonstrated that the ball travels faster horizontally when thrown at an angle of 30° than when thrown at an angle of 45°.

In Figure 7–3, the path of the projectile is shown as a true parabola, and it will be observed that the object returns to the horizontal at approximately the same angle at which it was projected. In actuality, the velocity and horizontal distance traveled will be reduced by air resistance, so that the path of the object will not be a true parabola. Because air resistance varies with the square of the velocity, the resistance is four times as great for an object traveling twice as fast as another similar missile. The lighter the object and the larger its surface area, the more it is affected by air resistance. Whereas with heavy, slow-moving objects like a 16-lb shot the air resist-

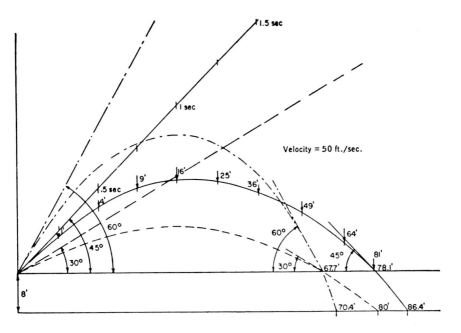

FIG. 7–3.   Path of an object projected at various angles at 50 ft/sec from a height of 8 ft (air resistance neglected). The parabolic path described by Galileo is evident. (From Broer, M.R.: Efficiency of Human Movement, courtesy W.B. Saunders Co.)

ance is negligible, light projectiles tend to drop to the ground quickly owing to a loss of horizontal velocity. For example, a baseball projected at 45°, which would travel 95 m in a vacuum, will actually travel only about 67 m, and its landing angle will be 55°.[2]

Curves. If a ball is thrown with a spin or hit off center so that it spins, aerodynamic effects may cause it to curve in its flight. The degree of curving will be positively related to three factors—the speed of the spin, the weight of the ball, and the roughness of its surface. The direction of the spin determines the direction in which the ball tends to curve.

An adequate mechanical analysis of curving requires reference to the complex laws of aerodynamics with consideration of different qualities of turbulence created on opposite sides of the spinning ball. The following is a more casual explanation: as the ball rotates, the rough surface creates a greater air resistance on the side of the ball that is turning toward its path through space, and a lesser air resistance on the side turning away from its path in space. This difference results in a force acting on the ball at right angles to its main direction, and the resulting lateral dis-

placement produces the curved path (Fig. 7–4).

Gravity tends to produce a parabolic downward curve in the path of the ball. Thus, in a down-curve (drop), gravity accentuates the curve; in a pure side-curve throw (in-shoot or out-shoot), gravity has no effect on the extent of lateral curving; and in an up-curve throw (up-shoot or hop), gravity tends to counteract the extent of curving, and vice versa. As a result, a drop is the easiest curve to throw, and an up-shoot is most difficult.

A new tennis ball, because of its light weight and fuzzy surface, curves much more readily than a baseball. The size, shape, and depth of the 336 dimples on a golf ball reflect the manufacturer's attempt to reduce draw while increasing lift.

Rebound Angles. Very roughly, we might assume that when an object, such as a ball, rebounds from a surface, the angle of incidence is equal to the angle of reflection. This is true only under idealized circumstances, such as when the surface is immovable, the ball is not spinning, and both objects are extremely hard. In practice these conditions are seldom met. Softer surfaces are compressible, so that some rolling or sliding of one object

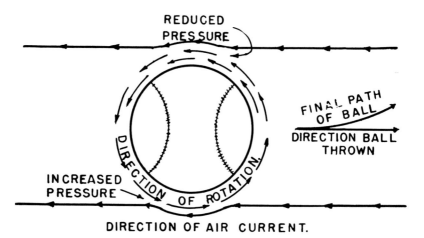

FIG. 7–4. A spinning ball is deflected from its straight path by dragging a "boundary layer" of air along with it in the direction of its rotation. This creates different pressures on opposite sides of the ball.

on the other may take place before rebound. The degree to which a surface resists deformation and tends to regain its shape quickly is expressed as that substance's coefficient of restitution. Billiard balls have a relatively high coefficient of restitution, and collisions between them are said to be relatively elastic. But when a billiard ball strikes a cushion, the relatively low coefficient of restitution of the cushion leads to an angle of reflection that is measurably less than the angle of incidence, and a similar situation exists when a compressible basketball strikes a relatively hard floor or backboard. Much more noticeable is the distortion of the rebound angle resulting from the spin of a ball. The direction of the deviation of the angle of reflection is obvious to anyone who has had experience with rebounding balls, and the effects are summarized in Figure 7–5.

Gyroscopic Action. The spin of an object in flight produces a stabilization against end-over-end tumbling and other erratic behavior. This effect is called gyroscopic action. The laws of gyroscopic action cannot be explained here, but it may be said that the result is beneficial to the flight paths of such sports implements as footballs and discuses.

Air Resistance. Small, heavy, smooth objects traveling at moderate speeds are affected very little by air resistance. Large, light, irregular objects traveling at fast speeds may be deterred significantly in their flight paths by air resistance. Thus, a baseball or shot is less affected, whereas a badminton bird or table tennis ball reacts significantly to air resistance.

The object's speed, referred to above, means its speed with respect to still air (rather than with respect to the ground). A head wind has the same effect as increasing the object's speed with respect to still air; a tail

FIG. 7–5. The effect of spin on the rebound angle of a ball striking a horizontal plane surface. When a tennis ball stroked with top spin applied with an average amount of force strikes the court, the ball acts to push the court backward. In accordance with Newton's third law, the court reacts with an equal and opposite reaction. This causes the rebound of the ball to be more forward and lower than would otherwise be the case. With no spin the ball should theoretically rebound at an angle equal to that of its approach. Actually it may be a bit lower since the ball comes off the court with a slight top spin because friction with the court stops the bottom of the ball, causing the top to move faster. A ball with backspin acts to move the court forward. The equal and opposite reaction of the court causes the rebound to be more backward and higher than would otherwise be the case. In actual play, of course, the relative coefficients of restitution of different balls and court surfaces greatly affect the results of the spin. (By permission of Tilmanis, G.: Advanced Tennis for Coaches, Teachers and Players, 1975.)

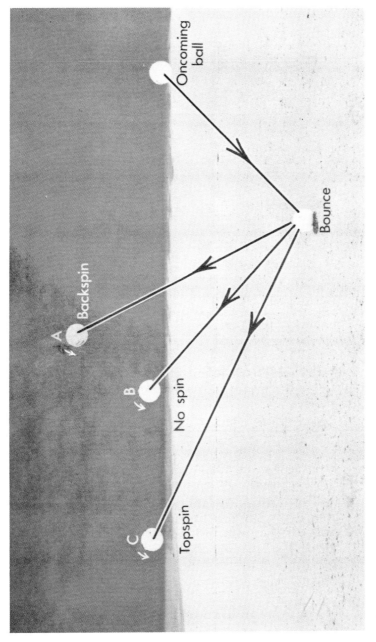

FIG. 7–5.   (Legend on facing page.)

wind, as decreasing the object's speed with respect to still air. The surface area of the human body is not great enough to cause great retardation due to air resistance at ordinary speeds of self-propulsion on a still day. Pugh concluded that air resistance accounts for about 7.5% of the net energy cost of running at middle distance speeds and about 13% of the cost of sprinting.[4]

On the basis of towing and wind tunnel experiences, Whitt[5] suggests that for a cyclist the air resistance may be calculated by the formula

Air resistance (lb force)
  = 0.0023 × frontal area (sq ft)
    × speed[2] (mi/hr)

This assumes an air density of 0.765 lb/ft[3].

In the event of a strong head wind, the relative speed of the body with respect to the airstream becomes large enough to cause significant retardation. Strong winds also affect the path of small objects such as a baseball or football. Records made in track and field events are disallowed if the runner is aided by a tailwind of greater than a stated magnitude.

Center of Percussion. Tennis and baseball players know from experience that hitting a ball at a certain spot on a racket or bat transfers the least initial shock to the hand of the player. In sports terminology this area is known as the "sweet spot"; in physics it is termed the center of percussion or center of oscillation of a compound pendulum.

The sweet spot is defined in two additional ways. Technically, one is the node of the amplitude of the first harmonic. It is located 4 or 5 in. toward the top from the center of percussion and is where the racket transmits the least amount of vibration to a player's hand. The other sweet spot is located where the center of restitution has its highest value and provides the maximal rebound. It is highest near the throat and lowest near the top of the racket.[6,7]

It has been reported that tennis players who hit the ball on the sweet spot do not develop elbow problems, whereas those who hit off-center do.[8]

STUDY QUESTIONS

1. Ascertain the world's records for running the various competitive distances from 100 m to 20,000 m. Prepare a graph showing the speed in m/sec for each event. How is the average speed affected by distance?

2. When a karate expert strikes with one arm, he simultaneously pulls the other one back. What principle is he seeking to invoke and for what purpose?

3. In punting into a head wind, what adjustment should the kicker make in the angle of projection of the ball? If kicking with a tail wind? Why?

4. The serve of Stan Smith has been timed at 136 mph; that of Margaret Court at 93 mph (measured by a different technique). The average man's serve is 82 mph; the average woman's, 68 mph. Assume that the ball is struck at a height of 9.5 ft and follows a linear trajectory until it lands in the service court at a point 58 ft horizontally away from the server. What is the linear displacement of the ball? Assuming average velocities cited above, what are the time intervals between impacts of the rackets and impacts of the balls with the ground? Actually, the balls fall off a linear trajectory because they are acted on by gravity during flight. Using the calculated time-of-flight estimates, how far will each player's ball fall under the influence of gravity? Which player's ball will have to be projected at the greater angle to the ground, and why?

6. In 1979, Doug Jones set a record by diving from a crane 165 feet above the water of Baltimore Harbor. What was his speed at the time of entering the water? (Ignore the effects of air resistance.)

7. What is the momentum of a 198-lb fullback moving at the rate of 23 ft/sec? Will his forward momentum be stopped if he is hit head-on by a 221-lb tackle moving at 19 ft/sec?

8. Assume a wrestler supine on the mat pushes upward against his opponent's head with a force of 100 kg. What is the effect on the wrestler himself? Why?

9. On June 19, 1963, Lt. Cliff J. Judkins, U.S.M.C., fell 4600 m into the ocean when his parachute failed to open. He received a compression fracture of the back, a hairline fracture of the pelvis, and two broken ankles. Assume the flier weighed 77 kg. What was his acceleration? The time of his fall? His speed at the time of impact? His velocity at the time of impact? The momentum with which he landed? The force with which he struck?

10. Tennis players contend that a ball with "heavy" top spin on it bounces higher than does a ball with top spin. This is contrary to the theoretical model shown in Fig. 7–5. What is the explanation of this apparent discrepancy? (Suggestion: Study Fig. 7–4.)

11. The *clavadistas*—those who pierce (the water)—at Acapulco, Mexico, dive into the ocean from the crest of a cliff called La Quebara, 41.5 m above the water. They must land 4 m out from the base of the cliff in order to miss the rocks. What distance do they have to travel? How long are they are in the air? What is the velocity with which they enter the water?

12. One of the fastest baseball pitches recorded was posted by Nolan Ryan, of the Los Angeles Angels, on August 20, 1974. The speed of the ball was 100.9 mph. Assume that the baseball weighed 5¼ oz. and that the above data also represent the mass and average velocity of the ball. Determine its momentum in g/m/sec. Assume that the ball left the pitcher's hand 55 ft from home plate. Disregarding the effects of gravity, air resistance, etc., how long a time does the batter have to see the ball before it reaches home plate?

REFERENCES

1. Untersharnscheidt, F., and Higgins, L.S.: Traumatic lesions of brain and spinal cord due to non-deforming angular acceleration of the head. Texas Rep. Biol. Med., 29:127, 1969.
2. Daish, C.B.: Learn Science Through Ball Games. New York, Sterling Publishing Co., 1972, pp. 15–16.
3. Burke, R.K.: Identification of Principles of External Mechanisms Affecting the Performance of a Selected Gymnastic Movement. Unpublished Master's Thesis, University of California at Los Angeles, 1950, p. 97.
4. Pugh, L.G.C.E.: The influence of wind resistance in running and walking and the mechanical efficiency of work against horizontal or vertical forces. J. Physiol., 213:255, 1971.
5. Whitt, F.R.: A note on the estimation of energy expenditure of sporting cyclists. Ergonomics 14:419, 1971.
6. Bernardo, S.: Physics of the sweet spot. Sci. Dig., 92:63, May 1984.
7. Andrews, J.G.: On the concept of the center of percussion. Med. Sci. Sports Exerc., 17:598, 1985.
8. Prevention and Treatment of Tennis Elbow. Phys. Sportsmed., 5:33, 1977.

RECOMMENDED READING

Briggs, L., Jr.: Effect of spin and speed on the lateral deflection (curve) of a baseball and the magnus effect for smooth sphere. Am. J. Phys., 27:589–596, 1959.
Brody, H.: Physics of the tennis racket. Am. J. Phys., 47:482–487, 1979.
Dapene, J.: A kinematic study of center of mass motion in the hammer throw. J. Biomech., 19:147, 1986.
Frankel, V.H., and Hang, Y-S.: Recent advances in the biomechanics of sport injuries. Acta Orthop. Scand., 46:484–497, 1975.
Hay, J.G.: The Biomechanics of Sports Techniques, 3rd Ed., Englewood Cliffs: Prentice-Hall, 1985.
Hay, J.G., et al.: A computational technique to determine the angular momentum of a human body. J. Biomech., 10:269–277, 1977.
Hooper, W.: Comment on "Maximizing the range of the shot put." Am. J. Phys., 47:748–749, 1979.
Lichtenberg, D.B., and Wills, J.G.: Maximizing the range of the shot put. Am. J. Phys., 46:546–549, 1978.
Schadewald, R.: It's 1–2–3 Strikes and Yer Out At the Old Ballistics Game! Sci. Dig., 86:56–61, 1979.
Walker, J.E.: Karate strikes. Am. J. Phys., 43:845–849, 1975.
Watts, R.G., and Sawyer, E.: Aerodynamics of a knuckleball. Am. J. Phys., 43:960–963, 1975.

II BASIC ANATOMY AND BIOMECHANICS OF SPECIFIC STRUCTURES

8 THE SHOULDER COMPLEX

MARK D. GRABINER

ANATOMIC CONSIDERATIONS

The mobility enjoyed by the upper extremity stems in part from the structures known as the shoulder girdle and the shoulder joint, or, more accurately, the glenohumeral joint. It is through this functional unit that the arm, forearm, wrist, and hand are connected to the axial skeleton and by control of this unit that the humerus can be positioned. Although structurally separate, the shoulder girdle and the glenohumeral joint are functionally inseparable.

The skeletal components of the shoulder girdle include two clavicles, two scapulae, and the sternum. These bones are responsible for the transmission of forces from the upper extremities to the body. This transmission of force, by necessity, follows a path defined by the joints associated with the shoulder girdle. The girdle is considered an open mechanical system—that is, the left and right sides are not directly connected and therefore can move independently. The indirect attachment between the left and right sides is through the manubrium of the sternum. The scapulae themselves are not connected to each other or to the vertebral column, although a connection or joint of sorts is considered to exist between the anterior surface of each scapula (subscapular fossa) and the tissues that lie between it and the ribs. This is often called the scapulothoracic articulation.[1]

The point of attachment of the scapulae to the clavicles is the acromioclavicular joint. It is a diarthritic gliding joint that in addition to being stabilized by the capsular ligaments is aided by two major ligamentous structures, the acromioclavicular and coracoclavicular ligaments. As with many anatomic structures, the name strongly suggests its location. The acromioclavicular ligament serves to strengthen the nonaxial acromioclavicular joint anteriorly; the coracoclavicular ligament, which connects the scapula to the coracoid process, provides the major protection for the joint. This ligament is composed of two structures, the conoid and trapezoid ligaments, which run from the superior aspect of the coracoid process to the inferior surface of the clavicle.

The triaxial, double diarthritic (gliding) sternoclavicular joint functions in all movements of the shoulder girdle. Though a double joint, the sternoclavicular joint functions as a triaxial ball-and-socket joint because the clavicle articulates with the manubrium of the sternum and also with the first rib. The clavicle, acting as a mechanical strut or arm, maintains the glenohumeral joint at its correct distance from the sternum. The articular surfaces of the medial ends of the clavicles are not anatomically contoured to the sternal point of attachment. An articular disk improves the degree of fit as well as acting as a shock absorber for forces transmitted from the shoulder region and helping to prevent dislocation of the joint. The disk is attached to the clavicle and the first costal cartilage. The sternoclavicular joint is also protected from excessive displacement by the costoclavicular ligament, which runs from the superior medial aspect of the first rib to the inferior medial surface of the clavicle (Figs. 8–1 and 8–2).

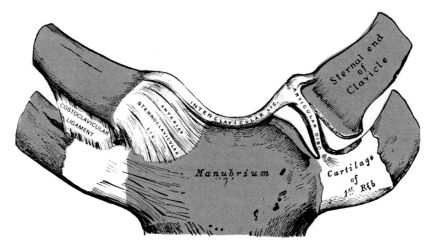

FIG. 8–1.   The sternoclavicular joints. Anterior aspect. (From Gray's Anatomy. 30th Ed. Philadelphia, Lea & Febiger, 1985, p. 367.)

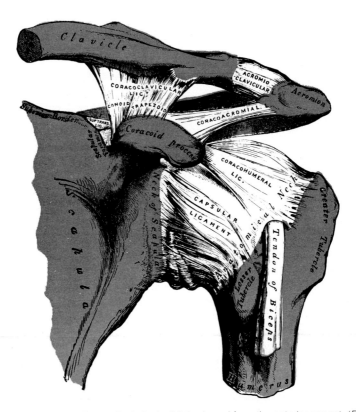

FIG. 8–2.   The left glenohumeral and acromioclavicular joints viewed from the anterior aspect. (From Gray's Anatomy. 30th Ed. Philadelphia, Lea & Febiger, 1985, p. 369.)

The glenohumeral joint consists of a nearly hemispherical humeral head and a relatively shallow glenoid fossa on the lateral aspect of the scapula. The glenoid labrum is a fibrous structure lining the perimeter of the glenoid fossa and serves, essentially, to deepen the articulation and thus improve its stability. The extreme mobility of the glenohumeral joint is achieved at the direct cost of stability, or resistance to displacement. The articular capsule, which completely surrounds the joint, is not a rigid structure and allows for a significant separation of the articulating surfaces during anterior and inferior humeral motion. The capsule attaches to the humeral neck inferiorly and to the bony rim of the glenoid fossa superiorly. Structurally, the joint is protected superiorly by the coracoacromial arch, formed by the coracoid process, the acromion process, and the coracoacromial ligament, which spans the distance between those two protuberances. Other ligaments, while not maintaining the joint surfaces in apposition, do protect the joint against displacement. The coracohumeral ligament runs from the coracoid process to the anterior aspect of the greater tubercle and serves to strengthen the joint capsule. The glenohumeral ligaments (superior, middle, and inferior) are also found in the anterior part of the joint and constitute part of the articular capsule. Although difficult to identify as individual ligaments, they run from the glenoid fossa to the lesser tubercle and the anatomic neck of the humerus.

JOINT MOVEMENTS

Movement of the shoulder girdle is generally described with respect to the scapula. The scapula may be elevated, depressed, abducted, adducted, upwardly rotated, downwardly rotated, and tilted both anteriorly and posteriorly. These movements do not generally occur independently nor do they occur in cardinal planes, because the scapulae follow the curvature of the thorax; however, the sagittal plane is considered to contain all but the tilt actions that occur in the frontal plane.

Elevation and depression represent upward and downward translation, respectively, of the scapula. Although rotation of the scapula, by definition, does not occur si-multaneously with elevation and depression, upward and downward rotation, characterized by a change in the angle of the glenoid fossa with respect to its normal position, generally accompanies elevation and depression, respectively.

Abduction and adduction occur when the scapula moves laterally away from or medially toward the vertebral column. These motions include anterior and posterior components in the frontal plane because of the thoracic curvature.

Movement of the inferior angle of the scapula away from or toward the thoracic surface is called posterior and anterior tilt, respectively. Posterior tilt is visible when the glenohumeral joint is hyperextended but in general has been shown to occur during normal excursion of the scapula through the frontal plane.[2]

Although shoulder girdle movement is defined with respect to the scapulae, it is noteworthy that the joint that is critical in all shoulder region movement is the sternoclavicular joint. As previously indicated, the strength of this joint depends on its ligamentous arrangement. The arrangement is such that dislocation of the joint is rare when a force is applied along the long axis of the clavicle; usually the bone will fail rather than be displaced. Because the sternoclavicular joint allows motion in essentially all planes, it permits circumduction, which is motion that describes a cone, the apex of which is the joint itself. Any triaxial joint allows circumduction.

Motion of the sternoclavicular joint in the transverse plane anteriorly is protraction, and the return movement is retraction; the range for each motion is approximately 15°. In the frontal plane the joint can allow 45° of elevation and 5° of depression. Rotation about the longitudinal axis of the clavicle may be 30 to 50°. Motion at the acromioclavicular joint is much more limited. The end of the clavicle may glide on the acromion and the scapula may rotate about the clavicle.

Movements of the shoulder girdle joints can be considered as supplementing the range of motion of the glenohumeral joint, which allows movement around all three axes and subsequently allows circumduction. Flexion and extension occur in the sagittal plane, the former being directed anteriorly. Abduction and adduction occur in the frontal plane, with abduction being directed laterally, initially moving the humerus away from the midline of the body. The hybrid movements of horizontal flexion and horizontal extension occur in a transverse plane. When the humerus is rotated about its long axis such that the medial surface, for example, moves anteriorly and then laterally, the movement is referred to as outward or lateral rotation. A rotation causing the same surface to move first posteriorly and then laterally is referred to as inward or medial rotation. Average values for glenohumeral flexion, hyperextension, abduction, horizontal flexion, horizontal extension, medial rotation, and lateral rotation are approximately 158°, 53°, 170°, 135°, 53°, 70°, and 90°, respectively.

Although movement of the glenohumeral joint is defined with respect to the humerus, movement of the humeral head with respect to the surface of the glenoid fossa occurs also. In rotation, the point of contact on the glenoid remains the same but the point of contact with the humerus varies. In rolling motion, the change in the point of contact occurs on both the humeral head and the glenoid fossa. Translation occurs when the contact point on the humeral head remains the same and that on the glenoid changes.[2] These types of movement cause the center of humeral rotation to change nearly continuously during motion.

All of the preceding movements named for each of the shoulder regions contribute to the extraordinary range of motion of the upper extremity as well as add to the complexity of the joint. Just as muscular contraction generally occurs as a function of agonist/synergist groups, so does motion at all the shoulder region joints serve to position the glenoid fossa so that the humerus can be moved accurately through its full range of motion. The nature of the interaction of the shoulder joint is a study in mechanical and neuromuscular coordination. For example, consider the relationships between the shoulder region joints as the glenohumeral joint passes through a relatively simple motion such as abduction through 180° (Fig. 8–3).

For this movement to be possible, the gle-noid fossa must move from its natural position to one in which it is directed superiorly. This means it has rotated upwardly. The upward motion of the lateral end of the scapula at the acromioclavicular joint increases the amount of upward rotation but in itself represents scapular elevation. The elevation of the scapula must by accompanied by a movement of the inferior angle of the scapula away from the vertebral column, which represents abduction. The overall motion of the scapula is associated with sternoclavicular elevation.

Inman and associates[3] indicated the complexity of the clavicular motion that accompanies humeral and scapular actions. They demonstrated that the range of scapular motion on the thoracic wall is possible only because of the motion at the acromioclavicular and sternoclavicular joints. Elevation of the humerus, in the form of either abduction or flexion, creates approximately 4° of clavicular elevation at the sternoclavicular joint for every 10° of humeral motion during the first 90° of humeral motion (Fig. 8–4). Above 90°, the clavicular elevation is negligible. Motion at the acromioclavicular joint has a total range of approximately 20° and occurs in the first 30° and after 135° of humeral abduction. Between these points there is almost no motion. The sum of movement at the acromioclavicular and sternoclavicular joints is equal to the range of motion at the scapula. The clavicle was also shown to rotate about its long axis and represents a fundamental factor of shoulder mobility. Indeed, Inman et al. showed that when this clavicular rotation is precluded, the range of motion of the shoulder complex is restricted to 110°.

Hart and Carmichael[4] reported that the humerus provides 90° and 120° of elevation for active and passive humeral motion, respectively. After 30° of abduction and 60° of flexion it was indicated that the ratio of scapular upward rotation to humeral movement was 1°/2°. For every 15° of humeral elevation there are 5° of scapular upward rotation and 10° of glenohumeral joint action.

MUSCLES OF THE SHOULDER COMPLEX

It is reasonable to present the musculature associated with the shoulder complex in the

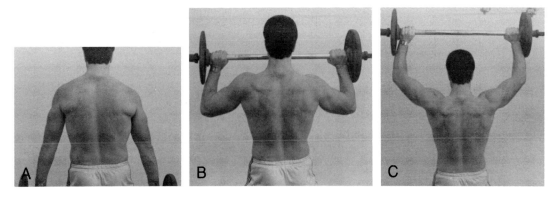

FIG. 8–3. Illustration of the mechanical and neuromuscular coordination of the components of the shoulder complex during a simple planar movement. *A*, Anatomic position. *B*, Midrange abduction. *C*, 120° abduction.

traditional fashion by dividing the region into the shoulder girdle and glenohumeral joint. It is critical to remember, however, the axiom that muscles rarely act individually, but rather in groups. Applying this notion to the shoulder, one can see the need for neuromuscular coordination between the two subregions that results in the complex mechanical behavior associated with positioning the humerus.

MUSCLES OF THE SHOULDER GIRDLE

Muscles of the shoulder girdle affect primarily the scapulae, causing rotations in the sagittal plane or frontal plane that, in turn, are associated with clavicular motion. These muscles are often divided into two groups, anterior and posterior, based on their locations with respect to the thorax.

Those muscles of the anterior group include the pectoralis minor muscle, subclavius muscle, and the serratus anterior muscle. The latter, by mass, actually falls more laterally and posteriorly (Fig. 8–5). The subclavius, a small muscle whose line of pull is predominantly along the axis of the clavicle, has been reported as serving primarily as a stabilizer for the sternoclavicular joint.[5] The Z and Y components of its pull may be considered negligible. The pectoralis minor muscle, inserting on the coracoid process, possesses a mostly Y-directed component, thereby serving predominantly to depress the scapula. Naturally, this depression is associated with some degree of downward rotation, but this rotation is due more to the mechanical axis about which the scapulae rotate (acromioclavicular joint) than to the tension generated by the muscle.

The serratus anterior muscle is a large muscle that can be separated functionally into at least two parts. Its function is related only to motion of the scapula. The superior portion of the muscle may passively support the scapula, elevate the scapula, and act as one part of a force couple (two parallel, oppositely directed, nonconcurrent forces that tend to cause rotation) in scapular rotation. The inferior portion of the muscle serves as part of the upward rotation force couple. During flexion of the humerus there is a greater anteriorly directed motion of the scapula on the thorax than during abduction of the humerus. As a result, the serratus anterior muscle plays a greater relative role in the movement than another member of the force couple, the trapezius.[6]

The muscles of the posterior shoulder girdle are the levator scapulae, rhomboid muscles, and trapezius muscle (Fig. 8–6). The levator scapulae and the rhomboid (major and minor) muscles are relatively simple muscles, creating tensions having X and Y components. These tensions serve to elevate and adduct the scapulae. The trapezius, however, spans a large area and has a complex origin and insertion. It is generally thought of as containing upper, middle, and lower portions. The trapezius plays a critical role in scapular positioning during flexion or abduction of the humerus.[6] Indeed, Yamshon and Bierman[7] reported on the significance of its

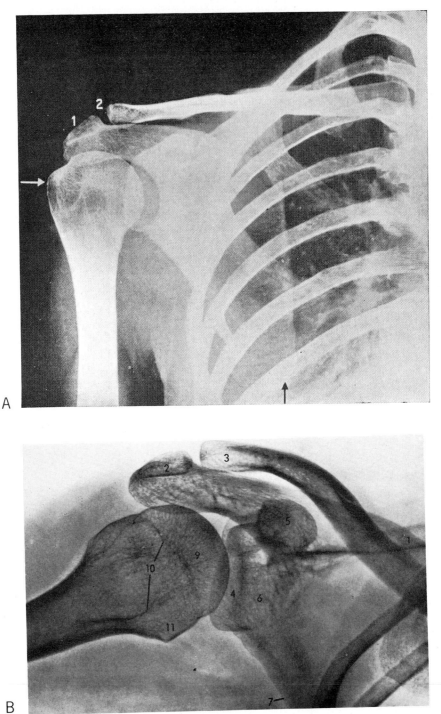

FIG. 8–4. *A* and *B*. Radiographs showing the shoulder complex as the glenohumeral joint is abducted and medially rotated. Note clavicular elevation. *1*, Spine of scapula; *2*, Acromion; *3*, Acromial end of clavicle; *4*, Glenoid cavity; *5*, Coracoid process; *6*, Neck of scapula; *7*, Lateral border of scapula; *9*, Head of humerus; *10*, Greater tubercle; *11*, Lesser tubercle. (From Gray's Anatomy. 30th Ed. Philadelphia, Lea & Febiger, 1985, pp. 234, 520.)

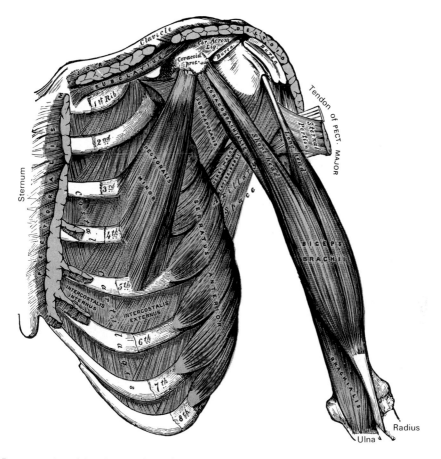

FIG. 8–5.   Deep muscles of the chest and anterior aspect of the arm, with the boundaries of the axilla. (From Gray's Anatomy. 30th Ed. Philadelphia, Lea & Febiger, 1985, p. 520.)

contribution in the first 90° of humeral elevation. Both range of motion and strength associated with the contraction of the trapezius are reduced by paralysis of this muscle.

MUSCLES OF THE GLENOHUMERAL JOINT

The musculature acting directly on the glenohumeral joint by virtue of humeral insertions may also be divided into anterior and posterior groups. The glenohumeral joint, demonstrating motion in three planes, is acted on by muscles that all possess some degree of X, Y, and Z force. These muscles play roles in both the motion and the protection of the glenohumeral joint.

Anteriorly, the superficial pectoralis major muscle, functionally separated into clavicular and sternal heads, is most visible topographically (Fig. 8–7). Both heads are active during horizontal flexion, though the clavicular head acts independently during glenohumeral joint flexion. During glenohumeral joint extension the sternal head is active. Initial glenohumeral position helps determine the flexion and extension roles of the two heads. Although the clavicular head is sometimes active during medial rotation[8] and the sternal head is active during adduction,[9] thereby making the muscle important in a broad spectrum of glenohumeral joint movement, surprisingly little disruption in everyday function is caused by radical mastectomy.[10] Other glenohumeral joint muscles adapt to the loss and provide stability. The anteriorly located coracobrachialis muscle, for example, too small to effectively substitute for the pectoralis major muscle in the role of movement, may supply a part of the required adduction stabilization force in the medial and inferior directions when the humerus is forced into abduction (Fig. 8–7).

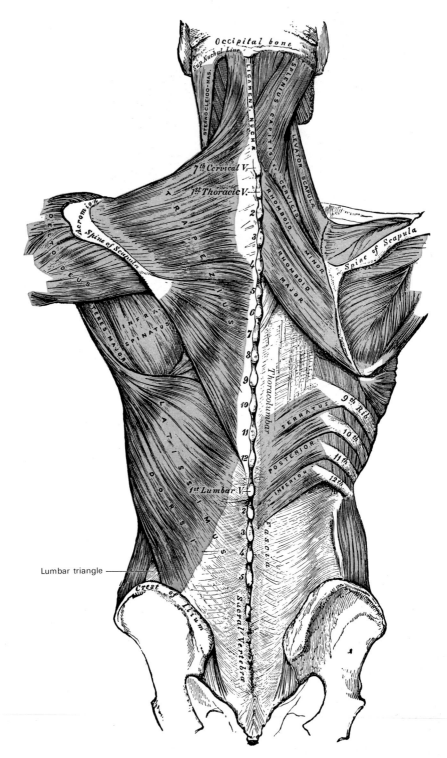

FIG. 8–6. Superficial and deep musculature of the posterior aspect of the trunk and shoulder complex. (From Gray's Anatomy. 30th Ed. Philadelphia, Lea & Febiger, 1985, p. 514.)

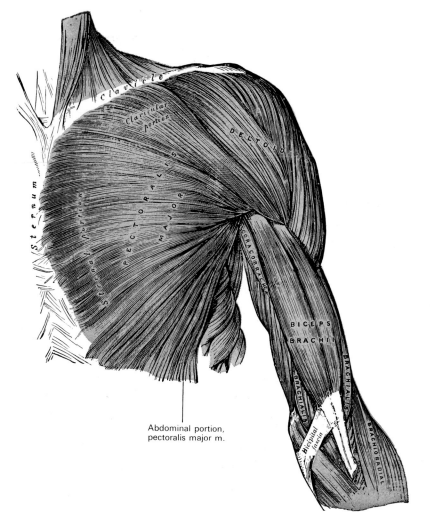

FIG. 8–7. Superficial muscles of the chest and anterior arm. (From Gray's Anatomy. 30th Ed. Philadelphia, Lea & Febiger, 1985, p. 519.)

The structurally complex deltoid, composed of anterior, middle, and posterior heads, becomes an accessory muscle with functional loss of the pectoralis major muscle. The three parts of the deltoid are active in nearly all humeral movement[7,9]; evidence suggests that the exceptions may be medial and lateral rotation.[6] All parts of the deltoid are important in adduction of the humerus. Inman et al. reported that the greatest [EMG] activity of the muscle was present between 90 and 180° of abduction or flexion, a relationship similar to that of supraspinatus muscle. This evidence may be interpreted as meaning that these muscles, contrary to previously held thought, do not act merely to initiate the movement of abduction.

The posteriorly located muscles of the glenohumeral joint include the latissimus dorsi, teres minor, infraspinatus, supraspinatus, and subscapularis muscles (Fig. 8–8). The latissimus dorsi and the teres major muscles have long been considered a functional pair, though the conditions under which the synergy occurs have often been unclear. Basmajian and De Luca[11] clarified the data, however. Essentially, teres major demonstrates no electrical activity, and therefore no active tension, when there is no resistance to movement. When resistance is encountered, however, this muscle will be electrically active whether the task is static or dynamic. The latissimus dorsi muscle is a very strong glenohumeral joint extensor and adductor as well as a "de-

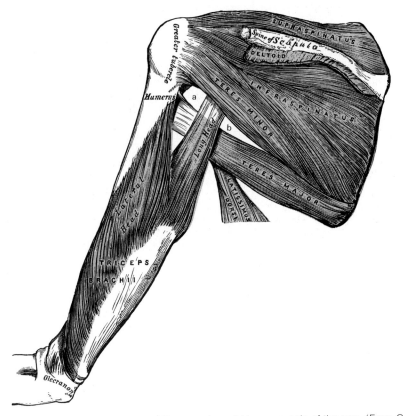

FIG. 8–8. Musculature on the posterior aspect of the scapula and triceps muscle of the arm. (From Gray's Anatomy. 30th Ed. Philadelphia, Lea & Febiger, 1985, p. 523.)

pressor'' of the humerus.[12] The supraspinatus muscle is also said to have as one of its major functions depression of the humeral head during glenohumeral elevation.

MECHANICAL CONSIDERATIONS OF INJURY TO THE SHOULDER COMPLEX

SHOULDER GIRDLE

The extreme range of motion of the shoulder complex, combined with the inherent instability of the region, makes it susceptible to a variety of injuries, ranging from mild to severe, that are common in the performance of everyday tasks as well as in athletic activities. Injuries associated with macrotrauma are those involving forces that exceed the mechanical properties of the tissues, whether bone, muscle, cartilage, tendon, etc.

The sternoclavicular joint, the only site of direct attachment of the upper extremity to the trunk, surprisingly does not have a very high rate of injury. The most common injury is sprain generated by a force that causes the shoulder to be displaced anteriorly. The medial end of the clavicle is forced medially, superiorly, and either anteriorly or posteriorly; either of the latter two movements places stress on the costoclavicular and sternoclavicular ligamentous. Rupture of these ligaments results in dislocation. In adults, dislocation and the ligamentous damage are said to be more probable than fracture of the clavicle; in preadolescents and adolescents, fracture is more likely, generally produced by a direct blow such as might be encountered in contact sports[13] (Fig. 8–9).

A common location of force resulting in injury to the acromioclavicular joint is the lateral margin of the acromion process, which displaces the acromion vertically downward while leaving the clavicle unmoved as it impinges on the first rib. A large percentage of acromiclavicular injuries, however, result

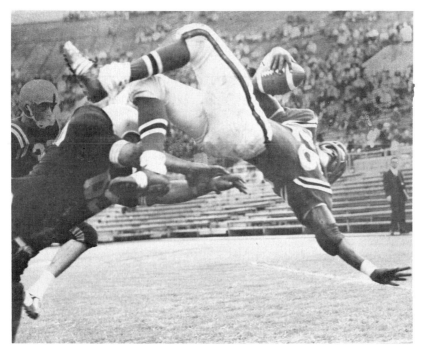

FIG. 8–9. Common mechanism of injury to the shoulder complex. The position has been suggested as being reflexive, due in part to labyrinthine and righting reflexes.[14] According to Smith and Stewart,[15] the acromion is driven inferiorly. The clavicle depresses only to the first rib, at which point either the acromioclavicular joint disrupts or the clavicle fractures. If fracture does not occur, the acromioclavicular ligaments are first stretched. Then, as the force continues, the coracoclavicular ligament is torn from the clavicle along with the muscle attachments of the deltoid and trapezius. Athletes term the resulting condition "knockdown shoulder."

from a fall on the outstretched arm being used to break a fall. On impact, the force is transmitted via the humeral shaft to the glenoid fossa and acromion process, which causes the entire scapula to be displaced with respect to the unmoved clavicle. These types of forces result in injury to the acromioclavicular and coracoclavicular ligaments (Figs. 8–10 and 8–11).

GLENOHUMERAL JOINT

The glenohumeral joint, like the shoulder girdle, is subject to injuries ranging from an annoying strain to dislocation and fracture. It has been reported that 20% of athletic injuries are associated with the glenohumeral joint, with wrestling, baseball, and other throwing events apparently having the greatest incidence.[16]

ROTATOR CUFF

The teres minor, infraspinatus, supraspinatus, and subscapularis muscles constitute a functional unit called the rotator cuff. In addition to creating a variety of torques about the glenohumeral joint, these muscles stabilize the joint, particularly against subluxation. The muscles strengthen the joint because of fibers that form part of the articular capsule. The weakest part of the capsule is said to be the inferior aspect, where reinforcement by rotator cuff muscles is minimal.

Saha[17] described dynamic stability of the glenohumeral joint as that required during movement, as opposed to static stability. The glenohumeral joint is most unstable anteriorly, to some degree inferiorly, and least of all posteriorly. Ovesen and Nielson[18] described the relative importance of the stabilizing structures that prevent anterior subluxation. Their focus was on the anterior aspect of the joint capsule and the subscapularis muscle. They reported that during the initial part of the range of motion for glenohumeral abduction, the subscapularis tendon and proximal third of the articular capsule limit external rotation. As abduction increases, the

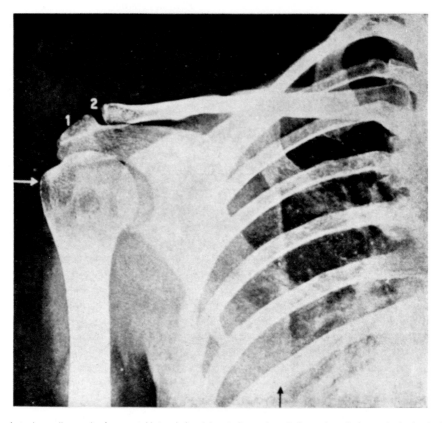

FIG. 8–10.   Anterior radiograph of a normal lateral shoulder girdle region. *1,* Acromion. *2,* Acromioclavicular joint. Lower arrow, inferior angle of scapula. Upper arrow, greater tuberosity. (Compare this picture to Figure 8–11.)

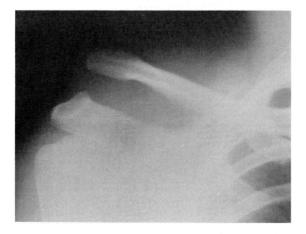

FIG. 8–11.   Example of type III disruption of the acromioclavicular and coracoclavicular ligaments and tearing of the deltoid and trapezius muscle attachments in a 19-year-old college football player. (Compare Fig. 8–10.) These injuries can be repaired. This player injured his right shoulder in his sophomore year and his left shoulder in his junior year. Both were repaired by the Stewart technique, and the player was selected in his senior year as the outstanding defensive back in the nation. (Courtesy Michale J. Smith, M.D., Marcus J. Stewart, M.D., and *Am. J. Sports Med.*)

distal portion of the capsule becomes the predominant limiter of external rotation.

Dynamic stability was reported to be dependent on the anthropometric development of the glenoid fossa, the tilt of the glenoid fossa, the angle of the head and neck of the humerus, and the strength of the rotator cuff. The glenohumeral joint's agonists are dependent on the help of the cuff muscles to position the humeral head with respect to the glenoid fossa so as to effect a full range of motion, as described earlier.[19]

The tilt of the glenoid fossa has also been attributed to the stability of the glenohumeral joint against inferior subluxation.[20] It was reported that, contrary to expectation, the vertically oriented muscles of the glenohumeral joint such as the deltoid and coracobrachialis muscles do not provide tension that protects the joint against downward pulls such as the one executed by one of the judo players in Figure 6–14. Rather, because of the horizontal and vertical components of the angle of the glenoid fossa, the humeral head moves laterally as it is forced inferiorly. The lateral movement stretches the supraspinatus muscle, and its activity, serving to stabilize the glenohumeral joint horizontally, also serves to prevent the inferiorly directed movement.

During everyday movement, the muscles of the rotator cuff are susceptible to repeated microtrauma (submaximal trauma) that may result in structural damage. Many times the source of damage is impingement against the coracoacromial arch when the glenohumeral joint is abducted or flexed. Indeed, impingement syndrome, which is not limited to ro-

tator cuff problems but includes bursitis and bicipital tendinitis, is the most common shoulder problem in sports medicine.[21] The problem is not, by any means, limited to athletics. Rotator cuff problems, for example, afflict more than 15% of the general population 40 to 50 years of age. In industrial workers, however, generalized pain in the shoulder region has been reported as having a prevalence of 30 to 40%.[22] Activities that involve heavy static loading of the shoulder complex muscles in conjunction with awkward positions have been related to this occupational cervicobrachial disorder. Clearly, any number of

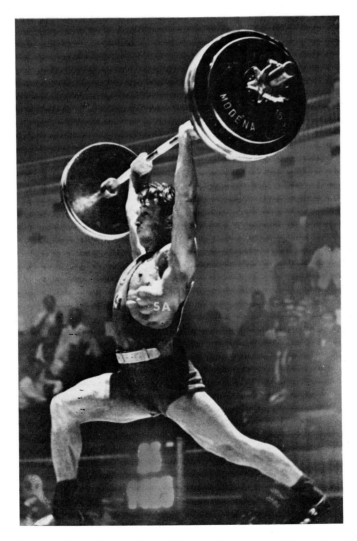

FIG. 8–12. Example of heavy static loading conditions of the shoulder complex that could lead to shoulder disorders. Pictured is Minaev, of the U.S.S.R., jerking 314 lb in winning the 132-lb weight-lifting title in the 1960 Olympic Games. This is an exceptionally fine photograph of the serratus anterior in action. (Kirkley, courtesy Iron Man.)

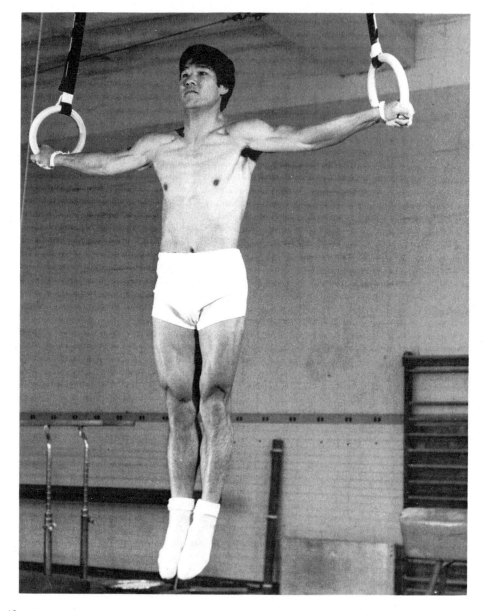

FIG. 8–13.   The iron cross being performed on the still rings. Shoulder girdle and shoulder joint muscles must contract intensively through their small moment arms to balance the torque generated by the mass of the body acting through the moment arm of the abducted upper extremities. The magnitude of the contractions and the various directions with which they act place great stress on the shoulder complex.

Sternal extremity   *Acromial extremity*

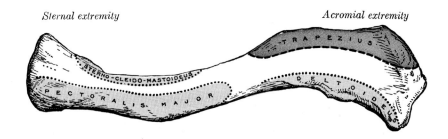

FIG. 8–14.   Left clavicle. Superior surface.

athletic events can be seen to fall within this description (Fig. 8–12).

Basically, impingement results because of the limited space below the coracoacromial arch for passage of certain parts of the rotator cuff. The impingment may be that of the supraspinatus or bicipital tendons. In the painful arc syndrome, the greater tubercle impinges against the coracoacromial arch. Impingement can be produced if the volume of the musculature is increased by either hypertrophy or edema resulting from injury (usually a time-dependent process associated with repeated microtrauma), and if the available space is decreased by bone growth that impinges on the tissue.[23]

Throwing is often associated with rotator cuff problems. Assessing the sequence of windup, propulsion, and follow-through, one can qualitatively identify the stresses placed on the cuff.[19] At the completion of the windup phase, at which time the glenohumeral joint is extended, abducted, and externally rotated, the anterior rotator cuff is most stressed. An intermediate phase, called the drag phase, is the period in which the direction of the motion is reversed by elastic recoil and by the forcible contraction of the interior

shoulder muscles, which increases the stress on the cuff. During the propulsive phase the glenohumeral joint may be found to go through 120° of medial rotation. At the latter stages of propulsion and during the follow-through it is the posterior aspect of the cuff that undergoes the most stress.

Consider the freestyle swimmer, who may abduct each shoulder up to 7200 times during a practice session, or the gymnast maintaining an iron cross on the still rings (Fig. 8–13), or the weight lifter, required to maintain an athlete-specific near-maximal weight in the overhead position during competition as opposed to repeating submaximal efforts during practice. In all of these cases, microtrauma to the cuff can result in inflammation that then may lead to edema, further impingement, and further microtrauma.

NEURAL INNERVATIONS

SHOULDER GIRDLE MUSCULATURE

trapezius: the spinal accessory nerve (spinal portion of CN XI) and branches from the anterior rami of C3 and C4.

levator scapulae: the cervical plexus sup-

Articular capsule   *Articular capsule*

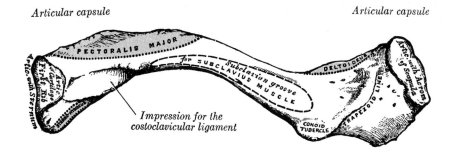

Impression for the costoclavicular ligament

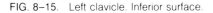

FIG. 8–15.   Left clavicle. Inferior surface.

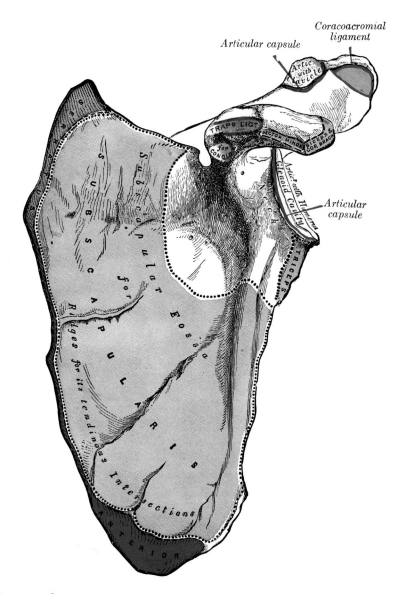

FIG. 8–16. Left scapula. Costal surface.

plying branches from C3 and C4 and the dorsal scapular nerve with fibers from C5.

rhomboid: the dorsal scapular nerve from the brachial plexus. The fibers come from C5.

serratus anterior: the long thoracic nerve from the anterior branches of C5, C6, and C7 before they enter the cervical plexus.

pectoralis minor: the medial anterior thoracic nerve originating in the brachial plexus. The fibers are from C8 and T1.

subclavius: from the brachial plexus, the fi-

bers of the nerve coming from C5 and C6.

SHOULDER JOINT

deltoid: the axillary nerve from the brachial plexus. The fibers are from C5 and C6.

supraspinatus: a branch of the suprascapular nerve from the brachial plexus. The fibers are from C5.

pectoralis major: the musculocutaneous nerve with fibers coming from C6 and C7.

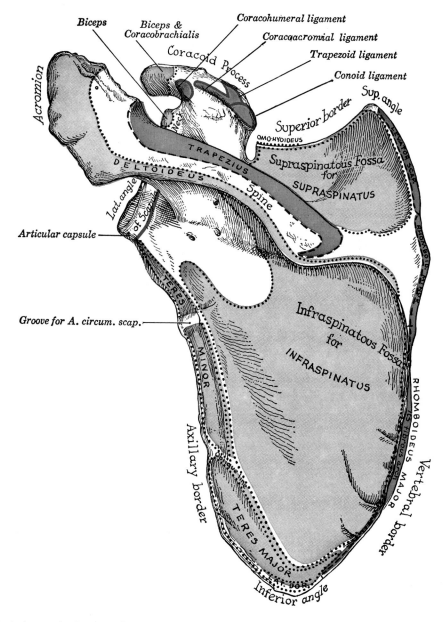

FIG. 8–17. Left scapula. Dorsal surface.

coracobrachialis: the musculocutaneous nerve with fibers from C6 and C7.

latissimus dorsi: the thoracodorsal nerve from the brachial plexus. The fibers come from C6, C7, and C8.

teres major: the lower subscapular nerve from the brachial plexus. Fibers come from C5 and C6.

infraspinatus: the subscapular nerve from the brachial plexus with fibers coming from C5 and C6.

teres minor: the axillary nerve with fibers coming from C5.

subscapularis: the subscapular nerves from the posterior cord of the brachial plexus.

STUDY QUESTIONS

1. Using Figs. 8–14, 8–15, 8–16 and 8–17 generate a list of origins for the shoulder complex muscles. Use the illustrations of the humerus at the end of Chapter 9 for insertions. For muscles originating on the posterior aspect of the thorax, sternum, and ribs, use Gray's Anatomy or some other text and compare your estimated origins and insertions with those provided. Where necessary, make adjustments to your responses.

2. Describe the differences in the motion at the shoulder complex produced by performing, both with the hands close together and with them wide apart, the following exercises: the bench press, the military press, and chin-ups.

3. Compare and contrast the major musculature that would contribute to performance in the above exercises.

4. What is the mechanism by which the latissimus dorsi muscle can serve as a humeral depressor (not the return movement from humeral elevation), an action that essentially remains undefined with respect to a plane and axis.

5. Justify the use by an archer of muscular endurance training that would specifically affect the anterior serratus to supplement shoulder girdle abduction.

6. Bull, de Freitas and Vitti[24] reported activity of the superior part of the trapezius muscle and levator scapulae during circumduction of the glenohumeral joint and pendular oscillation of the upper extremity. Present an explanation for these findings.

7. Via palpation, determine the approximate range of glenohumeral positions in which the clavicular and sternal heads play a role in flexion and extension, respectively. Explain the findings and make some practical applications.

REFERENCES

1. Matsen, F.A.: Biomechanics of the shoulder. *In* Basic Biomechanics of the Skeletal System. Edited by V.H. Frankel and M. Nordin. Philadelphia, Lea & Febiger, 1980.
2. Poppen, N., and Walker, P.: Normal and abnormal motion of the shoulder. J. Bone Joint Surg., *58-A*:195, 1978.
3. Inman, V.T., Saunders, J.B., and Abbott, L.C.: Observations on the function of the shoulder joint. J. Bone Joint Surg., *26*:1, 1944.
4. Hart, D., and Carmichael, S.: Biomechanics of the shoulder. J. Orthop. Sports Phys. Ther., *6*:229, 1985.
5. Reis, F.P., deCarmargo, A.M., Vitti, M., and de-Carvalho, C.A.F.: Electromyographic study of the subclavius muscle. Acta Anat., *105*:284, 1979.
6. Basmajian, J.V., and Deluca, C.J.: Muscles Alive. 5th Ed. Baltimore, Williams & Wilkins, 1985.
7. Yamshon, L.J., and Bierman, W.: Kinesiologic electromyography: the trapezius. Arch. Phys. Med., *29*:647, 1948.
8. deSousa, O.M., Berzin, F., and Berardi, A.C.: Electromyographic study of the pectoralis major and latissimus dorsi muscles during medial rotation of the arm. Electromyogr. Clin. Neurophysiol., *9*:407, 1959.
9. Scheving, L.E., and Pauly, J.E.: An electromyographic study of some of the muscles acting upon the upper extremity of man. Anat. Rec., *135*:239, 1959.
10. Flint, M.M., Drinkwater, B.L., and McKittrock, J.E.: Shoulder dynamics subsequent to radical mastectomy. EMG, *10*:171, 1970.
11. Basmajian, J.V., and DeLuca, C.J.: Muscles Alive. 5th Ed. Baltimore, Williams & Wilkins, 1985, pp. 220–221.
12. Jonsson, B., Olafsson, B.M., and Steffer, L.C.: Function of the teres major, latissimus dorsi, and pectoralis major muscles: a preliminary study. Acta Morphol. Scand., *9*:275, 1972.
13. O'Donoghue, D.H.: Treatment of Injuries to Athletes. Philadelphia, W.B. Saunders, 1976.
14. Carlsoo, S., and Johannson, O.: Stabilization of and load on the elbow joint in some protective movements. Acta Anat., *48*:224, 1962.
15. Smith, M., and Stewart, M.J.: Acute acromioclavicular separation. Am. J. Sports Med., *7*:62, 1979.

16. Nelson, C.L., et al.: Athletic injuries of the shoulder. Cleve. Clin. Q., *40*:27, 1973.
17. Saha, A.K.: Dynamic stability of the glenohumeral joint. Acta Orthop. Scand., *42*:491, 1971.
18. Ovesen, J., and Nielson, S.: Stability of the shoulder joint, cadaver study of stabilizing structures. Acta Orthop. Scand., *56*:149, 1985.
19. Penny, J.N., and Welsh, P.P.: Shoulder impingement syndromes in athletes and their surgical management. Am. J. Sports Med., *9*:11, 1981.
20. Basmajian, J.V., and Bazant, F.J.: Factors preventing downward dislocation of the shoulder joint: an electromyographic and morphological study. J. Bone Joint Surg., *41-A*:1182, 1959.
21. Jobe, F., and Jobe, C.: Painful athletic injuries of the shoulder. Clin. Orthop., *173*:117, 1983.
22. Herberts, P., Kadefors, R., Hogfors, C., and Sigholm, G.: Shoulder pain and heavy manual labor. Clin. Orthop., *191*:166, 1984.
23. Neer, C.S.: Anterior acromioplasty for the chronic impingement syndrome in the shoulder, a preliminary report. J. Bone Joint Surg., *54A*:41, 1972.
24. Bull, M.L., de Freitas, V., and Vitti, M.: Electromyographic study of the trapezius (pars superior) and the levator scapulae muscles in circumduction and pendular oscillation of the arm. Electromyogr. Clin. Neurophysiol., *24*:511, 1984.

9 THE ELBOW AND RADIOULNAR JOINTS

MARK D. GRABINER

ANATOMIC CONSIDERATIONS

In keeping with the ultimate purpose of the linkages constituting the upper extremity, that is, to allow positioning of the hands and fingers, the purpose of the elbow joint is to allow positioning of the wrist.[1] Though the elbow is typically classified as a diarthritic hinge joint, it is actually three joints enclosed in a common articular capsule: the humeroulnar joint, between the trochlear notch of the ulna and the trochlea of the humerus; the humeroradial joint, between the proximal surface of the radial head and the capitulum of the humerus; and the proximal radioulnar joint, formed by the radial head and the radial notch of the ulna. The elbow joint is stable because of the influence of both a strong bony architecture and a network of ligamentous tissue surrounding the joint.

The articular capsule completely covers the joint surfaces and includes the radial (lateral) collateral and ulnar (medial) collateral ligaments, which are thickened portions of the capsule proper. The radial collateral ligament crosses the elbow joint from its proximal attachment just distal to the lateral epicondyle of the humerus to its distal attachment at the annular ligament. The annular ligament serves to maintain the integrity of the proximal radioulnar joint. It holds the head of the radius in contact with the radial notch of the ulna. Were it not for the presence of this ligament, contraction of the biceps muscle of the arm would disarticulate this joint.[2] The ulnar collateral ligament consists of three portions that form a triangularly shaped band. The an-

terior portion runs from the medial epicondyle to the coronoid process; the posterior portion also attaches on the medial epicondyle but runs to the olecranon of the ulna. The transverse band connects the olecranon part of the posterior portion to the coronoid part of the anterior portion (Figs. 9–1 and 9–2).

The medial radioulnar joint is a ligamentous synarthrosis formed by the interosseous membrane holding together the shafts of the radius and ulna. The direction of the fibrous tissue is generally oblique. The oblique cord, the second ligament associated with the medial radioulnar joint and absent in some individuals, is a small, flat band that runs from the lateral aspect of the coronoid process to the radius.

The distal radioulnar joint is a diarthritic pivot joint between the head of the ulna and the ulnar notch. An articular capsule surrounds the joint and provides stability. Primarily, however, an articular disk, beneath the head of the ulna, holds the distal ends of the ulna and radius together (Fig. 9–3).

JOINT MOVEMENTS

The flexion and extension generally associated with the elbow joint occurs at the humeroulnar and humeroradial joints. The long axis of the ulna is not aligned with that of the forearm; that is, the forearm is directed somewhat laterally from the humeral axis, the deviation being known as the carrying angle. The carrying angle is usually 10 to 15° in males

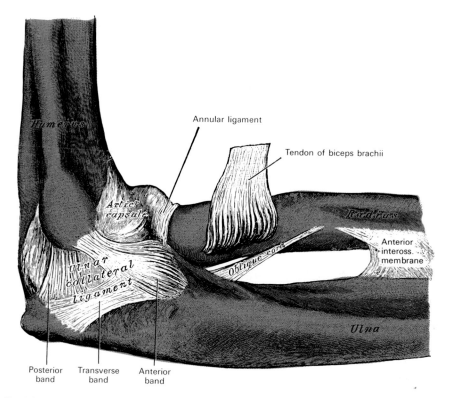

FIG. 9–1. The left elbow joint. Medial aspect. (From Gray's Anatomy. 30th Ed. Philadelphia, Lea & Febiger. 1985, p. 377.)

and 20 to 25° in females. The trochlea, being eccentrically shaped, has been reported to change the carrying angle during elbow flexion so that the misalignment between arm and forearm decreases.[3] The range of motion of flexion and extension is dictated primarily by the joint architecture and is approximately 140°.

When the radioulnar joints allow rotation of the forearm about its long axis, the radius pivots about the ulna. The movements of pronation (palm up to palm down) and supination (palm down to palm up) occur at the proximal radioulnar joint as the head of the radius moves about the ulna within the annular ligament (Figs. 9–3 and 9–4).

At the distal radioulnar joint, the end of the radius rotates about the head of the ulna. The range of motion for supination and pronation has been reported as 120 to 140°.[4]

MUSCLES OF THE ELBOW JOINT

FLEXORS

The biceps brachii, brachialis muscle, and brachioradialis muscle serve as the primary elbow flexor group (Figs. 9–5 and 9–6). They may be assisted in this function by other muscles that have a line of pull that falls anteriorly to the elbow axis of rotation. Such an example is the pronator teres muscle. Basmajian and DeLuca suggested that this muscle assists in elbow flexion only when the movement is resisted.[5] More recently, however, the pronator teres muscle has been shown to be active in elbow flexion much in the same pattern as the biceps brachii and brachioradialis muscle.[1] Basmajian and DeLuca[7] indicated that in the case of the major flexor group, the integrated action during voluntary motion has not been well-documented. For example, they found in an electromyographic investigation[8] that there was no predictable pattern of activation of these muscles; that is, which was the first, second, or third muscle to become active. Grabiner et al.[9] reported that the activity profiles of the biceps brachii and the brachioradialis muscle are different during isometric contraction.

Although activation levels remain the

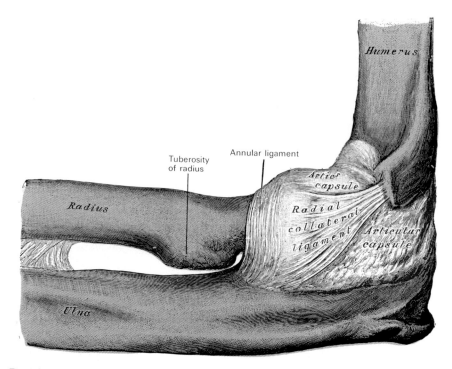

FIG. 9–2.   The left elbow joint. Lateral aspect. (From Gray's Anatomy. 30th Ed. Philadelphia. Lea & Febiger. 1985. p. 377.)

same, the biceps contributes less torque to elbow flexion when the radioulnar joints are pronated. The underlying mechanism is the radius' rotation around the ulna during pronation, which brings the insertion of the biceps closer to the axis of rotation. Indeed, as the radioulnar joints move from a supinated position to a pronated position, the moment arm of the biceps decreases from 1.964 cm to 1.271 cm, a decrease of 35%.[10] Muscular torque, being a multiplicative function of both tension (force) and moment arm, is similarly decreased.

The brachialis muscle has been referred to as a flexor par excellence of the elbow joint[11] and the workhorse among the elbow flexors.[7] Because it inserts on the ulna, its moment arm is not subject to changes during supination and pronation. It is active during all elbow flexions.[8]

The brachioradialis muscle is presently thought of as an accessory agonist whose contributions to elbow flexion are required during large flexion accelerations. This idea is fairly consistent with the spurt-shunt theory of MacConaill,[12,13] which predicted this role

based on the relationship of centripetal and centrifugal force to changes in angular velocity. The brachioradialis' supination and pronation roles[14] have been essentially dismissed, with the exception of resisted motion.

EXTENSORS

Only two muscles extend the elbow, the triceps brachii and the anconeus (Fig. 9–7). The medial and lateral heads of the triceps act only at the elbow joint. The long head, however, originating on the scapula at the inferior margin of the glenoid fossa, has an effect at both the glenohumeral joint and the shoulder girdle. The contribution of the long head to unresisted elbow extension is negligible.[13] This apparent control exerted by the central nervous system might be explained by the need to stabilize the scapula and humerus against the potential effects of the long head on those structures causing a decrease in the efficiency of movement (see Chapter 12). The long head is recruited against resistance. The lateral head, whose activity against unloaded movement is slightly greater than that of the long head, is also called upon to a greater

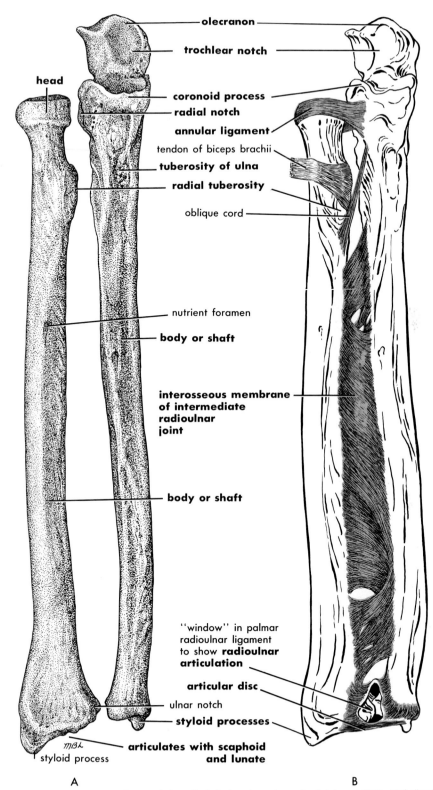

olecranon

trochlear notch

head

coronoid process

radial notch

annular ligament

tendon of biceps brachii

tuberosity of ulna

radial tuberosity

oblique cord

nutrient foramen

body or shaft

**interosseous membrane
of intermediate
radioulnar
joint**

body or shaft

''window'' in palmar
radioulnar ligament
to show **radioulnar
articulation**

articular disc

ulnar notch

styloid processes

**articulates with scaphoid
and lunate**

mβλ

styloid process

A   B

FIG. 9–3.   *A*, Anterior view of right radius and ulna. *B*, Anterior view of proximal, intermediate, and distal radioulnar articulations. (From Crouch, J.E.: Functional Human Anatomy. 4th Ed. Philadelphia, Lea & Febiger, 1985, p. 150.)

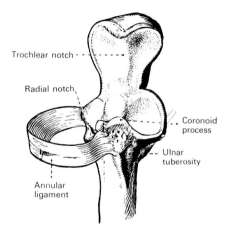

FIG. 9–4.   Proximal part of the ulna with the annular ligament of the proximal radioulnar joint. (From Gray's Anatomy. 30th Ed. Philadelphia, Lea & Febiger, 1985, p. 380.)

extent during resisted motion. The medial head has been identified as the prime agonist for elbow extension.

The anconeus muscle has been reported as always being active during active elbow extension.[16] This observation was later verified by Basmajian and DeLuca.[17] LeBozec, Maton, and Cnockaert[18] reported that the anconeus is quite active during slow movements; this may be another example of how the central nervous system systematically recruits entire muscles in an effort to influence efficiency.

MUSCLES OF THE RADIOULNAR JOINTS

PRONATORS

The two pronator muscles, the proximally located pronator teres and the distally located pronator quadratus, historically have provided confusing information (Fig. 9–8). Most authors prior to 1960 suggested that the pronation contributions by these muscles were equivalent and that the pronator teres would provide a maximum output with the elbow flexed through half of its range of motion. Basmajian and DeLuca[7] state categorically that elbow position has no effect on the activity of the pronator teres muscle. Addition-

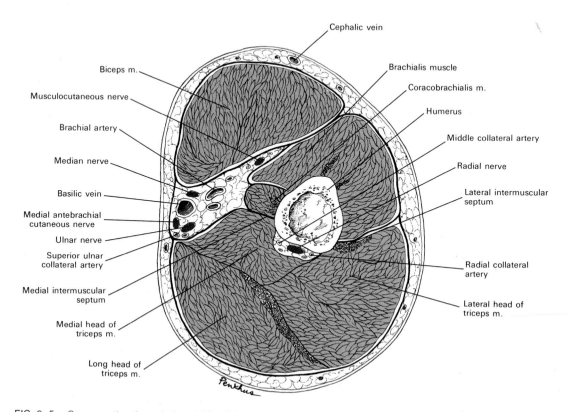

FIG. 9–5.   Cross section through the middle of the right arm. Viewed from the superior aspect. (From Gray's Anatomy. 30th Ed. Philadelphia, Lea & Febiger, 1985, p. 526.)

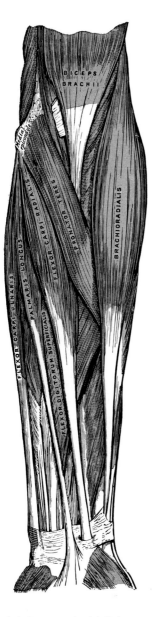

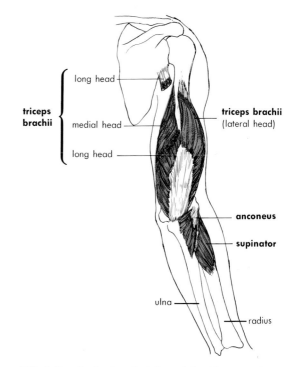

FIG. 9–7. Anatomic orientation of the triceps and anconeus muscles viewing the arm and forearm posteriorly. (From Crouch, J.E.: Functional Human Anatomy. 4th Ed. Philadelphia, Lea & Febiger, 1985, p. 230.)

tion of the elbow joint or the speed of movement. The biceps brachii is an assistant in supination when the elbow is flexed and the unresisted movement is fast, and in all resisted movements, regardless of elbow position.[16]

SPURT AND SHUNT MUSCLES

The concept of spurt and shunt muscles[12,13] was developed using the elbow joint and, although it has been the source of much debate,[20,21] is a good example of the interface between classical anatomic kinesiology and biomechanics. A spurt muscle, by definition, is one that possesses a line of pull across a joint such that it favors rotary force or torque. A shunt muscle, on the other hand, has a line of pull that is oriented predominantly along the long axis of a bone. The tension created by a shunt muscle, therefore, will be translated mostly into a joint stabilization force (Fig. 9–9). Naturally, the magnitude of the rotary and stabilizing components are changed as a joint moves through a range of

FIG. 9–6. Anterior aspect of left forearm. Superficial muscles. (From Gray's Anatomy. 30th Ed. Philadelphia, Lea & Febiger, 1985, p. 531.)

ally, although both muscles are recruited during fast or slow pronation, it is the pronator quadratus that is more consistently active.

SUPINATORS

Only two muscles may be consistently identified as radioulnar supinators. Of foremost importance is the supinator. It appears that the supinator independently initiates and controls supination, irrespective of the posi-

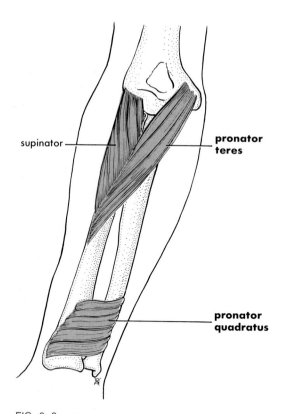

supinator

pronator teres

pronator quadratus

FIG. 9–8.   Pronator and supinator muscles of the right forearm. (From Crouch, J.E.: Functional Human Anatomy. 4th Ed. Philadelphia, Lea & Febiger, 1985, p. 233.)

motion. For example, although it is the classic spurt muscle, when extended the elbow theoretically causes the biceps to have a line of pull favoring joint stabilization.

Consider the elbow joint as it is flexed under the influence of the elbow flexors. Although the angular speed of flexion may remain constant, the direction of movement changes at every instant. These instantaneous changes in direction in actuality represent an acceleration caused by an unbalanced net resultant force directed toward the axis of rotation, a centripetal force. The magnitude of the centripetal force is calculated as any other force, $F = ma$. The acceleration, a, is the magnitude of the centripetal acceleration, given by v^2/r where v is the magnitude of the linear velocity of the center of gravity of the forearm. The distance of the center of gravity of the forearm to the elbow joint is the radius, r. If the mass and moment of inertia of the forearm is known, the centripetal force $F_c = mv^2/r$.

The linear velocity of the forearm may be expressed as the angular velocity, ω, multiplied by the radius of rotation, r. The equation then becomes $F_c = m(\omega r)^2/r$, which reduces to $m\omega^2 r$. It is clear, then, that as angular velocity increases, the requirement for centripetal force increases as a function of the square of angular velocity.

Centrifugal acceleration, that which acts away from the axis of rotation, exists contemporaneously with centripetal acceleration and is of equal magnitude but, as indicated, of opposite direction. It is associated with the tendency for the joint to become disarticulated by flying off at a tangent to the rotation, which it would do if not restrained by the centripetal force. The question MacConaill sought to answer was related to the source of the centripetal force's resistance to joint dislocation. Because of its anatomic location, a muscle such as the brachioradialis was thought of as a shunt muscle that was predisposed mechanically to create joint stabilizing force. It is logical that the spurt muscle itself cannot create enough centripetal force, because its primary responsibility is creating the force that can result in angular acceleration of the limb. If, for example, the biceps brachii were to have an angle of pull of 45°, which equalizes its rotary and stabilizing components of force, then the centripetal force required, based on a given mass, moment inertia, and flexion velocity about the elbow, could be estimated to require approximately 70 times that which is generated.

Electromyographic investigations[17] have lent support to the spurt-shunt concept. It was reported that the brachioradialis muscle was relatively quiet during slow elbow flexion both with and without resistance to movement, as well as during isometric contraction. During quick flexion, however, the brachioradialis was quite active, thereby elucidating the importance of angular velocity to the recruitment of shunt muscles. Stern,[21] however, demonstrated via mathematical modeling of the contractile characteristics of muscle and electromyography that spurt-shunt concepts are perhaps less than feasible. In fact, he demonstrated that the osseoligamentous structures at the elbow are strong enough to withstand up to 43 lb of disarticulating force without assistance from shunt muscles. Sur-

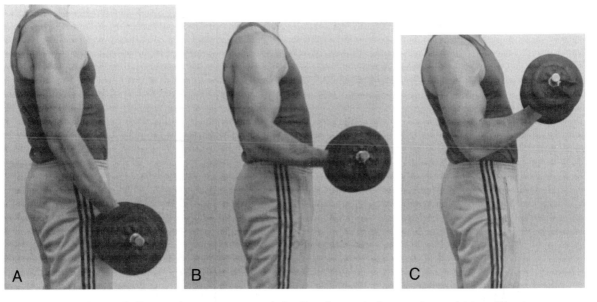

FIG. 9–9.   *A, B,* and *C,* Changes in moment arms and direction of muscular force vectors as joint position changes.

prisingly, he calculated that during a movement that could require shunt force, the biceps brachii provides more shunt force than
the brachioradialis muscle.

MECHANICAL CONSIDERATIONS OF INJURY TO THE ELBOW

Although the elbow is architecturally a stable joint and is supported ligamentously, injuries to it are common because of the magnitudes of the forces imposed on the elbow
joint in everyday living skills and tasks, not
to mention in a variety of athletic skills (Fig.
9–10). Although the elbow is difficult to
sprain (i.e., incur injury to a ligament) by flexion, hyperextension is often a cause of damage. During hyperextension of the elbow the
olecranon process impinges on the olecranon
fossa. Continued extension torque, if of sufficient magnitude, will cause the coronoid
process to be displaced posteriorly with respect to the trochlea. In this case, the resultant
sprain is to the anterior aspect of the collateral
ligament, generally the medial collateral ligament. If a hyperextension torque is continued beyond this point, the displacement of
the coronoid process may be large enough to
cause the distal end of the humerus to slide
over it until it is buttressed against the shaft
of the ulna, producing an elbow dislocation.

Concomitant to elbow dislocation is the rupture of the collateral ligaments.

Injuries do not have to occur as a function
of a macrotrauma. Indeed, many injuries occur over time as a result of repeated submaximal stress (microtrauma). Tennis elbow is a
condition similar to a lower leg (shank) afflic-
tion called shin splints. Both merely reflect
the area of injury rather than implying any
cause. Gruchow and Pelletier[22] indicate that
nearly half of all tennis players suffer from
tennis elbow at one time or another. Although
its cause is uncertain, factors such as age,
playing experience, playing time, ability, and
racket type have been clinically suggested as
possibilities. Some sports physicians believe
it occurs largely in players striving for an extremely hard serve and in those with a faulty
backhand. Grabiner et al.[23] suggest a possible
relation to overgripping. Nirchl and
Pettrone[24] suggest a mechanism related to the
overuse, damage, and incomplete or inappropriate healing of the origin of the short
radial extensor muscle of the wrist.
O'Donoghue[25] indicates that at least four conditions falling under the umbrella term tennis
elbow have, at least, a similar related cause—
an overuse syndrome that involves the gripping muscles coupled with ulnar and radial
flexion of the wrist. The discomfort or pain
associated with tennis elbow generally occurs

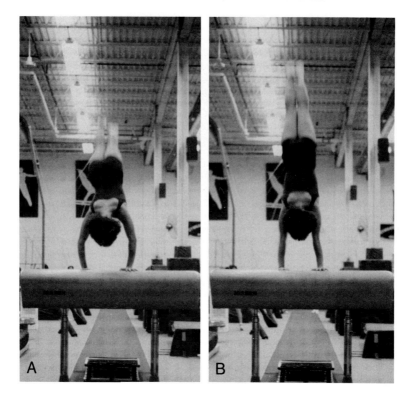

FIG. 9–10. *A* and *B*, Illustration of extreme forces applied to the elbow joint that affect different anatomic structures in disparate fashion. Note the tendency of the elbow to hyperextend in the latter part of the vault.

laterally and is magnified during gripping tasks and radioulnar pronation and supination. The four generalized conditions include epicondylitis of the supinator aponeurosis at the lateral epicondyle, radioulnar synovitis, strain of the aponeurosis, and radioulnar bursitis.

Treatments that have been suggested include changing the flexibility and the string tension of the racket, changing the stroke mechanics, and increasing the strength of the forearm muscles. Burton[23] demonstrated that both elastic and inelastic straps worn around the forearm increase pain-free grip strength in subjects suffering from tennis elbow. The straps had no such effect on healthy subjects, and their benefit as a treatment for tennis elbow rather than merely as a pain reliever has yet to be demonstrated.

Golfer's elbow usually refers to trauma about the medial epicondyle and often seems to involve the ulnar flexor muscle of the wrist (see Chapter 10). Medial epicondylitis is often called little leaguer's elbow and includes a number of symptoms. Medial loading of the elbow during pitching is often viewed as a primary cause. The loading occurs, in part, during the transition from the wind-up phase to the delivery phase, during which the shoulder joint may be observed to be maximally externally rotated.[27,28] In professional pitchers, reported problems at the elbow include muscle rupture, ligament sprain and rupture, ulnar traction spurs both with and without ulnar nerve involvement, loose bodies within the olecranon fossa and lateral compartment, and degenerative arthritis.[29] In children the most common injury to the pitching arm appears to be the medial epicondyle avulsion fracture. The medial epicondyle is a site of origin for the elbow flexor and pronator muscles, which undergoes stress during throwing. The avulsion fracture has been reported to be a function primarily of the forceful wrist flexion during the terminal stages of pitching rather than the valgus elbow stresses, which should be related intuitively.[29]

Larson has defined little leaguer's elbow as fragmentation, irregularity, mild separation, and enlargement or breaking of the medial

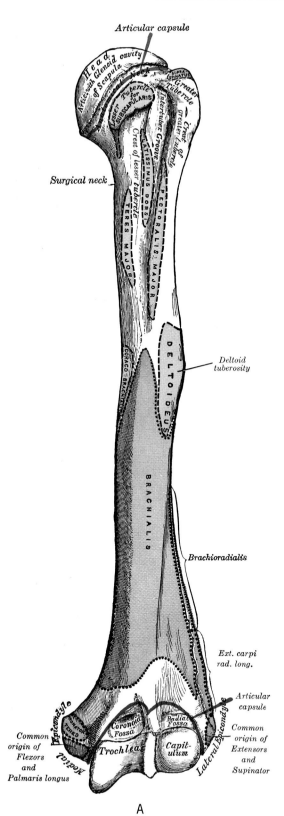

FIG. 9–11 *A,* Left humerus. Anterior view.

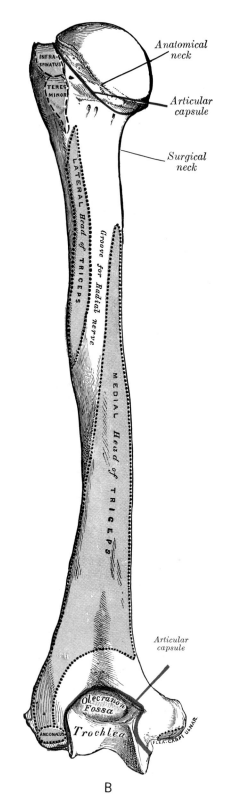

B

FIG. 9–11.   *B*, Left humerus. Posterior view.

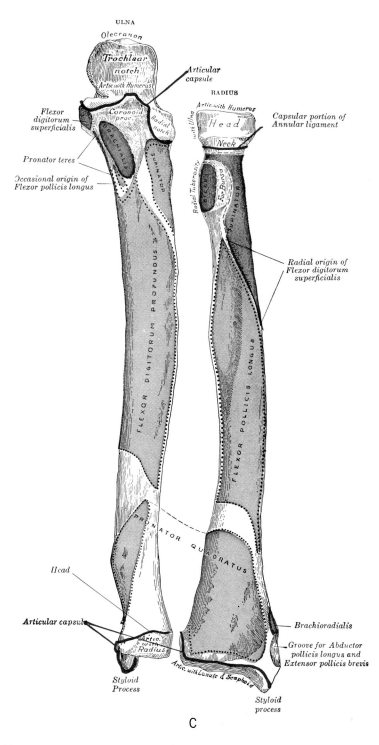

FIG. 9–11.   *C*, Left ulna and radius. Anterior aspect.

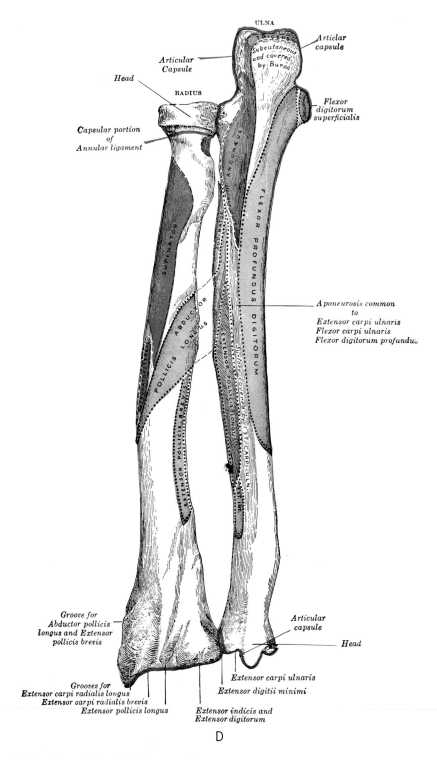

FIG. 9–11.   *D*, Left radius and ulna. Posterior aspect.

epicondyle of the elbow. These are merely various stages of the same reactive process that develops from stress. Lesions, seen on the lateral side of the elbow with much less frequency, are the result of compressive forces. While they are rare, they may be much more serious and may be indicative of osteochondritis dissecans, avulsion fracture, or osteochondritis of the radial head.[30]

NEURAL INNERVATIONS

biceps brachii: the musculocutaneous nerve from the brachial plexus. Fibers come from C5 and C6.

brachialis: primarily from the musculocutaneous nerve from the brachial plexus. The fibers come from C5 and C6. Sometimes present are branches from the radial and median nerves.

brachioradialis: a branch of the radial nerve from the brachial plexus. The fibers are from C5 and C6.

pronator teres: a branch of the median nerve containing fibers from C5 and C6.

triceps brachii: the radial nerve from the brachial plexus with fibers from C7 and C8.

anconeus: the innervation is identical to that of the triceps brachii, a branch of the radial nerve containing fibers from C7 and C8.

pronator quadratus: the anterior interosseous nerve, which branches from the median nerve. The fibers come from C8 and T1 by way of the brachial plexus.

supinator: the posterior interosseous branch of the deep radial nerve from the brachial plexus. Fibers come from C6.

STUDY QUESTIONS

1. Using Figs. 9–11A, 9–11B, 9–11C, and 9–11D, generate a list of origins and insertions for the muscles of the elbow joint. Compare your estimated origins and insertions to those from Gray's Anatomy or some other text and then, where necessary, make adjustments to your responses.

2. Present both mechanical and neuromuscular reasons for why chin-ups would be more difficult with a pronated grip (palm away from face) than with a supinated grip (palm toward face).

3. Present both mechanical and neuromuscular reasons for why chin-ups would be more difficult with a grip wider than shoulder width than with a shoulder-width grip.

4. What muscles at other joints could be categorized as spurt or shunt muscles?

5. Pauley, Rushing, and Scheving[31] reported sequential EMG activity in the three heads of the triceps muscle of the arm associated with progressive increase in finger flexion tension. Explain these findings.

REFERENCES

1. Matsen, F.A.: Biomechanics of the elbow. *In* Basic Biomechanics of the Skeletal System. Edited by V. Frankel and M. Nordin. Philadelphia, Lea & Febiger, 1980. pp. 243–253.
2. Gray, H.: Anatomy of the Human Body. Edited by C. Clemente. Philadelphia, Lea & Febiger, 1985.
3. Morrey, B.F., and Chao, E.Y.S.: Passive motion of the elbow joint: a biomechanical analysis. J. Bone Joint Surg., 58A:501, 1976.
4. Steindler, A.: Kinesiology of the Human Body Under Normal and Pathological Conditions. Springfield, C.C Thomas, 1976.
5. Basmajian, J.V., and DeLuca, C.J.: Muscles Alive. 5th Ed. Baltimore, Williams & Wilkins, 1985, p. 280.
6. Thepaut-Mathieu, C., and Maton, B.: The flexor function of m. pronator teres: a quantitative electro-

myographic study. Eur. J. Appl. Physiol., 54:116, 1985.
7. Basmajian, J.V., and DeLuca, C.J.: Muscles Alive. 5th Ed. Baltimore, Williams & Wilkins, 1985, pp. 277–280.
8. Basmajian, J.V., and DeLuca, C.J.: Muscles Alive. 5th Ed. Baltimore, Williams & Wilkins, 1985, p. 277.
9. Grabiner, M.D., Robertson, R.N., and Campbell, K.P.: Effects of fatigue on activation profiles and relative torque contribution of elbow flexor synergists. Med. Sci. Sports Exerc., 20:79–84, 1988.
10. An, K.N., et al.: Muscles across the elbow joint: a biomechanical analysis. J. Biomech., 14:659, 1981.
11. McGregor, A.L.: Synopsis of Surgical Anatomy. 7th Ed. Baltimore, Williams & Wilkins, 1950.
12. MacConaill, M.A.: Some anatomical factors affecting the stabilizing functions of muscles. Ir. J. Med. Sci., 6:160, 1946.

13. MacConaill, M.A.: The movement of bones and joints. 2. Function of the musculature. J. Bone Joint Surg., *31-B*:100–104, 1949.

14. Rasch, P., and Burke, R.: Kinesiology and Applied Anatomy. Philadelphia, Lea & Febiger, 1978.

15. Travill, A.A.: Electromyographic study of the extensor apparatus of the forearm. Anat. Rec., *144*:373, 1962.

16. DeHora, B.O.: "Musculus anconeus." Contribuicao ao estudo da sua arquitetura e das suas funcoes (In Portuguese). Thesis, University of Recife, Recife, Brazil, 1959. Cited in Basmajian, J.V., and DeLuca, C.J.: Muscles Alive. 5th Ed. Baltimore, Williams & Wilkins, 1985.

17. Basmajian, J.V., and DeLuca, C.J.: Muscles Alive. 5th Ed. Baltimore, Williams & Wilkins, 1985, pp. 287–288.

18. LeBozec, S., Maton, B., Cnockaert, J.C.: The synergy of elbow extensor muscles during dynamic work in man. Eur. J. Appl. Physiol., *44*:255, 1980.

19. Basmajian, J.V., and DeLuca, C.J.: Muscles Alive. 5th Ed. Baltimore, Williams & Wilkins, 1985, pp. 285–286.

20. Basmajian, J.V.: 'Spurt' and 'shunt' muscles: an electromyographical confirmation. J. Anat., *93*:551, 1956.

21. Stern, J.T.: Investigations concerning the theory of 'spurt' and 'shunt' muscles. J. Biomech., *4*:437, 1971.

22. Gruchow, H.W., and Pelletier, D.: An epidemiologic study of tennis elbow. Am. J. Sports Med., *7*:234, 1979.

23. Grabiner, M.D., Groppel, J., and Campbell, K.C.: Resultant ball velocity as a function of off-center impact and grip firmness. Med. Sci. Sports Ex., *15*:542, 1984.

24. Nirchl, R.P., and Pettrone, F.H.: Tennis elbow: the surgical treatment of lateral epicondylitis. J. Bone Joint Surg., *61A*:832, 1979.

25. O'Donoghue, D.H.: Treatment of Injuries to Athletes. Philadelphia, W.B. Saunders, 1976.

26. Burton, A.K.: Grip strength and forearm straps in tennis elbow. Br. Sports Med., *19*:37, 1985.

27. Hang, Y.S., et al.: Biomechanical study of the pitching elbow. Int. Orthop., *3*:217, 1979.

28. Shapiro, R.: Personal communication, 1986.

29. Gugenheim, J.J., Stanley, R., Woods, G.W., and Tullos, H.S.: Little league survey: the Houston study. Am. J. Sports Med., *4*:189, 1975.

30. Larson, R.L.: Little league survey: the Eugene study. Am. J. Sports Med., *4*:201, 1976.

31. Pauley, J.E., Rushing, J.L., and Scheving, L.E.: An electromyographic study of some muscles crossing the elbow joint. Anat. Rec., *159*:47, 1969.

10 THE WRIST AND HAND

MARK D. GRABINER

ANATOMIC CONSIDERATIONS

All of the linkages associated with the upper extremity might ultimately be associated with providing for the specialized movement function of the hand. The comparatively large area in the central nervous system dedicated to the control of the hand and the processing of information generated at the hand makes the hand a highly specialized organ. Fine motor tasks, such as those performed by a neurosurgeon, are performed with the same anatomic structure used by a karateist to smash wooden boards and bricks, a gross task whose major requirement is the transmission of force.

The hand is composed of 27 bones and over 20 joints. The bones, which are categorized into three groups, are the eight carpals, five metacarpals (which are numbered beginning with the thumb), and three rows of phalanges, totalling 14.

The carpals, classified as irregular bones, are in two rows of four. The proximal (first) row has the scaphoid, lunate, triquetral, and pisiform. The distal (second) row has the trapezium, trapezoid, capitate, and hamate. The five metacarpals have a proximal base, a body, and a distal head. The three rows of phalanges are the proximal, medial (middle), and distal rows, having five, four, and five members, respectively. The thumb does not have a medial phalanx. In general, the digits of the hands are numbered like the metacarpals but are commonly designated as thumb, index finger, middle or long finger, ring finger, and little finger.

The wrist joints are composed of the radiocarpal joints and the intercarpal joints. The former, a diarthritic condyloid joint, is formed by the distal end of the radius, an articular disk, and three of the four carpal bones in the proximal row. The distal end of the ulna and the pisiform bone are not involved in the wrist joint proper. The radiocarpal joint is separated from the proximal row of carpals by a fibrocartilage articular disk (Fig. 10–1). The three involved carpal bones form a smooth convex surface that receives the concave distal end of the radius and allows planar (nonaxial) motion to occur.

The intercarpal joints are divided into three groups:[1] the joints between the scaphoid, lunate, triquetral, and pisiform bones (the proximal row); the joints between the capitate, hamate, trapezoid, and trapezium (the distal row); and the midcarpal joint, the joint between the proximal and distal rows.

The ligaments of the radiocarpal joint include an extensive articular capsule and the palmar radiocarpal, dorsal radiocarpal, ulnar collateral, and radial collateral. The intercarpal joints are supported by a complex network of ligaments (Figs. 10–2, 10–3, and 10–4).

The distal row of carpal bones articulates with the five metacarpal bones. The carpometacarpal joints include those of the four medial fingers and that of the thumb. The latter is considered separately because of the significance of prehension. The carpometacarpal joint of the thumb is formed by the base of the first metacarpal and the trape-

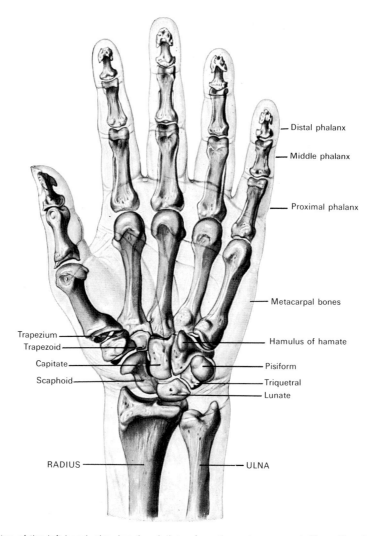

FIG. 10–1. Outline of the left hand, showing the skeleton from the palmar aspect. (From Benninghoff and Goerttler. Lehrbuch der Anatomie des Menschen, Urban and Schwarzenberg, 1975.)

zium. The carpometacarpal joints of the medial four fingers, however, are diarthrodial plane joints. The carpometacarpal joint of the thumb has a relatively loose articular capsule that is reinforced by the lateral (radial) palmar and dorsal (anterior and posterior oblique) carpometacarpal ligaments of the thumb. The ligaments of the carpometacarpal joints of the medial four fingers are the dorsal carpometacarpal ligaments, palmar carpometacarpal ligaments, and interosseous carpometacarpal ligaments.

All but the metacarpal bone of the thumb are connected to form the intermetacarpal joints associated with the dorsal, palmar, and interosseous metacarpal ligaments. The distal ends of the metacarpal joints form diarthro-dial ellipsoid joints with the proximal ends of the first phalanges, the metacarpophalangeal (MP) joints. These joints, which form the striking surfaces of the fully clenched fist, are covered dorsally by the expansions of the extensor tendons and are crossed on the palmar aspect by the flexor tendons. These joints are strengthened by the palmar, collateral, and deep transverse ligaments. The joints between the second and third phalanges are diarthrodial hinge joints, the interphalangeal (IP) joints. These joints are protected by the palmar and (two) collateral ligaments (Figs. 10–5 and 10–6).

JOINT MOVEMENTS

Combined joint action at the radiocarpal joint produces circumduction. The joint can

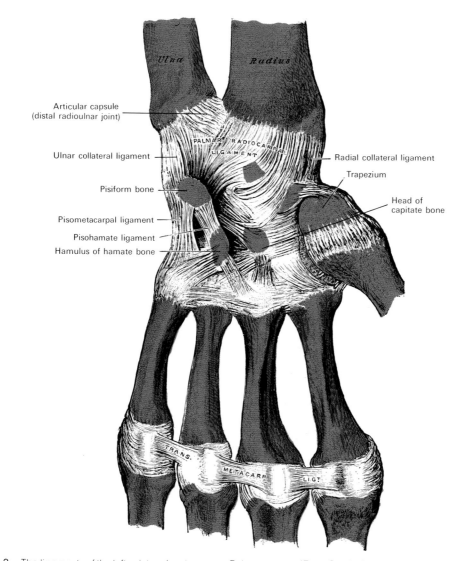

FIG. 10–2. The ligaments of the left wrist and metacarpus. Palmar aspect. (From Gray's Anatomy. 30th Ed. Philadelphia, Lea & Febiger, 1985, p. 382.)

allow all movement except rotation about its long axis. Motion in the frontal plane includes abduction, sometimes referred to as radial deviation or radial flexion, and adduction, sometimes referred to as ulnar deviation or ulnar flexion. In the sagittal plane the wrist can extend and flex. Flexion causes the palm to approach the surface of the forearm. Movement of the intercarpal joints is negligible.

The five carpometacarpal joints are of two types. The thumb's carpometacarpal joint is a saddle joint, allowing the thumb extensive and unique movement qualities. The remaining carpometacarpal joints are the diarthritic plane type. The second and third carpomet-

acarpal joints allow virtually no movement; the fifth, and to some degree the fourth, permit slight flexion, a movement observed when cupping the hands.[2]

The MP joint of the thumb is a diarthritic hinge joint allowing only flexion and extension. The remaining four MP joints are diarthritic condyloid joints with flexion-extension and abduction-adduction capabilities. Abduction is usually referred to as either radial deviation or radial flexion and is associated with the spreading of the fingers away from the middle finger. The reverse motion, adduction, is generally called ulnar deviation or ulnar flexion.

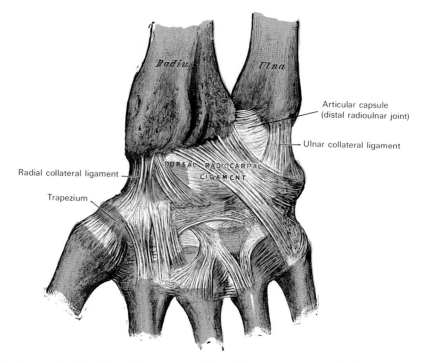

FIG. 10–3. The ligaments of the left wrist. Dorsal aspect. (From Gray's Anatomy. 30th Ed. Philadelphia, Lea & Febiger, 1985, p. 383.)

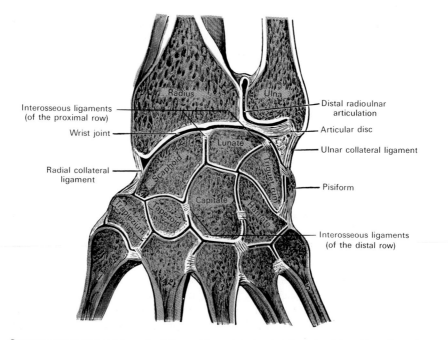

FIG. 10–4. Coronal section through the articulations at the wrist, showing the synovial cavities. (From Gray's Anatomy. 30th Ed. Philadelphia, Lea & Febiger, 1985, p. 383.)

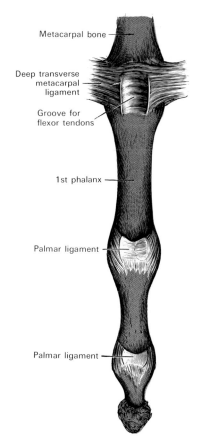

Metacarpal bone

Deep transverse metacarpal ligament

Groove for flexor tendons

1st phalanx

Palmar ligament

Palmar ligament

FIG. 10–5. The metacarpophalangeal and interphalangeal joints of a finger. Palmar aspect. (From Gray's Anatomy. 30th Ed. Philadelphia, Lea & Febiger, 1985, p. 389.)

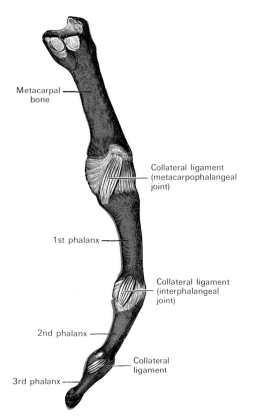

Metacarpal bone

Collateral ligament (metacarpophalangeal joint)

1st phalanx

Collateral ligament (interphalangeal joint)

2nd phalanx

Collateral ligament

3rd phalanx

FIG. 10–6. Metacarpophalangeal and interphalangeal joints of a finger. Ulnar or medial aspect. (From Gray's Anatomy. 30th Ed. Philadelphia, Lea & Febiger, 1985, p. 389.)

The thumb has one IP joint whereas the other fingers have two, a proximal interphalangeal (PIP) and a distal interphalangeal (DIP) joint. All the IP joints are diarthritic hinge joints that permit only flexion and extension. Ligamentous structures prevent hyperextension of these joints.

MUSCLES AND MOVEMENTS OF THE THUMB AND FINGERS

Six principal muscles act on the wrist, although the extrinsic muscles of the hand can act as assistant agonists. Soderberg[3] presents a convenient method for categorizing the muscles as a function of joint action, that is, flexion, extension, abduction, and adduction. Wrist flexion is predominantly a function of the synchronous action of flexor carpi radialis, flexor carpi ulnaris, and flexor digitorum superficialis.[4] It was reported that the flexor dig-

itorum profundus does not play a role in wrist flexion, although its position suggests a possible contribution, as do the positions of the palmaris longus and the flexor pollicis longus. These muscles in addition to the pronator teres (discussed in Chapter 9) compose what is referred to as the superficial flexor group of the forearm (Figs. 10–7, 10–8, and 10–9).

Soderberg[3] names three primary wrist extensors: extensor carpi radialis longus, extensor carpi radialis brevis, and extensor carpi ulnaris. However, Tournay and Paillard[5] indicate that except in the performance of fast wrist extension, the extensor carpi radialis longus is inactive. During fist-making the extensor carpi radialis longus is very active, whereas the extensor carpi radialis brevis is almost inactive.[6] By virtue of their position, extensors digitorum, digiti minimi, pollicis longus, and indicis may be considered assistant wrist extensors. A superficial extensor group of the forearm is composed of the ex-

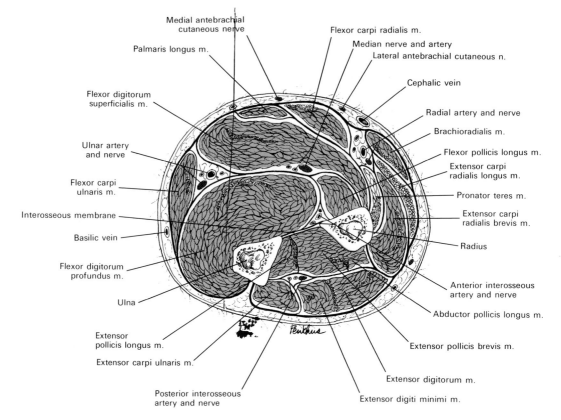

FIG. 10–7. Transverse section through the middle of the right forearm, viewed from above. (From Gray's Anatomy. 30th Ed. Philadelphia, Lea & Febiger, 1985, p. 530.)

tensors carpi radialis longus and brevis, extensor digitorum, extensor digiti minimi, extensor carpi ulnaris, and the elbow joint brachioradialis and anconeus muscles (Fig. 10–10).

The position of the fingers can influence the action of some of the above muscles of the wrist. *Gray's Anatomy* suggests that if the fingers are extended, the finger flexors can assist in wrist flexion, and vice versa for wrist extension. The properties of length-tension and of multijoint muscles would support this theory.

Radial and ulnar deviation (abduction and adduction) result from synergistic contraction of muscles that are responsible primarily for wrist flexion and extension. Abduction results from the contraction of the flexor and extensor carpi radialis. The extensor digitorum and flexor digitorum are active and may contract with extreme wrist adduction or abduction range of motion. Abduction may be assisted by the deep extensor group (abductor

pollicis longus, extensor pollicis brevis, extensor pollicis longus, extensor indicis, and the supinator) by virtue of their lines of pull (Fig. 10–11).

The intrinsic muscles of the hand are subdivided into three groups—those of the thumb, found on the radial side and responsible for the thenar eminence; those of the little finger, found on the ulnar side and responsible for the hypothenar eminence; and those in the middle of the hand and between the metacarpals. The 11 small intrinsic muscles of the hand are associated with movement of the fingers. They are categorized into three groups—the four lumbricals, the four dorsal interossei, and the three palmar interossei (Figs. 10–12 and 10–13). The lumbricals are located in the palm, and the interossei, between the metacarpals. All serve to flex the proximal phalanges and extend the middle and distal phalanges. Three muscles acting on only the little finger, the abductor digiti minimi, flexor digiti minimi brevis, and opponens digiti minimi, are also intrinsic hand muscles.

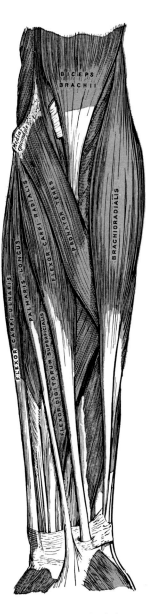

FIG. 10–8. Anterior aspect of left forearm. Superficial muscles. (From Gray's Anatomy. 30th Ed. Philadelphia, Lea & Febiger, 1985, p. 531.)

Thumb flexion occurs when the first metacarpal is moved across the palm; extension is the return movement. Thumb abduction from the anatomic position occurs as the first metacarpal moves away from the second in a plane perpendicular to that of the hand. Thumb adduction is the return movement. Opposition of the thumb to the fingers is a unique and critical action associated with the human hand and involves a combination of abduction, circumduction, and rotation that

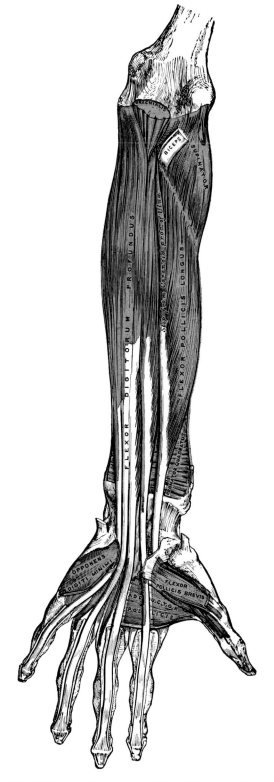

FIG. 10–9. Anterior aspect of the left forearm. Deep muscles. (From Gray's Anatomy. 30th Ed. Philadelphia, Lea & Febiger, 1985, p. 533.)

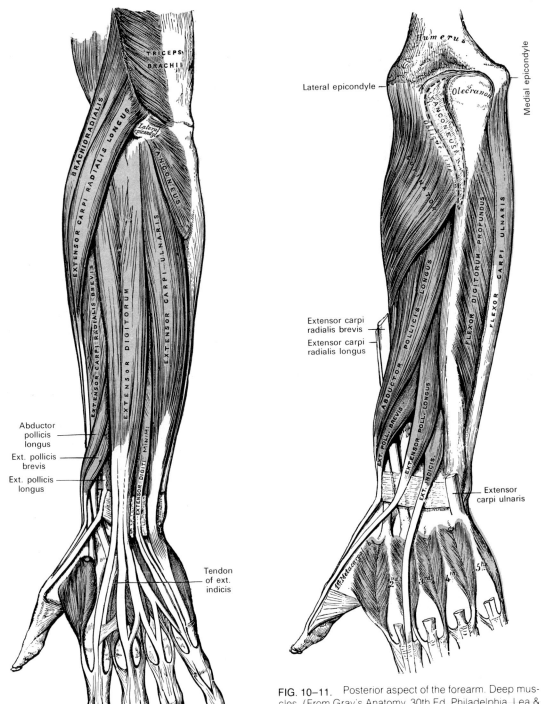

FIG. 10–10. Posterior aspect of the forearm and hand. Superficial muscles. (From Gray's Anatomy. 30th Ed. Philadelphia, Lea & Febiger, 1985, p. 536.)

FIG. 10–11. Posterior aspect of the forearm. Deep muscles. (From Gray's Anatomy. 30th Ed. Philadelphia, Lea & Febiger, 1985, p. 539.)

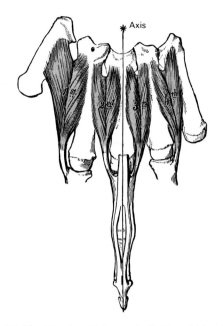

FIG. 10–12.   The dorsal interossei of left hand. Line down middle finger represents an imaginary axis. Abduction and adduction are determined according to this reference. (From Gray's Anatomy. 30th Ed. Philadelphia, Lea & Febiger, 1985, p. 555.)

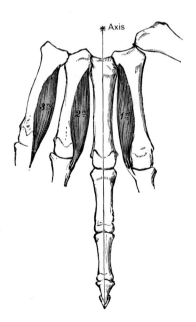

FIG. 10–13.   The palmar interossei of left hand. (From Gray's Anatomy. 30th Ed. Philadelphia, Lea & Febiger, 1985, p. 555.)

brings the tip of the thumb into a position facing, or in opposition to, the fingertips.

Eight muscles act on the thumb, four of which are intrinsic to the hand. The extrinsic muscles are the extensor pollicis longus, extensor pollicis brevis, abductor pollicis longus, and flexor pollicis longus. The four intrinsic muscles, originating at the thenar eminence, are the flexor pollicis brevis, opponens pollicis, abductor pollicis brevis, and adductor pollicis.

Movements of the thumb are a function of complex neuromuscular and mechanical interactions between the intrinsic and extrinsic muscles. A measure of the complexity and hence the importance of the thumb to normal hand function is reflected by the fact that the thumb's value has been estimated as between 40 and 50% of that of the entire hand.[2,7] Extension of the thumb joints is under the control of the extensor pollicis longus and brevis, which act on the phalanges and metacarpals. The opponens pollicis and abductor pollicis brevis are thenar muscles active during thumb extension.[8] The flexor pollicis longus, abductor pollicis longus, and flexor pollicis brevis control thumb flexion. However, the role of prime mover for MP joint flexion is a function of IP joint position. The flexor pollicis longus becomes the main agonist when the IP joint is flexed.[9] The flexor pollicis brevis plays an important role in positioning the unloaded thumb near the tips of the fingers, whereas the flexor pollicis longus is generally inactive. The flexor pollicis longus, however, appears to provide most of the force needed to counteract loads applied to the thumb in this position, irrespective of whether the distal phalanx is flexed or extended. The limiting factor in grip strength may indeed be a function of the inability of the thumb to oppose loads.[2]

Abduction of the thumb is contributed to by the extensor pollicis longus, flexor pollicis longus, flexor pollicis brevis, and adductor pollicis. The contribution of the flexor and extensor pollicis longus is required to work against a load and, in neutralizing the tendencies of the other muscles to flex or extend the thumb, provides a resultant adduction torque (Fig. 10–14).

The hypothenar muscles are the palmaris

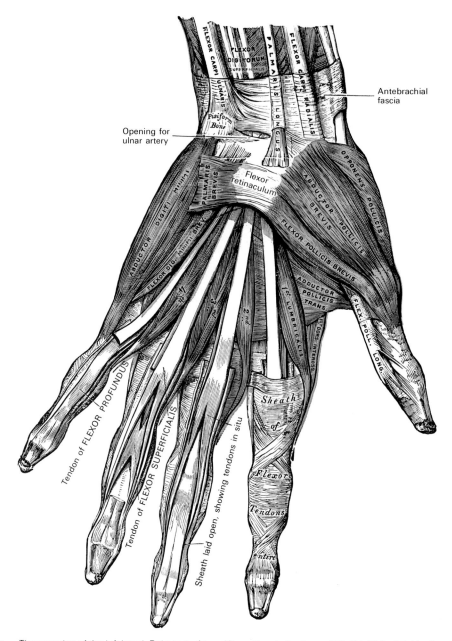

FIG. 10–14.   The muscles of the left hand. Palmar surface. (From Gray's Anatomy. 30th Ed. Philadelphia, Lea & Febiger, 1985, p. 553.)

brevis, abductor digiti minimi, flexor digiti minimi brevis, and opponens digiti minimi. The palmaris brevis is a small muscle with no bony attachments that creates no meaningful kinematics of the hand and is generally excluded from discussion regarding the group (Fig. 10–15).

Activity of the hypothenar muscles, excluding the palmaris brevis, is minimal during extension of the little finger.[8] Significant activity was observed in all three monitored muscles during abduction, and moderate activity in all three was also observed in flexion. The activity of the abductor digiti minimi during flexion of the little finger and during opposition of the thumb to the little finger suggests that abduction may be secondary to stabilization.

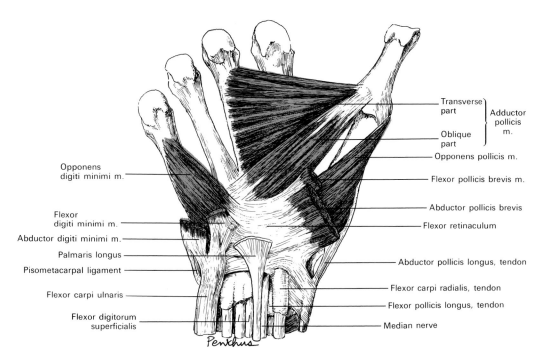

FIG. 10–15. A dissection of the palm of the right hand, showing the two parts of the adductor pollicis muscle, as well as the opponens pollicis and opponens digiti minimi muscles. (From Gray's Anatomy. 30th Ed. Philadelphia, Lea & Febiger, 1985, p. 552.)

When the thumb is softly placed in opposition to the sides and tips of each of the medial fingers, the thenar muscles are all more active than the hypothenar muscles.[8] Of the thenar muscles, the opponens is the most active and the flexor pollicis brevis is the least active. The most active hypothenar muscle is the opponens digiti minimi. As the force of opposition increases, the activity of the flexor pollicis brevis increases, becoming dominant. The opponens digiti minimi is still the most active hypothenar muscle under these conditions.

The fingers and their movements exemplify how knowledge of the type of joint and the direction of the line of pull of the involved muscles does not provide all of the information required to determine movement qualitatively. The complex dorsal expansion, or extension expansion, a highly specialized tendinous structure, is a major determinant with respect to finger motion (Fig. 10–16).

Though all the digits have an extensor expansion, the thumb's is somewhat modified. It consists of branching aspects of the insertions of the extensor muscles, interosseous muscles, lumbrical muscles, and some of the

thenar and hypothenar muscles. At the MP joint there is a hood that is formed by slips from the extensor muscle's tendon and that is wrapped partly around the sides of the proximal phalanx. This construction encloses the insertion of the interossei muscle. The lateral bands are found just distal to the hood and form the sides of the triangularly shaped extension expansion arising from the interossei. The lumbricals insert into the extension expansion at the shaft of the proximal phalanx distal to the lateral bands. The middle or central slip of the expansion is the main tendon of the extensor digitorum, which inserts on the dorsal aspect of the middle phalanx. This slip receives fibers of insertion from the interossei and lumbricals and it contributes to the lateral bands.

The extensor digitorum can extend to the distal as well as to the middle and proximal phalanges because of the extensor expansion. The lumbricals and interossei, however, found at the lateral bands and hood, cause flexion of the proximal phalanx at the MP joint and extension of the middle and distal phalanges.

The multijoint nature of the extensor digi-

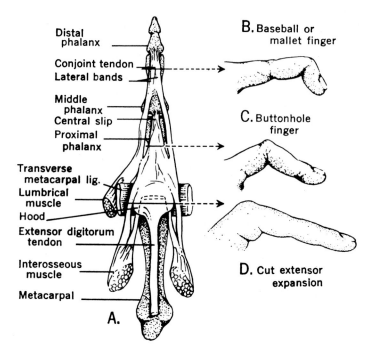

FIG. 10–16. *A*, Dorsal (extensor) expansion of the fingers. *B, C,* and *D,* The type of injury resulting from trauma to the expansion mechanism at the levels indicated: *B*, Severed conjoint tendon; *C*, Severed central slip; *D*, Severed extensor expansion. (Adapted from Entin, M.A.: Repair of extensor mechanism of the hand. Surg. Clin. North Am., April, 1960, p. 275.)

torum, flexor digitorum profundus, and flexor digitorum superficialis interferes with the ability to extend and flex the MP, PIP, and DIP joints simultaneously. However, positioning the wrist in flexion can stretch the extensor tendons and therefore contribute to the tension in the extensors and vice versa for the flexors. Extreme wrist positions, however, are not always possible or desirable (Fig. 10–17).

A question is raised then, regarding the mechanisms of the positions of full finger extension and flexion, as well as of the intermediate positions called the lumbrical and hooked positions (Fig. 10–18).

In the lumbrical position, the lumbricals and the dorsal and palmar interossei cannot simultaneously flex the MP joint and extend the PIP and DIP joints. In the hooked position, contraction of the long finger flexors is required for PIP and DIP flexion but also is associated with an undesired MP flexion torque. To negate the counterproductive torque, the extensor digitorum contracts but in so doing tends to cause PIP and DIP extension. These apparent inefficiencies can be

explained by the nature of the lever systems and the passive tension generated by stretched antagonists.

Rasch and Burke[2] present three general rules that may be used to explain the kinetics of the fingers. First, the lumbricals and interossei tend to be the dominant muscular system at the MP joint. Second, the extensor digitorum dominates the MP joint when the lumbricals are not active. Third, the long flexors dominate the PIP and DIP joints even when the extensor digitorum is active.

Full finger extension, then, is dominated by the extensor digitorum muscle at the MP joint, which stretches the lumbricals, which in turn contribute to PIP and DIP extension. In the lumbrical position, the lumbricals and interossei cause MP flexion, which stretches the tendon of the extensor digitorum muscle and subsequently causes extension of the PIP and DIP joints. In the hooked position both the extensor digitorum muscle and the long flexors contribute. The former dominates the MP joint and the latter two dominate the PIP and DIP joints. In full flexion, the long flexors dominate the MP, PIP, and DIP joints, but the

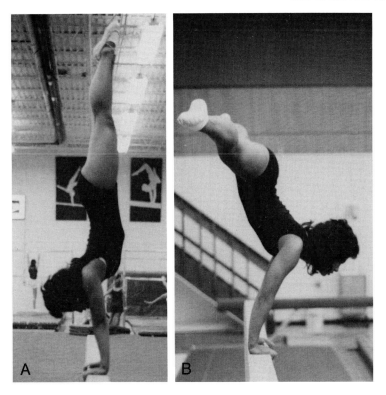

FIG. 10–17. *A* and *B*, Note the degree of the wrist extension as the gymnast supports herself. This position can aid in the development of phalangeal flexion torques.

stretch placed on the extensor expansion must be alleviated by some degree of wrist extension, or, in the very least, by avoiding wrist flexion (Fig. 10–19).

Prehensile movement may be generally considered as that category of hand movement in which the hand grasps an object (Fig. 10–20). Prehensile movements are classified as either power grip or precision grip. In the power grip, all of the extrinsic muscles contribute to force. The interossei and thenar muscles are used in the power grip, but the lumbricals (excluding the fourth) are not active.[11] Ohtsuki[12,13] reported on the contributions to grip strength by the four medial fingers. He indicated that the middle finger demonstrates the greatest contribution (33%) followed by the ring finger (27 to 28%), the index finger (24 to 25%), and little finger (15%). According to Ohtsuki, the anatomic arrangement of bones, in which the long axis of the middle finger is aligned with that of the capitate and radius, is not merely coincidental with his observations.

The gross motion and compressive force required in the precision grip are provided by

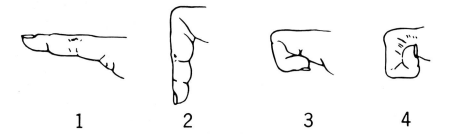

FIG. 10–18. Four basic positions of the finger. *1*, Full extension. MP extension, IP extension. *2*, Lumbrical position. MP flexion, IP extension. *3*, Hook. MP extension, IP flexion. *4*, Full flexion. MP flexion, IP flexion. (After Stack.[10])

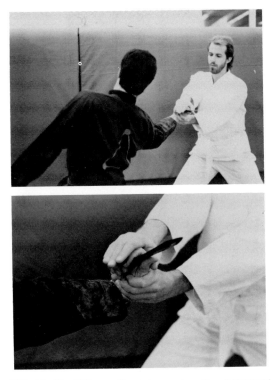

FIG. 10–19. Wrist positions shown place the phalangeal extensor mechanism on stretch, making it difficult to maintain a firm grip. This is a typical disarming technique against some types of hand-held weapons.

specific extrinsic muscles. Intrinsic muscles, however, provide the finely controlled aspects of the grip. If an object is to be rotated in the hand, the interossei are important to abduct and/or adduct the MP joints, and the lumbricals abduct and/or adduct and rotate the first phalanx. The interossei provide fine changes in compression, and the flexor pollicis brevis, opponens pollicis, and abductor pollicis provide adduction forces across the palm.

MECHANICAL CONSIDERATIONS OF INJURY TO THE WRIST AND HAND

About 7% of all sports injuries are to the hand.[2] Ligamentous and tendinous injuries, fractures, and dislocations are commonly associated with specific sports.[14] Karate, a sport that often emphasizes both "free fighting" and breaking techniques in which the hands are used to break wood, tiles, and bricks, might be expected to have a high incidence of hand injuries; structural changes caused by

forces applied and absorbed by the hand might be expected much in the same way as they occur in the foot of female ballet dancers.[15] The hands of some karateists can reach velocities of 14 m/sec and generate forces of over 650 lb.[16] However, Crosby[17] reported that long-term practitioners of karate did not seem to be predisposed to either osteoarthritis or tendinitis in the hand. This finding is consistent with Larose and Sik,[18] who reported that as a result of karate-specific hand conditioning, practitioners generally showed no changes in bone structure, degeneration of the metacarpal heads, or dystrophic soft-tissue calcification. Not surprising is the reported risk in karate of fractures and dislocations of the phalanges and metacarpals. Rasch and Burke[2] wrote that these injuries occur predominantly at the fourth and fifth metacarpals because in the closed fist, the fourth and fifth metacarpals, unlike the second and third, are not supported externally by the thenar eminence.

Trauma to various aspects of the upper extremity proximal to the wrist and hand often can result in distal dysfunction. Three nerves of the upper extremity, the ulnar, medial, and radial, are often subjected to injury and directly influence hand function. Injuries to the elbow can affect the ulnar nerve as it courses between the medial epicondyle and olecranon, where it is covered by only fascia and skin. Abduction and adduction of the fingers and flexion of fingers four and five are affected by ulnar nerve injury. The median nerve is the nerve for the radial side of the forearm and hand. One of the many branches of this nerve supplies most of the muscles of the thenar eminence, and injury to the nerve can profoundly affect thumb function. The radial nerve supplies the extensor muscles of the arm and forearm. Spiraling down the humerus from the brachial plexus, it can be damaged as a result of shoulder complex injuries such as dislocations and fractures, thereby affecting motion at the wrist and hand.

The carpal tunnel is a relatively constricted area located on the anterior aspect of the wrist through which passes the eight flexor tendons, the flexor pollicis longus, and the median nerve. The tunnel itself is composed on three sides by the carpal bones and on the

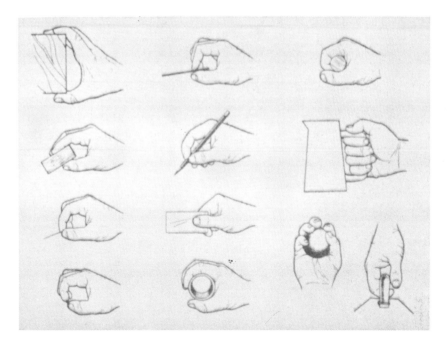

FIG. 10–20. Twelve basic types of grasp. (Courtesy of Artificial Limbs. After Schlesinger.)

fourth by the volar carpal ligament. Carpal tunnel syndrome is a result of compression that can be initiated by micro- or macro-trauma, tenosynovitis (inflammation of a tendon sheath) of the flexor tendons, fracture, or dislocation of any of the carpal bones. Basically, swelling of the tunnel contents or a constriction of the tunnel proper impinges on the median nerve. The results can be a range of symptoms in the distribution of the median nerve, from tingling of the index and long fingers to atrophy of the thenar muscles.

NEURAL INNERVATIONS

palmaris longis: the median nerve with its fibers coming from C6 and C7 by way of the brachial plexus.

flexor carpi radialis: the median nerve, with its fibers coming from C6 and C7 by way of the brachial plexus.

flexor carpi ulnaris: the ulnar nerve from the brachial plexus. Fibers are from C8 and T1.

flexor digititorum superficialis: the median nerve from the brachial plexus. Fibers come from C7, C8, and T1.

flexor digitorum profundus: the anterior interosseous nerve, the fibers of which come from the brachial plexus by way of the ulnar and median nerves. Fibers are from C8 and T1.

extensor carpi radialis longus: the radial nerve from the brachial plexus. Fibers come from C6 and C7.

extensor carpi radialis brevis: a branch of the radial nerve with fibers C6 and C7.

extensor carpi ulnaris: posterior interosseous branch of the deep radial nerve from the brachial plexus. Fibers are from the C6, C7, and C8.

extensor digitorum: posterior interosseous branch of the deep radial nerve from the brachial plexus. Fibers come from the C6, C7, and C8.

extensor digiti minimi: posterior interosseous branch of the deep radial nerve of the brachial plexus. Fibers arise from the C6, C7, and C8.

extensor pollicis longus: posterior interosseous branch of the deep radial nerve from the brachial plexus with fibers from C6, C7, and C8.

extensor indicis: posterior interosseous branch of the deep radial nerve of the brachial plexus. Fibers arise from the C6, C7, and C8.

abductor pollicis longus: posterior interos-

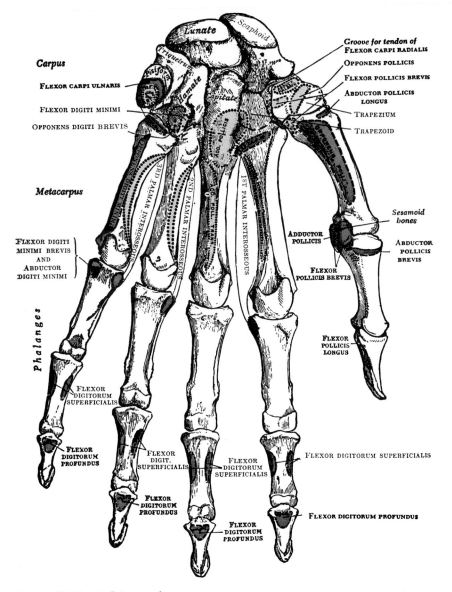

FIG. 10–21.   Bones of left hand. Palmar surface.

seous branch of the deep radial nerve from the brachial plexus with fibers from C6 and C7.

extensor pollicis brevis: posterior interosseous branch of the deep radial nerve from the brachial plexus with fibers from C6 and C7.

lumbricals: the first two lumbricals from the third and fourth digital branches of the median nerve, containing fibers from C6 and C7; the third and fourth lumbricals from branches of the palmar branch of the ulnar nerve, containing fibers from C8.

dorsal interossei: the palmar branch of the

ulnar nerve with fibers coming from C8 and T1 by way of the brachial plexus.

palmar interossei: the palmar branch of the ulnar nerve with fibers coming from C8 and T1 by way of the brachial plexus.

abductor digiti minimi: the deep branch of the ulnar nerve from the brachial plexus with fibers from C8.

flexor digiti minimi brevis: the deep branch of the ulnar nerve from the brachial plexus with fibers from C8 and T1.

opponens digiti minimi: the deep branch of the ulnar nerve from the brachial plexus with fibers from C8 and T1.

flexor pollicis longus: the anterior interos-

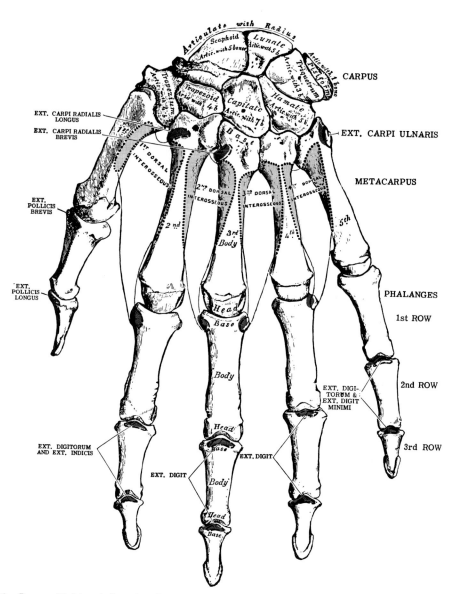

FIG. 10–22. Bones of left hand. Dorsal surface.

seous nerve from the median nerve. Fibers come from C8 and T1.

flexor pollicis brevis: superficial head supplied by fibers from the median nerve; deep head supplied by fibers from the ulnar nerve.

abductor pollicis brevis: the median nerve with fibers from C6 and C7.

abductor pollicis: the deep palmar branch of the ulnar nerve. Fibers come from C8 and T1.

opponens pollicis: the median nerve with fibers from C6 and C7.

STUDY QUESTIONS

1. Using Figs. 10–21 and 10–22, generate a list of origins and insertions for the intrinsic muscles. Use Figure 9–11 for the origin of the extrinsic muscles. Compare your estimated origins and insertions to those from *Gray's Anatomy* or some other text and then, where necessary, make adjustments to your response.

2. Using the photo of the gymnast doing a handstand on the balance beam (Fig. 10–17), calculate the flexion torque required at the wrists if the mass of the gymnast is 50 kg and the COG fall 7.5 cm anterior to the hands. What is the tension required in the wrist flexor if the average moment arm length is 1.9 cm?

3. What muscles/muscle groups are stressed differently when doing push-ups or a bench press exercise with a wide versus a narrow hand position with respect to the body and with the arms moving through a sagittal versus transverse plane?

4. Describe anatomically and with respect to muscle properties why it is difficult to completely flex the wrist and extend the fingers simultaneously

5. Describe anatomically and with respect to muscle properties why the fingers tend to abduct when extended fully.

REFERENCES

1. Gray, H.: Anatomy of the Human Body. 30th Ed. Edited by C.D. Clemente. Philadelphia, Lea & Febiger, 1985.
2. Rasch, P.J., and Burke, R.K.: Kinesiology and Applied Anatomy. Philadelphia, Lea & Febiger, 1978.
3. Soderberg, G.L.: Kinesiology—Applications to Pathological Motion. Baltimore, Williams & Wilkins, 1986.
4. Backdahl, M., and Carlsoo, S.: Distribution of activity in muscles acting on the wrist: an electromyographic study. Acta Morphol. Neerl. Scan., 4:136, 1961.
5. Tournay, A., and Paillard, J.: Electromyographie des muscles radiaux a l'état normal. Rev. Neurol., 89:277, 1953 (In French).
6. Basmajian, J.V., and DeLuca, C.J.: Muscles Alive, 5th Ed. Baltimore, Williams & Wilkins, 1985.
7. Wadsworth, C.T.: Clinical anatomy and mechanics of the wrist and hand. Orthop. Sports Phys. Ther., 4:206, 1983.
8. Basmajian, J.V., and DeLuca, C.J.: Muscles Alive. 5th Ed. Baltimore, Williams & Wilkins, 1985, pp. 296–309.
9. Johnson, D.R.: An electromyographic study of the extrinsic and intrinsic muscles of the thumb. Unpublished Master's thesis, Queen's University, Canada, 1970.
10. Stack, H.G.: Muscle function in the fingers. J. Bone Joint Surg., 44-B:899, 1962.
11. Long, C., Conrad, P.W., Hall, E.W., and Furler, S.L.: Intrinsic-extrinsic muscle control of the hand in power grip and precision handling. J. Bone Joint Surg., 52A:853, 1976.
12. Ohtsuki, T.: Inhibition of individual fingers during grip strength exertion. Ergonomics, 24:21, 1981.
13. Ohtsuki, T.: Decrease in grip strength induced by simultaneous bilateral exertion with reference to finger strength. Ergonomics, 24:37, 1981.
14. McHue, F.C.: Athletic injuries of the proximal interphalangeal joint requiring surgical treatment. J. Bone Joint Surg., 52A:937, 1970.
15. Sammarco, G.J.: The foot in ballet and modern dance. In Disorders of the Foot. Edited by M.H. Jahss. Philadelphia, W.B. Saunders, 1980.
16. Feld, M.S., McNair, R.E., and Wilk, S.R.: The physics of karate. Sci. Am., 240:150, 1979.
17. Crosby, A.C.: The hands of karate experts: Clinical and radiological findings. J. Sports Med., 19:41, 1985.
18. Larose, M.D., and Sik, K.D.: Karate hand conditioning. Med. Sci. Sports, 1:95, 1969.

11 THE VERTEBRAL COLUMN

MARK D. GRABINER

Movement of the upper extremities, the lower extremities, or both in any type of activity entails the transmission of internal and external forces to the central supporting column of the body, the vertebral column. Forces from the upper extremities are transmitted at the sternoclavicular joints and ribs. Forces from the lower extremities are transmitted through the hip joints to the bony pelvis prior to reaching the vertebral column by way of the lumbosacral joint. The vertebral column provides support for the upright posture, provides a protective yet flexible sleeve for the delicate spinal cord, provides sites for the attachment of muscles, and serves to transfer and attenuate loads from the head and trunk to the lower extremities and vice versa. The vertebral column's accomplishment of its purposes is notable from an engineering standpoint. It must be structurally flexible; it must undergo tension, compression, shear, bending, and torsion forces even under heavy load; it must be hollow to allow nerves and blood vessels to pass through it protected but to emerge from it at various levels without being damaged even during movement; and it must function adequately for a lifetime.[1]

ANATOMIC CONSIDERATIONS

The vertebral column is composed of 33 vertebrae, 24 of which are joined to form a flexible column. From superior to inferior they are classified as cervical (C1–C7), thoracic (T1–T12), lumbar (L1–L5), sacral (S1–S5), and four coxygeal. The sacral and coxygeal vertebrae are called false vertebrae because in the adult they are fused to form the sacrum and coccyx. The remaining vertebrae, cervical, thoracic, and lumbar, are called true vertebrae because they remain unfused throughout life (Fig. 11–1).

As can be seen in Figure 11–1, the vertebral column possesses curvatures in each of the three regions. The thoracic curve, called primary, is present at birth, whereas the cervical and lumbar curves are called secondary because they develop in response to forces exerted on infants' bodies. These forces arise when an infant begins to hold up its head and when it begins to sit up on its own. Females generally possess a more marked lumbar curve than males. A normal lateral curvature of the vertebral column is present in the thoracic area. The direction of the curve correlates with the dominant hand of an individual.

As might be expected, components of the vertebral column differ structurally because of the differences in the magnitudes of the forces affecting them. The vertebrae do have general characteristics, however, except for the highly specialized first and second cervical vertebrae, the atlas and axis. Figures 11–2 and 11–3 illustrate typical vertebrae selected from the middle of the thoracic region. The vertebral foramen, through which passes the spinal cord, is bounded anteriorly by the vertebral body and posteriorly by the vertebral arch. This arch is formed by two pedicles and laminae. The pedicles arise from the ver-

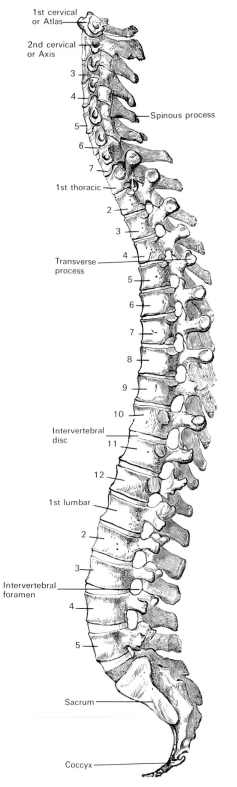

1st cervical or Atlas

2nd cervical or Axis

3

4

5

6

7

Spinous process

1st thoracic

2

3

4

Transverse process

5

6

7

8

9

10

Intervertebral disc

11

12

1st lumbar

2

3

Intervertebral foramen

4

5

Sacrum

Coccyx

FIG. 11–1.   Lateral view of the vertebral column. Observe the cervical, thoracic, and pelvic curvatures. (From Gray's Anatomy. 30th Ed. Philadelphia, Lea & Febiger, 1985, p. 127.)

tebral body, whereas the laminae arise from the pedicles. A spinous process projects posteriorly from its origin at the junction of the laminae, and two transverse processes project posteriorly and laterally from where they arise at the junctions of the pedicles and laminae. Two pairs of articular processes, superior and inferior, unite adjacent vertebrae. Spinal nerves at each segmental level exit from the vertebral column by way of the intervertebral foramina, which are bounded by the vertebral notches (superior and inferior) of adjacent vertebrae.

The vertebral column is supported and protected from forces in part by the articular structures. The two types of joints in the vertebral column are cartilaginous synarthritic joints and gliding diarthritic joints. The former type are found along the vertebral column from the axis to the sacrum and are composed of fibrocartilaginous disks between the bodies of adjacent vertebrae. These disks are contiguous with layers of hyaline cartilage on the inferior and superior surfaces of the bodies and are classified as symphyses. The shape of the disk is a function of the vertebral bodies that it separates, whereas its thickness varies with its location in the column as well as between different sections of the same disk. In the thoracic region the disks are of nearly uniform thickness, whereas in the cervical and lumbar areas they are thicker anteriorly, which difference contributes to the regional curves.[2] Fully 25% of the length of the vertebral column may be attributed to the disks. Although not freely movable, disks allow for limited motion in three planes.

Intervertebral disks are composed of two main structures. The nucleus pulposus is a gel-like mass located centrally in the disk. It is bounded by a layer of strong fibrocartilage called the anulus fibrosus (Fig. 11–4).

Disks degenerate with age in association with a reduction in their capacity to bind with water. This reduced water-binding quality is related to decreased elasticity (the ability to return to normal shape following a distortion caused by an applied force), which influences the capability to store energy and distribute loads, and therefore the ability to resist loading.

The diarthritic joint found in the vertebral

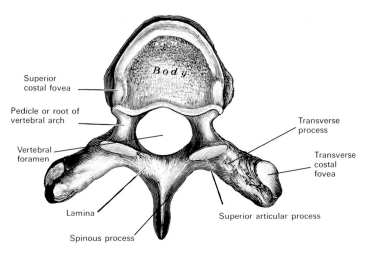

FIG. 11–2.   A typical thoracic vertebra, cranial aspect. (From Gray's Anatomy. 30th Ed. Philadelphia, Lea & Febiger, 1985, p. 129.)

column is the synovial joint between the articular processes of adjacent vertebrae. The articular capsules of these joints are thin and quite loose, attaching to the margins of the articular processes. The flexibility (the ability of a joint to traverse a range of motion) of the vertebral column is directly related to the orientation of these joints with respect to one another. The orientation changes from level to level.

Ligamentous support for the column comes from six structures. The anterior longitudinal ligament runs from the axis to the sacrum along the anterior surfaces of the vertebral bodies. It adheres to the disks and protruding margins of the bodies but is not firmly attached to the middles of the bodies. The posterior longitudinal ligament also runs from the axis to the sacrum but along the posterior surfaces of the bodies within the vertebral foramen (Fig. 11–5). The ligamenta flava connect the laminae of adjacent vertebrae along the entire length of the vertebral foramen. The ligamenta flava consist of yellow elastic tissue whose extensibility (the ability to lengthen) and elasticty allow for separation of

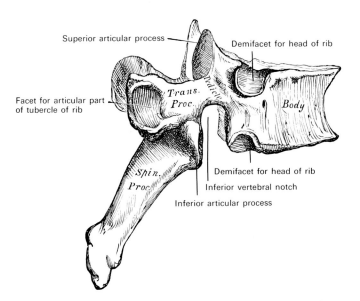

FIG. 11–3.   A typical thoracic vertebra, right lateral view. (From Gray's Anatomy. 30th Ed. Philadelphia, Lea & Febiger, 1985, p. 135.)

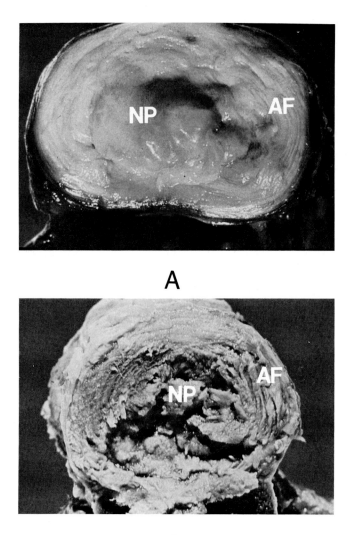

FIG. 11–4. Intervertebral disk composed of the nucleus pulposus (NP) and the anulus fibrosus (AF). *A*, Normal disk; *B*, Severely degenerated disk. (From Frankel, V.H., and Nordin, M.: Basic Biomechanics of the Skeletal System. Philadelphia, Lea & Febiger, 1980, p. 257.)

the laminae during vertebral column flexion. The supraspinal ligament connects the tips of the spinous processes from C7 to the sacrum. It is a strong fibrous cord whose fibers, depending on the cord's location, can span up to four vertebrae. Superior to C7 it is continued as the ligamentum nuchae, a fibroelastic membrane that represents in man a vestige of a major elastic ligament found in some types of grazing animals. In these types of animals, the ligamentum nuchae is important in providing passive cervical support against flexion caused by the effect of gravity on the mass of the head. The interspinal ligament connects adjacent spinous processes.

JOINT MOVEMENTS

Movement of the vertebral column is a function of both the "triaxial" synarthritic intervertebral disks and the diarthritic gliding facet joints. The orientation of the facet joint to both the horizontal and the vertical dictates both the type and magnitude of motion that can be experienced by any vertebral unit. A vertebral unit consists of two adjacent vertebrae and the related connective structures such as the disk and ligaments.[3] Movements of the vertebral column can be described with respect to the various distinct anatomic regions that make up the column.

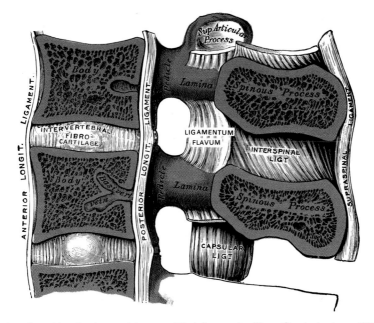

FIG. 11–5. Sagittal section of two lumbar vertebrae and their ligaments. (From Gray's Anatomy. 30th Ed. Philadelphia, Lea & Febiger, 1985, p. 347.)

The first two cervical vertebrae are highly specialized structures dedicated to the carriage of the cranium. The frequency of neck injuries in football is often blamed on the fragility of the first and second cervical vertebrae. The first, called the atlas, has no body but is a bony ring surrounding the vertebral foramen. On its upper surface it has two large concave articular surfaces that accommodate the occipital condyles of the skull. These atlanto-occipital joints allow considerable flexion and extension of the head. The joint has a loose capsule but is spanned by the anterior, posterior, and lateral atlanto-occipital ligaments. The second vertebra, called the axis, has a short peg, called the dens, which extends vertically from its body into the vertebral foramen of the atlas, where a very large ligament separates it from the spinal cord. This process serves as a pivot around which the atlas rotates rather freely, making it possible to rotate or shake the head from side to side. Movement in these two joints is relatively free compared to the other intervertebral articulations.

In the rest of the cervical region, however, the facet joints are inclined up to 45° from the transverse plane (anterior to posterior) and lie, in general, oriented with the frontal plane.

Because of this particular alignment, the cervical region facet joints allow flexion and extension in the sagittal plane, lateral flexion in the frontal plane, and rotation in the transverse plane. Range of motion for flexion and extension varies from approximately 5 to 17° degrees, lateral flexion from 5 to 10°, and rotation from 8 to 12° for each facet joint.[4]

In the thoracic region, facet joints are at angles of up to 60° to the transverse plane and 20° to the frontal plane. These joints allow lateral flexion ranging from 7 to 10° per segment and rotation of from 2 to 10°. The upper eight segments (T1 to T8) allow up to 9° of rotation, but this amount is reduced to about 2° in the lower four thoracic segments. Flexion and extension, further restricted by the ribs, is limited to about 3 to 4° in the upper ten segments, but may reach 10° in the lower segments. Thoracic vertebral range of motion is also influenced by the thickness of the intervertebral disks.

In the lumbar region the facets can be perpendicular to the transverse plane and up to 45° to the frontal plane. Because of this alignment, rotation in the transverse plane is severely restricted, to 2° per segment in all but the last (L5 to S1), which may allow up to 4°. Flexion and extension range from 12° at the most superior lumbar vertebrae to 20° at the most inferior. Lateral flexion ranges from 3 to 8° per segment.

Any motion of the vertebral column as a unit is a function of a series of motion segments. Interindividual variance is so great that "normal" values are difficult to define, although the range of motion is highly related to both age and sex.[3] Certainly, however, it is also a function of the level of activity that specifically requires and taxes extreme vertebral range of motion (Fig. 11–6).

LOW-BACK PAIN

The lumbar region of the spine is the part most susceptible to athletic injury.[5] Indeed 80% of the world's population at some time encounters back pain, probably in the lumbar region,[6] three times more frequently than upper-back pain.[7]

Causes of low-back pain have been classified into five major categories:[8] intra-abdominal disorders, abdominal/peripheral vascular disease, psychogenic disorders, neurogenic sources such as cerebral, spinal cord, or peripheral nerve lesions, and spondylogenic sources, which are related to the vertebral column and associated anatomic structures.

A question that is often raised with respect to low-back disorders is why the lumbar region seems to be predisposed to injury. Two fundamental factors are the inherent weakness of the structure itself and the forces or loads it encounters during everyday living tasks and recreational/athletic activities. The sources of the loads to which the spine is subjected include body weight, externally applied loads, and the contraction of muscles.

LOADS EXPERIENCED BY THE VERTEBRAL COLUMN

Back pain, especially in the lumbar region, is so prevalent in athletics, occupational environments, and even domestic situations that related biomechanical research has been ongoing worldwide. In athletics, the activities that can lead to back injuries have been categorized as weight-loading, rotation-causing, and back-arching.[5] Athletic activities can fall within one or more categories.

Weight-loading sports are those that tend to compress the spine. In addition to weight lifting, vertically jarring sports such as jogging and horseback riding are included. Although serious spinal injuries are infrequent in joggers, Guten[9] reported factors associated with high risk based on a sample of ten runners who had suffered herniated ("slipped") disks. In addition to previous disk ailments were cited middle age, low levels of flexibility, body height less than 6 ft, and changes in running mechanics. Crossen[10] associated back

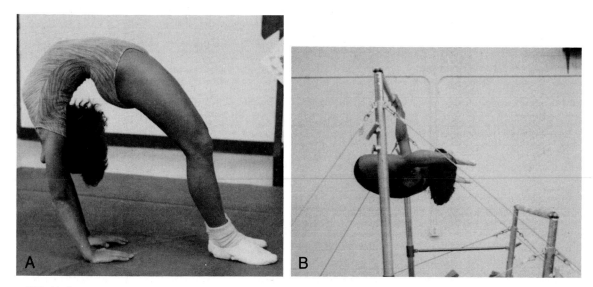

FIG. 11–6.   *A* and *B*, Extreme range of motion of the vertebral column is a prerequisite of success in female gymnastics.

pain in runners with inflammation of the sciatic nerve caused by "tight" gluteal and low-back muscles, a factor cited by Guten. Imbalance between the strength of the back and of the abdominal musculature may also be a source of problems. An imbalance can create, among other things, a shift of the pelvic posture, thereby altering the lordotic curve and subsequently stressing the disk. Fair[11] has related the high rate of low-back injury in female athletes to absence of [adequate] strength in the back and abdominals, in addition to other factors.

Rotation-causing activities are those during which the vertebral column is subjected to forceful twists. Racket sports and golf are included in this category. Stover, Wiren, and Topaz[12] suggest that in golf the hyper-rotation during the backswing and follow-through, along with the large muscular forces required to generate high clubhead speeds, is potentially dangerous. The aerial maneuvers executed by gymnasts and divers certainly fall within this category.

Activities in the back-arching category include volleyball, rowing, and swimming (breaststroke and butterfly). Also, it has been suggested that contemporary rowing style and training techniques increase the strains on the back. Hyperextension injuries during various weight training exercises and techniques followed by the extreme trunk flexion have been identified as possible injury mechanisms.[13] Flexion injuries may result from a combination of the degree of flexion, the velocity of the movement, vigorous contraction of antagonists, and the number of repetitions required in practice and competition (Fig. 11–7).

For simplified biomechanical analyses, the vertebral column can be treated as a rigid body rotating about its axis, found at the lumbosacral joint (L5-S1). Consider some of the forces acting on this type of model during the elementary postures of standing and lifting, given a man of 891 N (200 lb) standing erect. If 50% of body weight lies above the lumbosacral joint, one could assume a compressive force of 445.5 N (100 lb). However, in the normal individual, the superior surface of S1 is tilted anteriorly between 30 and 40° (the sacral angle) (Fig. 11–8). This tilt introduces

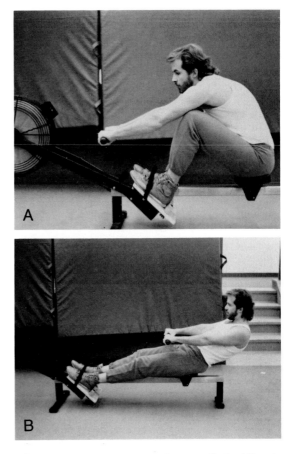

FIG. 11–7.   Note the presence of extreme flexion (*A*) and extension (*B*) range of motion in this activity. Usually large forces are associated with the motion.

a shear force of up to 341.25 N (76.6 lb). The compressive forces act predominantly on the anulus fibrosus through the compression of the nucleus pulposus. The shear forces affect mainly the intervertebral foramen, sometimes called the neural arch, the area between the adjacent inferior and superior articular processes.

If the man now flexes the vertebral column so that the angle is 45°, it is clear that the moment arm of the center of gravity of the upper body, and the moment arm of any external weight in the hands or elsewhere, increases. This means that if the upper body is to be held in a position of static equilibrium, the torque exerted by the vertebral extensors (erector spinae) must be equal to this forward rotational tendency. The required torque can be seen to increase as the angle of the trunk

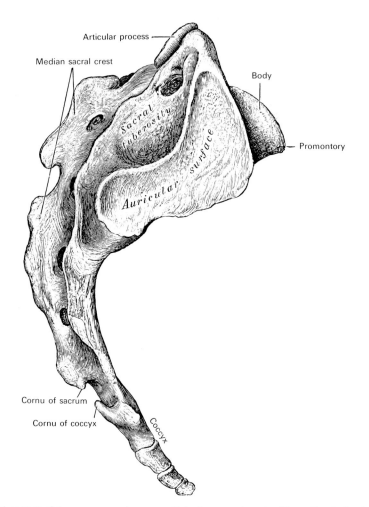

FIG. 11–8. Lateral aspect of the sacrum and coccyx. Note the sacral angle. (From Gray's Anatomy. 30th Ed. Philadelphia, Lea & Febiger, 1985, p. 141.)

approaches 90° when the moment arm is at its maximum.

As the angle of the trunk increases beyond 90° and as the center of gravity is brought closer to the axis of rotation, the moment arm begins to decrease. Therefore, the contribution of the trunk extensors required to counter this torque also decreases. However, after a certain point in the range of motion of vertebral and associated hip flexion, "flexor relaxation" may be observed. (It should be noted here that only 60° of vertebral column flexion are possible without hip/pelvis contributions. After 60° the range of motion is a function of anterior pelvic tilt.) First observed by Floyd and Silver[14,15] and subsequently affirmed by Pauly[16] and Wolf, et al.,[17] the erector spinae demonstrate electrical silence. Gra-

biner, Campbell, and Azcueta[18] verified the electrical silence and illustrated the strong relationship between activity and external torques, which is a function of the moment arm of the trunk, head, and arms.

When the flexor relaxation has occurred, the passive osseoligamentous structures have been said to be responsible for the stabilization of the vertebral column.[14] (The stretched erector spinae, however, and the underlying deep posterior group create passive tension despite electrical silence in accord with their length-tension properties.) Because the moment arm of the postvertebral ligaments is small,[19] the need for forces of this magnitude can be potentially damaging to the ligaments. The loss of at least some muscular control at the extreme positions provides important biomechanical information regarding various lifting tasks, both symmetric and asymmetric.

MUSCLES OF THE VERTEBRAL COLUMN

The muscles acting on the vertebral column can initially be divided into two categories, anterior and posterior. Muscles in both categories exist in bilateral pairs, although they can and do function independently (unilaterally). As a general rule, muscles of the anterior category cause flexion of the vertebral column, whereas muscles of the posterior category are responsible for extension. One muscle, the quadratus lumborum, is considered to act as a pure lateral flexor. Within each of the general categories the muscles may be further divided kinesiologically, in terms of the region they most directly affect.

ANTERIOR GROUP—CERVICAL FLEXORS

The prevertebral group of muscles consists of the longus colli and longus capitis, the rectus capitis anterior, and the rectus capitis lateralis (Fig. 11–9). These are deep muscles that cause flexion of the head and cervical vertebrae (except for the longus colli, which acts only on the cervical vertebrae) when contracting bilaterally. Unilateral contraction of these muscles causes lateral flexion of the cervical vertebrae or rotation of the head. The eight hyoid muscles cause cervical flexion against a resistance greater than that of the segment, but primarily are used in swallowing.

The superficial sternocleidomastoid, a two-headed muscle, also flexes the head and cervical vertebrae. Acting unilaterally, the cervical vertebrae will flex laterally and the head will rotate to the opposite side (the terms opposite side and same side as they relate to causing rotation will be used to indicate the side with respect to the unilaterally contracting muscle).

The scalene muscles (anterior, middle, and posterior) can be considered with the anterior category but in fact lie more laterally. Although important in respiration, they also flex the cervical vertebrae or, if unilaterally activated, laterally flex the cervical vertebrae (Figs. 11–10 and 11–11).

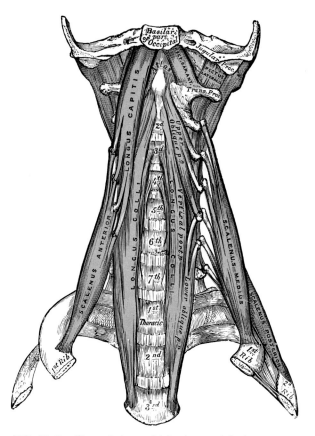

FIG. 11–9.   The anterior and lateral prevertebral muscles. (From Gray's Anatomy. 30th Ed. Philadelphia, Lea & Febiger, 1985, p. 462.)

ANTERIOR GROUP—LUMBAR FLEXORS

As indicated previously, the degree of thoracic region flexion and extension is extremely restricted. Therefore, only the lumbar region is presented. Because of the thoracic region's limitations to movement in the sagittal plane, the large range of cervical flexion-extension does not influence the lumbar region.

The group of muscles responsible for lumbar flexion is generally referred to as the abdominals. They have no direct connection to the vertebral column. Some are further distinguished in that they do not possess bony attachments at either end. Furthermore, in addition to the critical joint actions they effect (that is, lumbar flexion), they are important in the constriction of the abdominal cavity and its contents. This latter function increases intra-abdominal pressure, which in addition to being associated with elimination of waste products (defecation and micturition) also re-

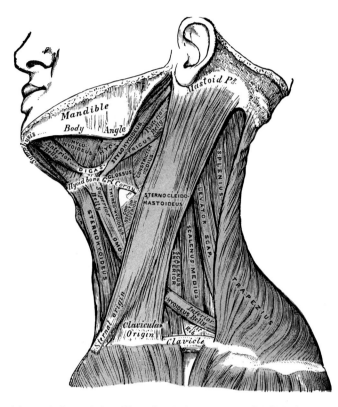

FIG. 11–10.   Muscles of the neck. Lateral view. (From Gray's Anatomy. 30th Ed. Philadelphia, Lea & Febiger, 1985, p. 458.)

duces the loads experienced by the lumbar vertebrae during particular activities. A discussion of this function follows the introduction of the musculature.

The rectus abdominis, as its name implies, runs vertically down the abdomen, its right and left parts being separated by the tendinous linea alba. By virtue of its vertically oriented line of pull, it is a prime agonist for spinal flexion and a lateral flexor when it is activated unilaterally.

The internal and external obliques (Fig. 11–12) cover the anterior and lateral portions of the abdominal wall between the rectus abdominis anteriorly and the latissimus dorsi muscle/thoracolumbar fascia posteriorly. The fibers of these muscles run nearly perpendicularly to one another, a feature that is reflected by a major difference in their unilateral actions.

When both sides of the external obliques contract simultaneously, the Z and X components of their pull are neutralized. When only one side of the muscle is activated, how-

ever, vertebral flexion results and, in addition, a lateral flexion and trunk rotation, in this case to the opposite side. With the exception of the direction of the rotation, the same is true for the internal obliques. During a unilateral contraction of this muscle the rotation of the trunk is to the opposite side. The transverse abdominis, the deepest muscle of this group, does not have a function associated with motor performance because of its line of pull and tendinous connections. All of these muscles, however, have a common anatomic connection or relation to one another in that the aponeurotic sheaths of the external and internal obliques and the transverse abdominis form the sheath of the rectus abdominis.

POSTERIOR GROUP—VERTEBRAL EXTENSORS

Approximately 140 individual muscles are involved in the motor function of the vertebral column. For purposes of general move-

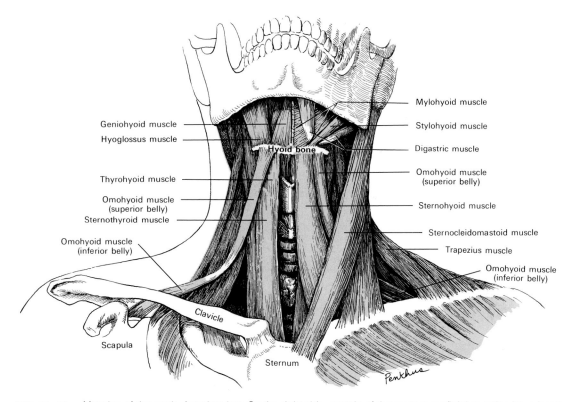

FIG. 11–11.   Muscles of the neck. Anterior view. On the right side, certain of the more superficial muscles have been removed. (From Gray's Anatomy. 30th Ed. Philadelphia, Lea & Febiger, 1985, p. 466.)

ment analysis, separating the spinal extensors into specific groups simplifies the topic without causing a significant loss of understanding. Two major groups of muscles compose the posterior group (or vertebral extensors), the erector spinae and the deep posterior group.

The erector spinae group, or the sacrospinalis muscle, originates as a large fleshy mass in the sacral area; as it ascends the vertebral column, it divides into three main columns (Figs. 11–13 and 11–14). The split, occurring in the upper lumbar level, results in the formation of the iliocostalis muscle, the longissimus muscle, and the spinalis muscle (still considered globally as the erector spinae). In the thoracic and lumbar regions, the sacrospinalis muscle is covered by the thoracolumbar fascia. This structure is particularly relevant considering the prevalence of low-back syndrome and the relationship of greater abdominal muscle strength to the reduction of loads on the vertebral column. The transverse abdominis and the lower portion of the origin

of the internal oblique arise from this fascia. Additionally, the lower portion of the origin of the external oblique is juxtaposed with a part of the latissimus dorsi, the latter of which is also incorporated in the fascia.

The iliocostalis muscle branch, the most lateral of the three columns, further divides into three regional parts, the iliocostalis lumborum, thoracis, and cervicis. The names strongly suggest their anatomic placement. The intermediate column (longissimus) and the medial column (spinalis) both split into three regional parts, the thoracis, cervicis, and capitis. All of these muscles serve to extend the vertebral column at various levels. Unilateral contraction of the iliocostalis muscle and the longissimus thoracis will cause lateral flexion and rotation to the same side. Lateral flexion and rotation of the cervical vertebrae and head are produced by the longissimus cervicis and capitis, respectively, when one side contracts. Spinalis thoracis and cervicis contracting unilaterally also cause lateral flexion. Spinalis capitis is generally associated

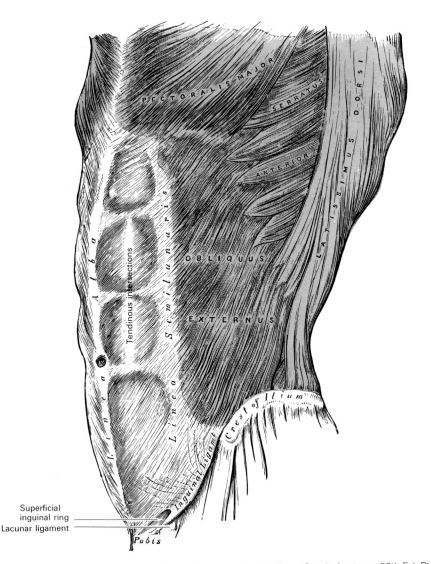

FIG. 11–12.   *A* and *B*, Superficial musculature of the abdomen and trunk. (From Gray's Anatomy. 30th Ed. Philadelphia, Lea & Febiger, 1985, p. 486, p. 489.)

structurally and functionally with semispinalis capitis.

The splenius muscles (cervicis and capitis) are often considered as a part of the erector spinae group. Both serve as cervical vertebrae extensors and can cause rotation of those vertebrae and the head.

The deep posterior spinal group includes the intertransversii, interspinales, rotatores, and multifidus, all of which serve to extend the vertebral column (Figs. 11–15 and 11–16). Acting unilaterally, these muscles can cause lateral flexion and rotation to the opposite side. It is important to note that, as is the case with all muscles, the degree to which these unilateral actions occur depends on the torque generated by the contraction. These muscles generally possess very small moment arms. For example, to the erector spinae acting at the L5-S1 joint has been attributed a moment arm of 24 mm.[20] Based on the muscle's observed line of pull, these resultant lateral flexion and rotary movements might very well be considered to be merely biomechanically predicted movements as opposed to significant movements.

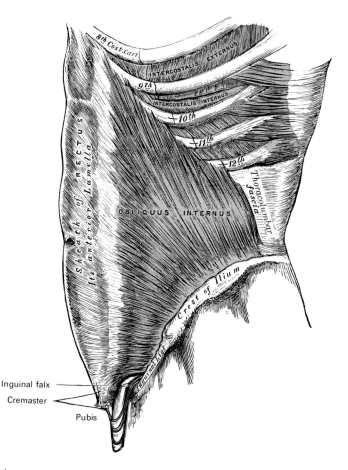

FIG. 11–12.   *Continued.*

ROLE OF THE ABDOMINAL MUSCULATURE IN THE REDUCTION OF VERTEBRAL LOADS

The lumbar vertebrae and their associated disks are subjected to very large forces during the course of everyday activity. Generally, fracture of the vertebral body will occur before rupture of a healthy disk.[21] Various researchers have estimated or measured the magnitudes of these forces. Because of the frequency of injuries to the back and the subsequent economic repercussions, vertebral column mechanics have been studied extensively. Some authors, seeking to quantify normally encountered forces on the vertebral column, have used biomechanical models. One model[22] estimated the compressive forces at L5 to be 10,000 N. Others have reported more conservative values of 4250 N compression.[7] In dynamic models, in which

forces resulting from inertia and acceleration must be considered, peak compressive forces of 7000 N have been reported.[23] Kumar and Davis[24] suggested that, as a general rule, dynamic lifts can be considered at least twice as stressful as static holds for the same resistance. Naturally, shear forces increase with compressive forces, and if loading is asymmetric, rotational forces are introduced.

The loads on the vertebral column, especially the lumbar region, should be kept as low as possible. Bartelink[25] hypothesized regarding the role of intra-abdominal pressure (IAP) in relieving vertebral loads. He observed clinically that individuals suffering from ruptured disks and nerve root compressions often displayed tense (contracted) abdominal musculature. Similarly, Morris and associates[26] proposed that the thoracic and abdominal cavities, under the compressive action of the abdominals, become quasi-static

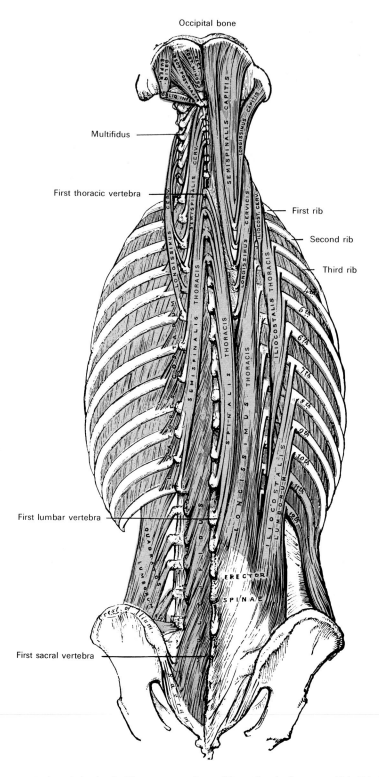

FIG. 11–13. Deep muscles of the back. The erector spinae. (From Gray's Anatomy. 30th Ed. Philadelphia, Lea & Febiger, 1985, p. 467.)

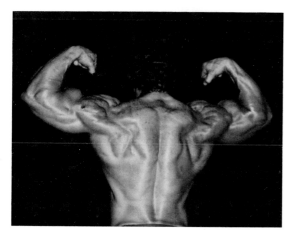

FIG. 11–14. Example of muscular hypertrophy associated with intensive weight training. Note the erector spinae of Roy Duval, former Mr. World. (Photo by Klemens.)

cylinders. These cylinders, supported by the perineum, were said to be capable of resisting part of the forces of the loaded trunk, essentially contributing to the required extensor torque. This is a biomechanical protective mechanism.

The relationship between strong abdominals and a healthy back has long been of interest to kinesiologists. An intuitive cause-effect relationship exists among abdominal muscle contraction, compression of the abdominal contents, and an increase in the IAP. The greater the IAP and the more rigid the thoracoabdominal cylinder, the greater the fraction of vertebral load shared, and the greater the reduction of the vertebral loads.

Davis[18] reviewed the importance of IAP with respect to evaluation of loads on the lumbar spine. The IAP versus time during lifting tasks has been characterized and the relationship between IAP and lumbar forces has been defined. Consistent with dynamic modeling of the back, peak IAP values associated with motion of the load and the trunk occur at the onset and termination of a lifting maneuver. These peaks are absent during static holds.

Ekholm and associates[27] reported on the activity of the abdominal muscles (rectus abdominis and external obliques) and the erector spinae demonstrated by four subjects during different lifting techniques. They showed that electromyographic activity of the erector spinae closely followed the calculated L5-S1 torque curves. It should be noted that the erector spinae EMGs have been shown to be strongly related to invasively measured intradiskal pressure and IAP.[28] Intradiskal pressure is measured directly by inserting pressure-sensitive transducers into the in vivo disk.

In the study by Ekholm et al.[27] the vertically oriented rectus abdominis was essentially inactive in four of five subjects. One subject, however, demonstrated a rectus abdominis activity profile that paralleled the L5-S1 torque calculations. This particular subject was tall and athletically trained, whereas the other subjects were classified as untrained. Similarly, Morris et al.[26] had previously reported rectus abdominis activity in tall subjects lifting heavy weights (approximately 441 N or 99 lb), demonstrating a consistent pattern and suggesting a potential training/learning or anatomically defined effect. External oblique muscles demonstrated low levels of EMG activity but, qualitatively, did vary well, with the torque calculations. This covariance, too, is consistent with the report by Morris et al.,[26] which showed more pronounced activation of these muscles during vertebral column loading.

Generally, the relationships among abdominal muscle activation, increases in IAP, and possible subsequent reduction of vertebral loads support the hypothesis regarding the reduction of lumbar loads by the abdominal muscles, though contradictory reports exist. Ekholm et al.[27] cite a study by Hamberg et al.[29] in which a coincidence between the peaks of IAP and abdominal muscle electromyograms did not occur. Krag et al.[30] also reported data suggesting a failure of IAP to reduce lumbar loads. It remains a reasonable argument that strong abdominals preemptively safeguard the low back against the myriad potentially hazardous activities in addition to maintaining a proper pelvic posture and avoiding the time-related and gravity-related sagging of the abdominal contents.

BASIC THORACIC MECHANISMS

The major purpose of the thorax, composed of the thoracic vertebrae, twelve corresponding pairs of ribs, the costal cartilages, and the sternum, is protection of the major respira-

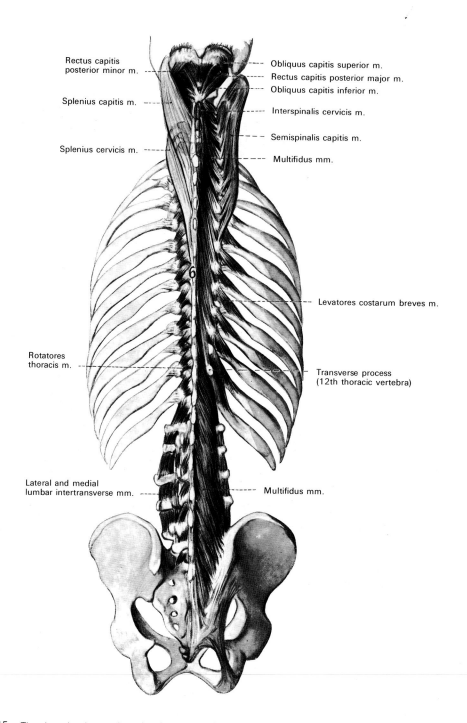

Rectus capitis
posterior minor m.

Splenius capitis m.

Splenius cervicis m.

Obliquus capitis superior m.
Rectus capitis posterior major m.
Obliquus capitis inferior m.

Interspinalis cervicis m.

Semispinalis capitis m.

Multifidus mm.

Levatores costarum breves m.

Rotatores
thoracis m.

Transverse process
(12th thoracic vertebra)

Lateral and medial
lumbar intertransverse mm.

Multifidus mm.

FIG. 11–15.   The deep back muscles, showing some of the transversospinal and interspinal intertransverse muscles. (From Benninghoff and Goerttler, Lehrbuch der Anatomie des Menschen. 11th Ed. Vol. 1. Urban & Schwarzenberg, 1975.)

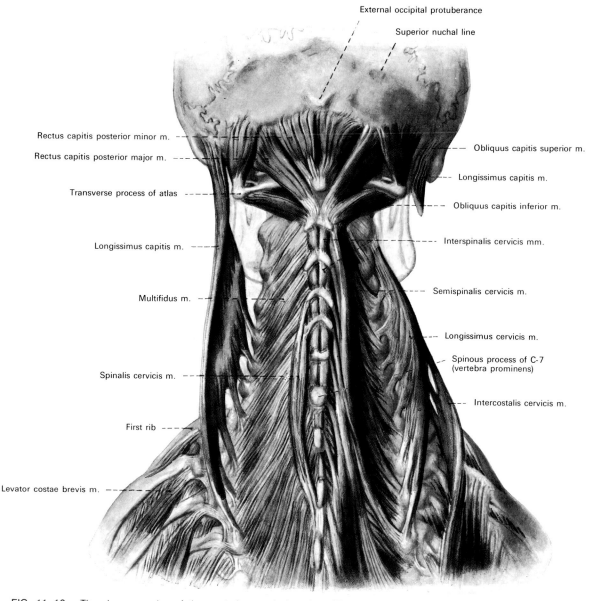

FIG. 11–16. The deep muscles of the posterior cervical region. (From Benninghoff and Goerttler, Lehrbuch der Anatomie des Menschen. 11th Ed., Vol. 1. Urban & Schwarzenberg, 1975.)

tory and circulatory systems components (Fig. 11–17).

Motion of the thorax is concerned primarily with respiration. The restricted range of thoracovertebral motion, as it relates specifically to the complexity and number of tasks underlying human motion, makes it of less concern than either the cervical and lumbar regions. Motion of the thorax is defined predominantly by elevation and depression of the ribs and, under various conditions, in-

cludes the participation of muscles previously discussed and others that merit consideration (Fig. 11–18). The primary muscles of respiration are generally considered to be the diaphragm and the intercostals. The scalene, sternomastoid, pectoral, serratus anterior, and abdominal muscles have been considered to be both agonists and accessory muscles.

In humans, the diaphragm is the foremost inspiratory muscle. With activation and subsequent contraction, the diaphragm expands

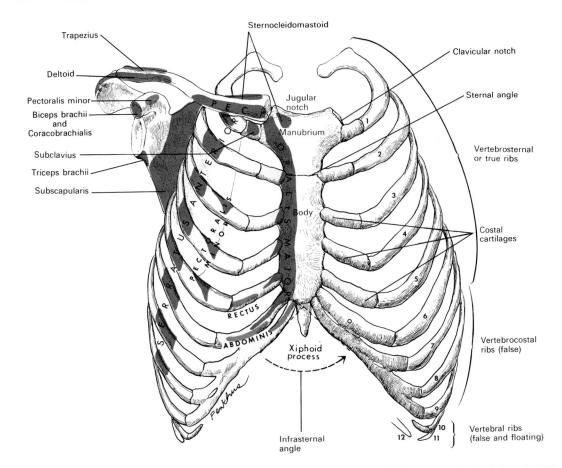

FIG. 11–17. Protective structure of the thorax. Observe the costal cartilages and their manner of articulation with the sternum. Suprasternally note the jugular notch on the superior border of the manubrium, lateral to which articulate the clavicles. The intrasternal angle is formed by the midline articulation of the costal margins of the two sides. Muscle origins are in red, insertions in blue. (From Gray's Anatomy. 30th Ed. Philadelphia, Lea & Febiger, 1985, p. 151.)

the base of the thorax by moving the ribs superiorly and laterally. This movement occurs by the forces transmitted through its central tendon (insertion) to its origin, which attaches nearly entirely around the inner surface of the body cavity. The range of diaphragmatic movement is approximately 1.5 cm during quiet respiration and 12.0 cm during deep respiration.

The internal obliques and external intercostals are active during expiration and inspiration, respectively. These muscles function according to the interspace at which they are located. The lower intercostals are essentially quiet during quiet breathing but are recruited as breathing becomes more vigorous. The recruitment occurs superiorly to inferiorly.

The abdominal muscles that serve as vertebral flexors and assist in generating IAP are anatomically situated such that they can aid in expiration. Indeed, it is well accepted that in humans the abdominals are the primary expiratory muscles.[31] The rectus abdominis is much less important than the internal oblique, external oblique, or transverse abdominis. All forced expiratory functions such as coughing and regurgitation, however, recruit all of these muscles. One role of the abdominals is to restrict the depth of maximum inspiration.

SPECIFIC DEFECTS
contributed by P. Rasch

The flexibility of the spinal column is sometimes reflected by the development of undesirable deviations.

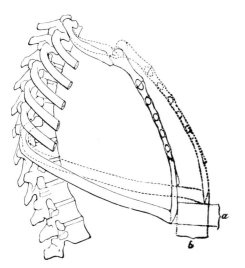

FIG. 11–18.   Enlargement of the chest by elevation of the ribs.

Kyphosis. Kyphosis and abducted scapulae are distinctly different, the former being an increased posterior convexity of the thoracic spine and the latter being a forward deviation of the shoulder girdle. One begets the other, however, and the two commonly appear together as an integrated defect.

Resistant or structural kyphosis, or any such defect accompanied by acute pain, indicates probable disease or hereditary defect of a more serious nature. Corrective exercises should never be given in such cases except when prescribed by a physician.

Lordosis. Lordosis is an increased posterior concavity of the normal lumbar or cervical curve, accompanied by a forward tilt of the pelvis.

The simpler type of hollow back is assumed temporarily whenever one carries a weight in the arm held in front of him, as when a waiter carries a heavy tray of dishes. The muscles of the lower back are shortened and the abdominal muscles are elongated. When this position is assumed habitually, too much weight is thrown on the posterior edges of the bodies of the lumbar vertebrae, and there is a marked tendency to develop abducted scapulae in compensation for the backward shifting of the body weight. Individuals who are more flexible than the average person have only to acquire the ability to assume the right position

of the spine and then to practice it until the habit is established.

When the pelvis is tilted too far forward, the back muscles and flexors of the hips are shortened while the abdominal muscles and hamstrings are elongated. It will do no good to correct the imbalance of trunk muscles alone or of hip muscles alone; both groups must be adjusted and controlled to keep the pelvis in its proper degree of inclination.

Exercises to correct lordosis will not be of any use when the pelvis is inclined too far forward. None will help to elongate the flexors of the hips. If the iliofemoral ligaments are short, they will tilt the pelvis forward in spite of all the muscles can do to prevent it. When the flexors of the hips and iliofemoral ligaments are just a little short, it may be possible to stretch them in the following manner: lie supine, knees extended, and try to press the lumbar part of the back close to the floor. Possibly putting one hand there and trying to press the back against it will help. The work has to be done by the hamstrings, glutei, and abdominal muscles, against the resistance of the extensors of the lumbar spine, flexors of the hips, and iliofemoral ligaments. A variation that will sometimes help is to flex the knees a few degrees, sliding the feet along the floor toward the hips; then press the back down against the floor and hold it there while slowly extending the knees. This uses the extensors of the knees, along with the hamstrings and abdominal muscles, to stretch the flexors of the hips and the iliofemoral ligaments.

Making an intelligent decision as to when a lordotic back needs correction is a matter of some difficulty. Scandinavian authors appear convinced that backs with greater than average lordotic curves are stronger and, vice versa, that stronger backs are more lordotic, than the average.

Flat Back (Lumbar Kyphosis). Flat back involves an abdominal decrease in the normal lumbar curve. The angle of obliquity of the pelvis is reduced, as the hamstrings are too short and the flexors of the hip and the iliofemoral ligaments are too long. It is commonly associated with the round shoulders, flat chest, and protruding abdomen characteristic of the clinical picture of fatigue. The

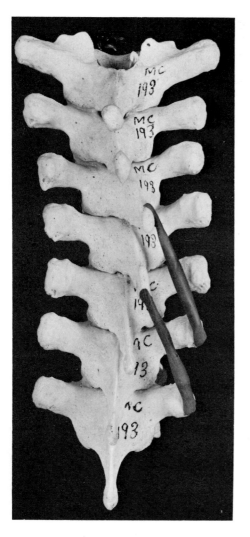

FIG. 11–19.   This illustration of a segment of the spinal column demonstrates the manner in which the unopposed action of the deeper muscles of the spine (semispinalis, multifidus, and rotatores) causes the vertebrae to rotate into a scoliotic position when the muscles of the opposite side are paretic. (Photo by Allbrook.)

condition is difficult to correct, but attention to increasing the strength and tone of the abdominal and erector spinae muscles may prove rewarding.

Lateral Curvature. Lateral curvature of the spine, which in pronounced stages is called *scoliosis,* is a sideward deviation. It represents a combination of lateral deviation and longitudinal rotation. One might expect that the muscles on the concave side of the curve would be stronger than those on the convex side, and this is what would be observed if the curve were due to unopposed action of the longitudinal muscles. However, electromyographic studies have shown that in the majority of cases the muscles on the concave side are weaker than normal. This is attributed to the fact that imbalance of the deeper muscles (semispinal, multifidus, and rotators) is the main factor in producing the deformity. These deep muscles are important rotators. When those of one side are paretic, the unopposed action of the muscles of the opposite side rotates the vertebrae into a scoliotic position[27,28] (Fig. 11–16).

In some cases, however, the muscles on the convex side are atrophied and those on the concave side are contracted. Whether the changes that then take place can be explained on the basis of muscle imbalance alone is controversial.[28] Roaf believes that lordosis is a lengthening of the anterior longitudinal ligaments and a shortening of the posterior components.[29–31] Under the influence of the abdominal muscles, gravity, respiration, and other factors, a rotation of the vertebrae develops and a lateral curvature appears. The complexities involved in scoliotic defects should make it obvious that physical educators and therapists should not attempt to "correct" them without the advice and guidance of a qualified physician.

Lateral curvature lessens the ability of the spine to support the body weight, distorts the body cavities, crowds the organs out of place, and in advanced cases causes pressure on the spinal nerves where they pass out of the vertebral canal. Scoliosis usually begins with a single C-curve. This may be to either side, but because most people are right-handed, the muscles on the right side of the body are generally stronger and the convexity tends to develop to the left. The condition tends to be more prevalent in girls and among ectomorphic types, but it is not confined to either. The curvature may extend the whole length of the spine or it may be localized. A C-curve may tilt the head sideways, in which case there is a reflex tendency to right it until the eyes are again level. Over a period of time this righting reflex creates a reversal of the C-curve at the upper spinal levels, producing an S-curve. Further attempts at compensations may appear, creating additional undulations in the curve (Fig. 11–19).

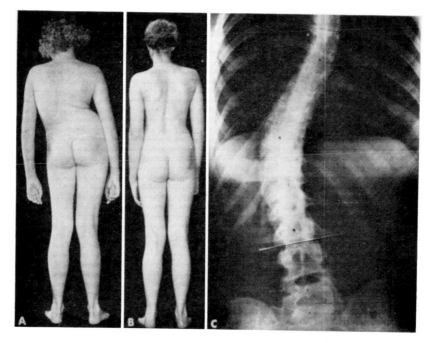

FIG. 11–20. *A,* Severe thoracolumbar curve after poliomyelitis in a 14-year-old girl. *B,* The same girl 2 years later, following correction by turnbuckle cast and spinal fusion from the seventh thoracic to the third lumbar vertebra. *C,* X-ray of spine of this patient at age 18. (Reprinted with permission from Risser, J.C.: Scoliosis, past and present. J. Bone Joint Surg., *76A:*167–199, 1964.)

In the early stages scoliosis may be *functional,* or *postural.* These terms indicate that the curve can be obliterated by voluntary effort or by hanging from the hands. In the later stages the condition becomes *resistant,* or *structural,* and the curve can no longer be so obliterated. Once a structural curve is established, corrective exercises may produce a compensatory curve rather than an abolition of the primary curve.

Scoliosis may be caused by numerous unilateral conditions, including hereditary defects in structure; deterioration of vertebrae,

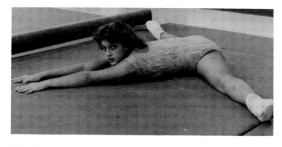

FIG. 11–21. The pancake, a gymnastic maneuver requiring extreme flexibility. Another such maneuver is the back walkover (see Fig. 11–6).

ligaments, or muscles as the result of infections or disease; unilateral paralysis of spinal muscles; unilateral short leg; unilateral flatfoot or pronation; and imbalance of muscular development as the result of occupation or habit.

Preliminary studies of children in early adolescence have revealed that 11% show symptoms of scoliosis. The majority of the curves were thoracolumbar. Nineteen states have passed laws requiring the screening of school children for signs of scoliosis, but the problem remains severe. The Scoliosis Research Society estimates that 700,000 children between ages 10 and 14 are affected by some degree of scoliosis. Because it progresses with growth and there is no way to predict the extent to which it will develop in a given patient, early identification and treatment is essential.

Until recently, structural scoliosis was corrected by use of a body cast and spinal fusion (Fig. 11–20). The newest development in the treatment of simple C-curves in children is the use of electronic devices that stimulate the weak back muscles during a patient's sleep.

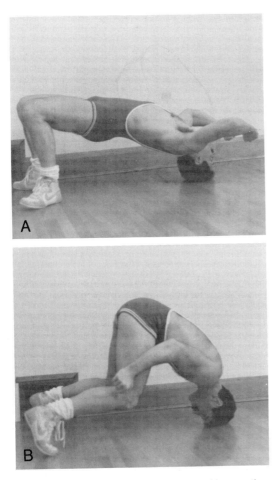

FIG. 11–22. *A,* A defensive maneuver used by wrestlers when they are in danger of being pinned. Typically, the offensive wrestler would have his mass somewhere over this individual's upper thorax. *B,* Another often-used neck bridging position common in wrestling.

Since the 1960s, resistant cases often have been treated with a Harrington rod implant. A metal rod with a ratchet mechanism is attached to the vertebrae above and below the curve and the curve is straightened by lengthening the rod with the ratchet. Other surgical techniques require that the vertebrae be wired to one or two rods, or use a combination of the two methods.

It would appear that the role of the kinesiologist is decidedly limited in the treatment of such cases, but Roaf[31] comments that successful techniques must combine the patient's own muscular efforts with an external force over an extended period of time. Unless joint mobility and good muscular coordination are achieved, true postural control cannot be achieved.

NEURAL INNERVATIONS

longus colli: branches from the ventral rami of C2 to C6.

longus capitis: branches from C1, C2, and C3.

rectus capitis anterior: fibers from the anterior rami of C1 (and possibly C2).

rectus capitis lateralis: a branch of the loop between C1 and C2.

sternocleidomastoid: the spinal part of the accessory and branches of the anterior rami of C2 and C3.

scalenus anterior: branches from the anterior rami of C5 and C6 (and sometimes C4).

scalenus medius: branches from the anterior rami of C3 through C8.

scalenus posterior: branches of the ventral primary divisions of the last three cervical nerves.

quadratus lumborum: branches of C12 and L1.

rectus abdominis: branches of I7 through I12.

external oblique: branches of I8 through I12, the iliohypogastric nerve, and the ilioinguinal nerve.

internal oblique: branches of I8 through I12, the iliohypogastric nerve, and the ilioinguinal nerve.

transverse abdominis: branches from I7 through I12, the iliohypogastric nerve, and the ilioinguinal nerve.

iliocostalis lumborum: posterior rami of the spinal nerves

iliocostalis thoracis: posterior rami of the spinal nerves

iliocostalis cervicis: posterior rami of the spinal nerves

longissimus thoracis: posterior rami of the spinal nerves

longissimus cervicis: posterior rami of the spinal nerves

longissimus capitis: posterior rami of the spinal nerves

spinalis thoracis: posterior rami of the spinal nerves

spinalis cervicis: posterior rami of the spinal nerves

spinalis capitis: posterior rami of the spinal nerves

splenius cervicis: posterior rami of the lower cervical nerves

splenius capitis: lateral branches of the posterior rami of the middle and lower cervical nerves.

intertransversarii: anterior and posterior rami of the spinal nerves.

interspinales: posterior rami of the spinal nerves

rotatores: posterior rami of the spinal nerves.

multifidi: posterior rami of the spinal nerves.

diaphragm: the phrenic nerve from the cervical plexus with fibers mostly from the fourth but also from the adjacent cervical nerves.

intercostalis interni: the intercostal nerves.

intercostalis externi: the intercostal nerves.

STUDY QUESTIONS

1. Present discussion describing why females generally possess a larger lumbar curve than males and why the direction of the thoracic curve in the frontal plane should be related to the dominant handedness of the individual.

2. Analyze Figures 11–21 and 11–6 and discuss the ligaments and muscles responsible for maintaining the integrity of the vertebral column.

3. Wrestlers often perform what is called a "neck bridge" (Fig. 11–22). What passive and active structures in the cervical region are stressed during both front and back neck bridges and during the transition to one from the other?

4. Observe the origins and insertions of the internal and external obliques and, using the concept of moment of inertia as a premise, develop an argument based on mechanical principles as to why each of these muscles causes an oppositely directed trunk rotation. Similarly, describe why the transverse abdominis does not cause any trunk movement.

5. Weight lifters may often be observed to wear broad belts around their waists. Similarly, girdles, primarily cosmetic in nature but also used for support, are very much in use by certain populations. Discuss the role of these devices mechanically and neuromuscularly in terms of what and how they may contribute to vertebral support and any detrimental effects of their chronic use.

6. Discuss why maximal inspiration requires an anatomic limit and possible mechanisms by which the abdominals may serve in this capacity.

REFERENCES

1. Jayson, M.: Backache: a matter of structural distress. New Scientist, 71:320, 1976.
2. Gray, H.: Anatomy of the Human Body, 30th Ed. Edited by C.D. Clemente. Philadelphia, Lea & Febiger, 1985.
3. Lindh, M.: Biomechanics of the lumbar spine. In Basic Biomechanics of the Skeletal System. Edited by V.H. Frankel and M. Nordin. Philadelphia, Lea & Febiger, 1980.
4. White, A.A., and Punjabi, M.M.: Clinical Biomechanics of the Spine. Philadelphia, J.B. Lippincott, 1978.
5. Alexander, M.J.: Biomechanical aspects of lumbar spine injuries in athletes: a review. Can. J. Appl. Sports Sciences, 10:1, 1985.
6. Toufexis, A.: That aching back! Time, 114:30, 1980.
7. Troup, J.G.: The risk of weight-training and weight-lifting in young people; functional anatomy of the spine. Br. J. Sports Med., 5:27, 1970.
8. Schellinger, D.: The low back pain syndrome. Med. Clin. North Am., 68:1631, 1984.
9. Guten, G.: Herniated lumbar disc associated with running. Am. J. of Sports Med., 9:155, 1981.
10. Crossen, D.: Getting back to running. Runners World, 15:72, 1980.
11. Fair, J.: Low back pain in women athletes. Coaching Women Athletes, 5:64, 1979.
12. Stover, C.N., Wiren, G., and Topaz, S.R.: The modern golf swing and stress syndrome. Phys. Sports Med., 4:43, 1976.
13. Stallard, M.C.: Backache in oarsmen. Br. J. Sports Med., 14:105, 1980.
14. Floyd, W.F., and Silver, P.S.: The function of the erector spinae in flexion of the trunk. Lancet, 1:133, 1951.
15. Floyd, W.F., and Silver, P.S.: The function of the erector spinae muscles in certain movements and postures in man. J. Physiol. (Lond.), 129:184, 1955.
16. Pauly, J.E.: An electromyographic analysis of certain

movements and exercises—some deep muscles of the back. Anat. Rec., *155*:223, 1966.

17. Wolf, S.L., Basmajian, J.V., Russo, C.T., and Kutner, M.: Normative data on low back mobility and activity levels. Am. J. Phys. Med., *58*:217, 1979.

18. Grabiner, M.D., Azcueta, S., and Campbell, K.R.: Flexion relaxation revisited: clinical applications. Biomechanics XI, in press.

19. Davis, P.R.: The role of intra-abdominal pressure in evaluating stresses on the lumbar spine. Spine, *6*:90, 1981.

20. Nemeth, G., and Ohlsen, H.: Moment arm lengths of trunk muscles to the lumbosacral joint obtained in vivo with computed tomography. Spine, *11*:158, 1986.

21. Eie, N.: Load capacity of the low back. J Oslo City Hosp., *16*:73, 1966.

22. Morris, J.M.: Biomechanics of the spine. Arch. Surg., *107*:418, 1973.

23. Frievalds, A., Chaffin, D.B., Garg, A., and Lee, K.S.: A dynamic biomechanical evaluation of lifting maximum acceptable loads. J. Biomech., *17*:251, 1984.

24. Kumar, S., and Davis, P.R.: Spinal loading in static and dynamic postures: EMG and intra-abdominal pressure study. Ergonomics (London), *26*:913, 1983.

25. Bartelink, D.L. The role of abdominal pressure in relieving pressure on the lumbar intervertebral discs. J. Bone Joint Surg., *39*:718, 1957.

26. Morris, J.M, Lucas, D.B., and Bresler, B.: Role of the trunk in stability of the spine. J. Bone Joint Surg., *43A*:327, 1961.

27. Ekholm, J., Arborelius, V.P., and Nemeth, G.: The load on the lumbo-sacral joint and trunk muscle activity during lifting. Ergonomics (London), *25*:145, 1982.

28. Ortengren, R., Andersson, G., and Nachemson, A.: Studies of the relationships between lumbar disc pressure, myoelectric back muscles activity, and intra-abdominal (intra-gastric) pressure. Spine, *6*:98, 1981.

29. Hamberg, J., et al.: Activation of abdominal muscles and intra-abdominal pressure—before and after training of the abdominal muscles. Byg ghalsans Forskningsstifteise, *4*: 1978 (In Swedish).

30. Krag, M.H., Byrne, K.B., Gilbertson, L.G., and Haugh, L.D.: Failure of intraabdominal pressurization to reduce erector spinae loads during lifting tasks. Presented at the North American Conference on Biomechanics, Montreal, Canada, August, 1986.

31. Roaf, R.: The basic anatomy of scoliosis. J. Bone Joint Surg., *78B*:786–792, 1966.

12 THE HIP JOINT

MARK D. GRABINER

ANATOMIC CONSIDERATIONS

The hip joint is a diarthrodial ball-and-socket joint that, unlike the glenohumeral joint (another ball-and-socket articulation), possesses inherent architectural stability. It is formed by the insertion of the head of the femur into the acetabulum of the os coxae (hip bone). The acetabulum itself is formed by the union of the three pelvic bones, the ilium, the ischium, and the pubis. These bones, each of which makes up approximately one-third of the acetabulum, are not completely ossified until the middle of the second decade of life. The acetabular cavity is positioned such that it faces laterally, inferiorly, and anteriorly as it receives the femoral head (Fig. 12–1).

The articular capsule of the hip joint is extremely strong and dense. It attaches to the rim of the acetabulum and at the neck of the femur. Anteriorly, where the greatest strength is required, the capsule is much thicker than it is posteriorly, where it is thin and loose. Reinforcing accessory ligaments found at the external-anterior aspect of the capsule include the iliofemoral, the pubofemoral, and the ischiofemoral ligaments. The iliofemoral ligament restrains hip extension and can also limit rotation of the femur around its long axis. The ligament is a factor in preventing the trunk from rotating backward during standing thus reducing the need for muscular contraction to maintain erect posture. The pubofemoral ligament restricts hip abduction as well as extension and outward rotation (Fig. 12–2). The ischiofemoral ligament, located more posteriorly than the

others, limits inward rotation of the hip (Fig. 12–3).

The acetabular labrum, for which an analogous structure exists at the glenohumeral joint, is a fibrocartilaginous rim that lines the margin of the acetabulum, serving to deepen the socket, thereby improving the stability of the joint. Additionally, the labrum protects the edge of bone. Specific sex-related differences exist in the geometry of the human pelvis. In addition to the well-known differences in pelvic width and height between males and females, the femoral head is significantly smaller (by 30%) in females than males. Though the small head would be expected to result in greater stress on the female hip joint,[1] the labrum plays a crucial role in reducing force at the joint and perhaps retarding the onset or occurrence of stress-related injuries or disorders. The acetabular notch, a discontinuity in the structure, is spanned by the transverse acetabular ligament. When this ligament is considered as an extension of the acetabular labrum, the labrum completely envelops the joint (Fig. 12–4).

JOINT MOVEMENTS

Despite the inherent stability afforded to the hip joint by virtue of its architecture and ligamentous support, the hip joint demonstrates a large degree of mobility. The motions allowed by the hip, described with respect to the femur, include flexion and extension in the sagittal plane, abduction and adduction in the frontal plane, and internal (medial, in-

193

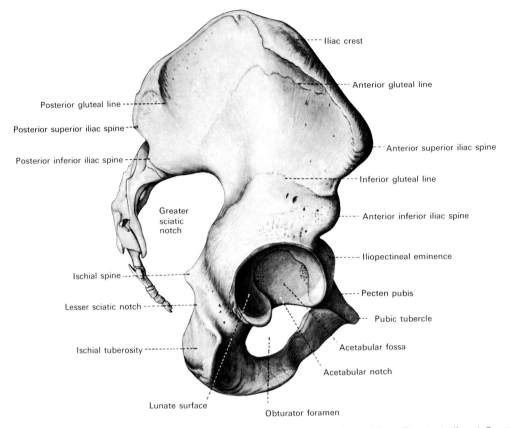

FIG 12–1   Right hip bone with sacrum and coccyx. External or lateral surface. (From Benninghoff and Goerttler, Lehrbuch der Anatomie des Menschen. 11th Ed., Vol. 1. Urban & Schwarzenberg, 1975.)

ward) and external (lateral, outward) rotation in the transverse plane.

The positioning of the shaft of the femur, by way of the femoral neck, some distance away from the bony pelvis helps prevent restrictions to the range of motion of the hip joint that could result from impingement. The neck-shaft angle allows the shaft of the femur to be positioned more laterally from the pelvis. In the frontal plane, with respect to the long axis of the femur, the normal neck-shaft angle is approximately 125°. Deformity in which the angle is larger, termed coxa vara, and deformity in which the angle is smaller, termed coxa valga, cause changes in the transmission of forces both to and from the femur.

A second angle, that of anteversion, is the angle at which the neck projects from the femur in the anteroposterior direction. Although large variation exists among individuals, the normal value is approximately 12 to 14°.[2]

The hip joint can move independently of the pelvic girdle but can be complemented by pelvic tilts. Unlike the open system of the shoulder girdle, the closed system of the pelvic girdle makes moving the right side independently of the left impossible. In the upright position, the superior and inferior apertures of the pelvis form angles to the horizontal plane of approximately 50 to 60° and 15°, respectively. This angle is called the inclination of the pelvis[2] (Fig. 12–5).

Pelvic tilts are rotations measured with respect to the pelvic inclination and are classified with respect to the hips and lumbosacral joints. Forward tilt is associated with hip flexion and lumbosacral hyperextension. Backward tilt is associated with the opposite motions, hip extension and lumbosacral flexion. Right lateral tilt involves left lateral flexion of the lumbosacral joint, abduction of the right hip, and adduction of the left hip. Left lateral tilt involves the same motions to the opposite sides.

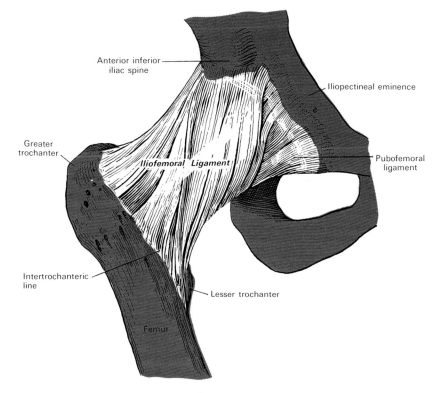

Anterior inferior iliac spine

Iliopectineal eminence

Greater trochanter

Iliofemoral Ligament

Pubofemoral ligament

Intertrochanteric line

Lesser trochanter

Femur

FIG. 12–2. Right hip joint viewed anteriorly. (From Gray's Anatomy. 30th Ed. Philadelphia, Lea & Febiger, 1985, p. 391.)

The hip joint demonstrates its largest range of motion in the sagittal plane, in which flexion can be found to go to 140° and extension to 15°. Abduction can also go to 30°, and adduction is just slightly less than this, to 25°.[3,4] Adduction must be associated with some flexion. The degree of hip flexion will affect the magnitude of medial and lateral rotation. In an extended position, in which the restraining effects of the ligamentous tissues are manifested, the ranges of internal and external rotation are reduced to 70° and 90°, respectively.

MUSCULATURE OF THE HIP JOINT

There are 22 muscles that act on the hip joint. Several classification schemes have been presented, but a straightforward method is merely to identify those muscles that make major contributions to each of the possible hip joint actions.

The members of the flexor group include the psoas and iliacus, the primary agonists, and rectus femoris (Fig. 12–6). The psoas (major and minor) plays a major role not only as a hip flexor but also as a hip joint stabilizer. Because the origin of the psoas is the bodies and the intervertebral disks of T12-L5, the psoas probably has some influence on the lumbar vertebrae,[4] that is, hyperextension. The iliacus muscle, like the psoas, plays a predominant role in hip flexion under almost any condition and range of motion. The potential influence of the psoas at the lumbar curve is not an issue, however, as the iliacus muscle originates on the inner surface of the ilium. Any other hip actions ascribed to this muscle can only be minor. The rectus femoris, a member of the quadriceps femoris group, is the only muscle of the group that acts on the hip. A major hip flexor, rectus femoris has been said to assist in external rotation and abduction. Based on its line of pull, one would expect that these contributions are small.

The extensor group at the hip includes the hamstring muscles, semimembranosus muscle, semitendinosus muscle, and long head of the biceps femoris (Fig. 12–7). The biceps femoris, which are two separate origins, each

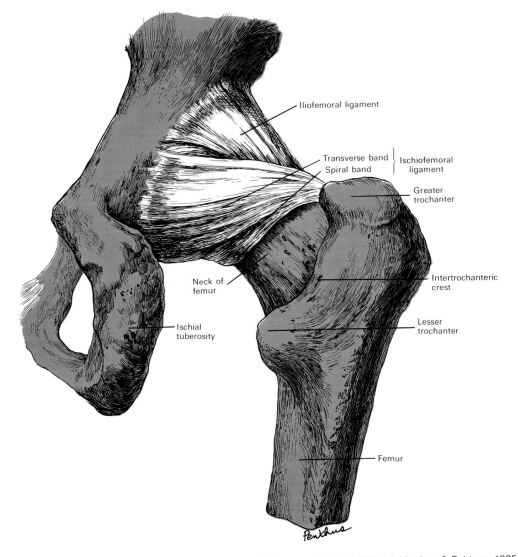

Iliofemoral ligament

Transverse band
Spiral band
} Ischiofemoral ligament

Greater trochanter

Neck of femur

Intertrochanteric crest

Ischial tuberosity

Lesser trochanter

Femur

FIG. 12–3. Right hip joint viewed posteriorly. (From Gray's Anatomy. 30th Ed. Philadelphia, Lea & Febiger, 1985, p. 392.)

having a separate nerve supply, are active in ordinary hip extension, whereas the semimembranosus and semitendinosus muscles are active in extension against resistance. The biceps femoris suffers a large number of hamstring pulls, perhaps as a result of incoordination in the actions of the fibers composing the two muscles.

The gluteus maximus muscle (Fig. 12–8) also is a strong extensor during heavy or moderate efforts in addition to being an external rotator and, depending on the aspect of the muscle under consideration (superior versus inferior), either an abductor (of the flexed hip) or an adductor (against an abduction resistance). Although not an important postural muscle,[5] it is moderately active during eccentric trunk flexion and very active in concentric trunk extension. During standing, trunk rotation can elicit activity of the gluteus maximus muscle on the side opposite to the rotation, a motion that essentially represents a lateral hip rotation.[6]

The adductor group of the hip is composed of the gracilis (Figs. 12–6 and 12–7), adductor longus, adductor brevis, adductor magnus, and pectineus muscles (Fig. 12–9). Found on the medial aspect of the thigh, the adductors

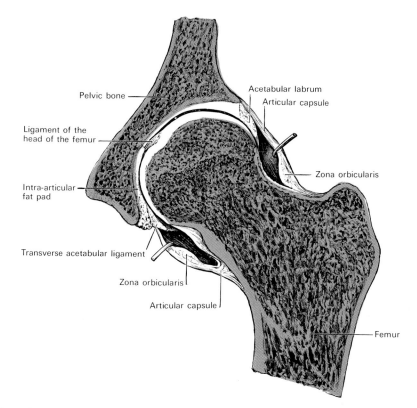

FIG. 12–4. Coronal section through the hip joint. (From Gray's Anatomy. 30th Ed. Philadelphia, Lea & Febiger, 1985, p. 394.)

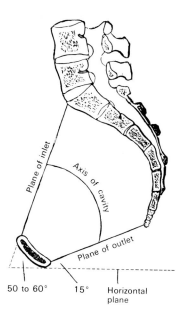

FIG. 12–5. A sagittal diagram of the female pelvis showing that the plane of the pelvic inlet forms an angle of 50 to 60° with the horizontal plane, while the plane of the outlet forms an angle of 15°. Observe the curvature of the pelvic axis between the planes of inlet and outlet. (From Gray's Anatomy. 30th Ed. Philadelphia, Lea & Febiger, 1985, p. 272.)

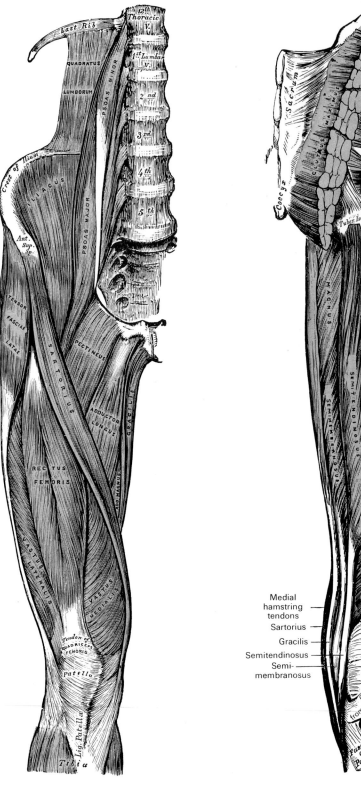

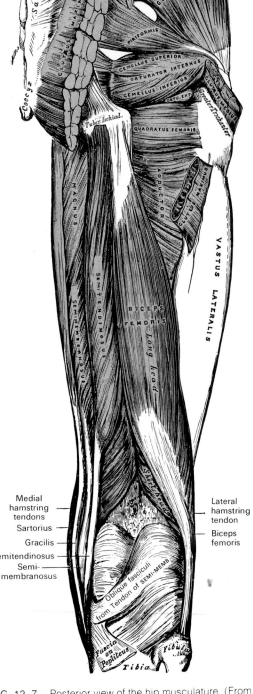

FIG. 12–6.   Anterior view of the hip musculature. (From Gray's Anatomy. 30th Ed. Philadelphia, Lea & Febiger, 1985, p. 558.)

FIG. 12–7.   Posterior view of the hip musculature. (From Gray's Anatomy. 30th Ed. Philadelphia. Lea & Febiger. 1985. p. 567.)

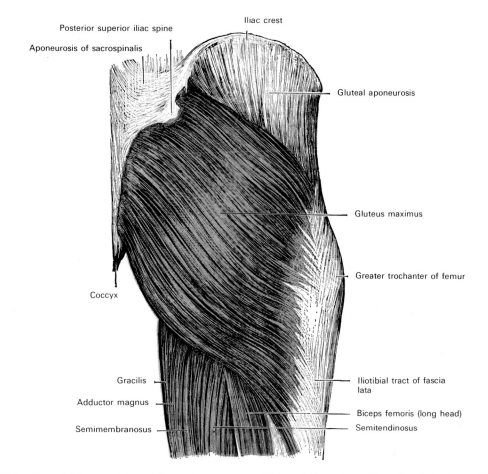

Posterior superior iliac spine

Iliac crest

Aponeurosis of sacrospinalis

Gluteal aponeurosis

Gluteus maximus

Greater trochanter of femur

Coccyx

Gracilis

Iliotibial tract of fascia lata

Adductor magnus

Biceps femoris (long head)

Semimembranosus

Semitendinosus

FIG. 12–8.   Superficial musculature of the posterior superior thigh and hip regions. (From Gray's Anatomy. 30th Ed. Philadelpha, Lea & Febiger, 1985, p. 566.)

form most of the muscle mass in that area, creating somewhat of a contradiction of the structure-function relationship. One would expect that a muscle group of this size would play a critical role in locomotion, stance, and general movement, yet the movement of adduction is somewhat less than critical. One explanation for the size of the adductor mass is that at least two secondary joint actions at the hip occur for each adductor, as well as potential knee actions. In addition to the obvious role of adduction, medial rotation is ascribed to the adductor longus and adductor magnus muscle.[7] The adductor longus has been observed to demonstrate activity during hip flexion.[8] Dancers and gymnasts are said to be subject to tearing of the fibers of this muscle near its tendinous attachment to the pubis while performing splits.

The abductor group is composed of several muscles that act predominantly in other joint actions. Few activities require forceful hip abduction. The gluteus medius muscle is considered a prime mover for this action and plays an important role in stabilizing the pelvis during locomotion and in preventing the Trendelenburg sign (lateral pelvic tilt or hip drop). Other muscles that can assist in abduction when the motion is resisted, when the hip is in a particular position, or under both circumstances include the gluteus minimus, the gluteus maximus, the rectus femoris, the sartorius muscle, and the tensor fascia latae. The role of the tensor fascia latae depends highly on the rotation (internal or external) of the hip.[9]

The abductor mechanism includes both the gluteus medius and maximus[10] and is related to the need for the pelvic rim to be pulled toward the greater trochanter during the

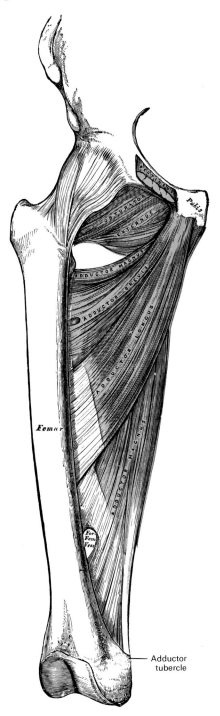

FIG. 12–9. Deep muscles of the medial femoral region. (From Gray's Anatomy. 30th Ed. Philadelphia, Lea & Febiger, 1985, p. 565.)

stance phase of locomotion. The abductors of the support leg prevent the dropping of the pelvis to the contralateral side, which would be caused by the weight of the body mass above the hip and the inertial characteristics of the swing leg.

Numerous previously presented muscles contribute to the internal or external rotation of the femur about its long axis. The gluteus medius and minimus, tensor fascia latae, adductor longus and magnus, and the gracilis muscle can all serve to internally rotate the femur.[4] Soderberg[10] indicated the primary agonists to be the gluteus medius and minimus. Based only on these two muscles and the estimation that the "power" of the rotators is about 33% that of the external rotators, Soderberg suggested they are relatively unimportant.

External rotation is a function of a part of the gluteus maximus, the rectus femoris, and a group of six muscles generally grouped as the outward rotators (Fig. 12–7). The group, including the piriformis muscle, the internal obturator, the external obturator, the quadriceps femoris, and the superior and interior gemellus muscles, basically performs only outward rotation, although the piriformis muscle, the internal obturator muscle, and the gemelli can help abduct the flexed hip.[2]

Two-Joint (Multijoint) Muscles

Multijoint muscles are those that cross a number of joints and create significant kinetics at those joints. The muscles of the lower extremity are often used as anatomic examples and research topics with respect to the specific mechanisms of their control by the central nervous system and the resultant joint actions. Markee et al.[11] suggested that two-joint muscles might act at one end without influencing the other; this hypothesis was contradicted by Basmajian and DeLuca.[12] The general rule regarding a two-joint muscle (with ony one head) is that it pulls both of its tendons nonselectively toward the belly of the muscle, thereby influencing both joints. A two-joint muscle cannot act as a one-joint muscle without the assistance of other muscles and unless one of the joint actions is stabilized by other muscles. The kinetic effect of the muscle on the second joint is decreased.

A simple example of multijoint muscle activity is the psoas paradox, in which the psoas muscle, while flexing the hip, causes hyperextension of the lumbosacral region through anterior pelvic tilt, even though the psoas is considered a trunk flexor. The paradox, the extension/flexion role reversal, can be observed during exercises such as straight-leg sit-ups and double-leg raises. The lumbar vertebrae are pulled anteriorly and inferiorly by the contraction of the psoas. Simultaneous contraction of the abdominals prevents the anterior tilt of the pelvis unless the abdominals are fatigued or weak, in which case the pelvis does not rotate anteriorly and the lumbar vertebrae are not hyperextended.

Lombard's paradox is defined as the "activity of a two-joint muscle when the required torque at one joint is in the opposite direction to that caused by the muscle."[13] This is easily demonstrated when rising from a chair, a condition during which contraction of the quadriceps femoris and the hamstrings is evident. In this case the extensor torque at the hip by the hamstrings is in excess of the flexor torque at the hip by the rectus femoris. Similarly, at the knee, the extensor torque of the quadriceps dominates the flexor torque of the hamstrings. This inequity has raised questions regarding metabolic economy during conditions of Lombard's paradox.

During some combinations of joint actions, motions created by two-joint muscles are more efficient than they would be if created by uniarticular muscles. During running, for example, just prior to heel contact the hip extensors perform positive work on the hip at the same time that they perform negative work on the shank to decelerate the extension at the knee. Fortunately, the hamstrings can perform both functions simultaneously at a small metabolic cost. Elftman[14] estimated the energy expenditure for two- and one-joint muscles to perform this task to be 2.61 and 3.97 horsepower, respectively. Performance by a two-joint muscle represents an energy savings of over 34%.

Tendinous action, belt-like action, and pulley action are characteristics attributed to two-joint muscles because these muscles cannot

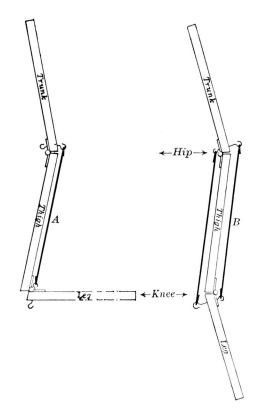

FIG. 12–10. Lombard's paradox. *A*, Hamstring extending hip and flexing knee. *B*, Hamstring with aid of tendon action of rectus femoris, extending both joints.

cause a full range of motion simultaneously at each joint on which they act.[15] An example of the mechanism of tendinous action using a three-segment model of the trunk, thigh, and shank is presented in Figure 12–10.

The contraction of the "hamstrings," represented in Figure 12–10A by an elastic band, causes both knee flexion and hip extension. In Figure 12–10B, a taut cord is placed in the model to represent the rectus femoris. The fact that the cord is taut indicates some degree of muscle stiffness due, in part, to the cord's rectus femoris activation. When the hamstrings contract and the hips extend, rotation of the pelvis will displace the origin of the rectus femoris posteriorly, which will transmit tension through the cord and cause knee extension. In a sense, some of the hamstring tension is transmitted to the rectus femoris through the pulley of the bony pelvis. Remember that a pulley is a simple machine that alters the direction of a force application. Note that knee extension is opposed by the knee flexion torque of the hamstrings. It is the vectoral sum of the torques that will determine the resultant angular motion.

Gregiore and associates[16] investigated energy flow from the hips through the knee and the ankle during vertical jumping. Their model reflects the tendinous action of the involved two-joint muscles. Additionally illustrated is a characteristic of two-joint muscles that allows the muscles to exert concentric force without necessarily shortening significantly, which would result in a loss of contractile force. This exertion of force is related to the concepts of concurrent and countercurrent movement patterns.

When the hip and knee flex simultaneously, such as in the preparatory move of a karate kick, or extend simultaneously, as in the attack phase of the kick, the muscle contracts yet does not lose as much of its length as two uniarticular muscles would if performing the same action. In Figure 12–11B, as the rectus femoris shortens at one end to flex the hip, it lengthens distally as the knee flexes; this is an example of a concurrent movement pattern with respect to the muscular contraction.

In a countercurrent movement pattern, one two-joint muscle of an antagonistic pair shortens at both ends while the other lengthens. Simultaneous hip flexion and knee extension shorten the rectus femoris at both ends while stretching the hamstrings at both ends. A punt is a example of this type of movement (Fig. 12–12).

MECHANICAL CONSIDERATIONS OF INJURY TO THE PELVIC AND HIP REGIONS

PELVIS

The iliac crest is particularly susceptible to injury because of its superficial location (as is the case for the sacrum) and the mass of soft tissues in the immediate area. Contusions such as "hip pointers" include periostitis (inflammation of the periosteum) of the iliac crest, strain, and muscular avulsions.[13] More serious, of course, are fractures of the ilium, which are infrequent because most sports involving forces that could result in this type of

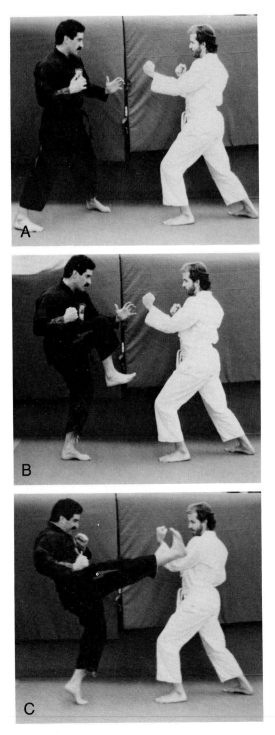

FIG. 12–11.   *A*, *B*, and *C*, An example of a concurrent movement pattern.

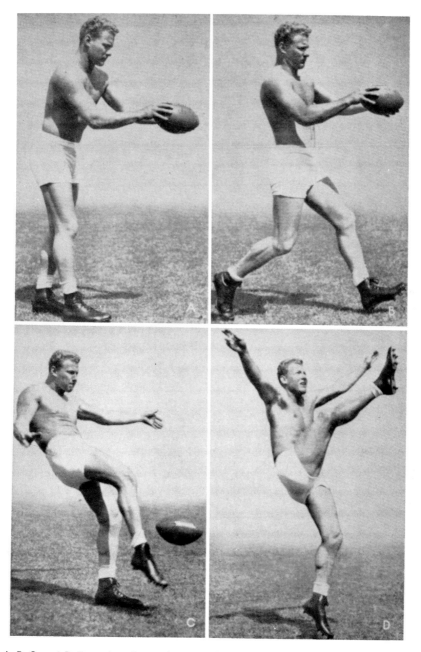

FIG. 12-12.   *A, B, C,* and *D,* Examples of a countercurrent movement pattern.

injury require protective padding.[17] Intense running and jumping may often cause fractures of the anterior superior iliac spine.

HIP JOINT

The hip joint is extremely stable and has a large range of motion. Whereas for athletes the knee seems more susceptible to very se-

rious injury, for the nonathletic population there are some startling statistics regarding hip fractures. For example, osteoporosis, a degenerative bone condition mostly affecting females over age 45, is the cause of 1.3 million fractures each year. Of these fractures, 200,000 are at the hip, and 40,000 of these will cause complications leading to death.[18] Hip fractures, then, represents the leading cause of death in older individuals in the United States.[19] Hip fractures occur less frequently in blacks over age 45 than in whites of that age, though the reasons underlying this difference are not clear.

Soft-tissue injury in the hip region is a much more common occurrence in athletic than in nonathletes. Stretch-related injuries are often reported, particularly with respect to muscle and nerve. Other factors making this region susceptible to injury are the extreme range of motion, the powerful muscular contractions associated with the region during activities such as the various forms of locomotion, and the abrupt directional and positional changes common in athletic and recreational activities.

For example, hamstring strain has been attributed to powerful quadriceps contraction associated with delay in the relaxation of the antagonistic hamstrings. In some types of martial arts, kicks above chest level are associated with a flexion and medial rotation of the hip that may strain the outward rotators. Horseback riders and especially dancers and gymnasts often injure the adductor muscles, because dance and gymnastics often call for activities involving front and side splits (Fig. 12–13). A particular dance movement called a hinge in which the hips and trunk are extended has been associated with damage to the femoral nerve.[20] During the extreme hip extension the superior pubic ramus can act as a fulcrum over which can be stretched the femoral nerve, which travels in a groove between the psoas and iliacus muscles.

Two factors that can aid in reducing hip or thigh injuries are related to reducing the imbalance of strength between antagonistic sets of muscles and maintaining flexibility. The quadriceps femoris and hamstring groups demonstrate varying ratios during growth. Comparison of strength measurements for children grouped by age supports the hypothesis that the greater the departure from an optimal strength ratio, the greater the possibility for injury.[21] Values for the optimal ratio vary. Rasch and Burke[22] suggested that the strength ratio of quadriceps to hamstrings must not fall below the critical threshold 70:30. Klein suggested that imbalance greater than 10% predisposes to (knee) injury. His

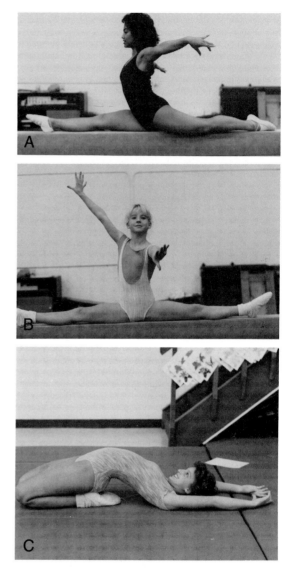

FIG. 12–13.   *A*, Front split; *B*, Side split; *C*, Hinge. Observe the differences in the positions of the hips and therefore in the tissues that are placed under stress.

statistics are impressive; of 515 college football players, none of those who demonstrated a strength ratio of greater than 4% but less than 10% was injured. Of the 79.5% of the players that were injured, all had strength imbalances of greater than 9.8%, and all of the injuries were on the weak side.[21]

Other research reports disagree. In one study, after 172 high-school football players were tested for isokinetic strength imbalances, no relationship was evident between (knee) injuries and a difference of 10% or more between quadriceps and hamstrings strength.[23] Although equity of strength is perhaps an unreasonable goal, the preferred ratio is as close to it as possible.

NEURAL INNERVATIONS

psoas major-minor: branches of the femoral nerve from the lumbar plexus, which contains fibers from L2 and L7.

iliacus: branches of the femoral nerve from the lumbar plexus, which contains fibers from L2 and L3.

sartorius: two branches from the femoral nerve containing fibers from L2 and L3; one branch serves the proximal portion, and a second branch serves the distal portion.

rectus femoris: the femoral nerve with fibers coming from L2, L3, and L4.

biceps femoris: the long head is supplied by two branches from the tibial portion of the sciatic nerve and contains fibers from S1, S2, and S3; the short head is served by branches from the peroneal portion of the sciatic nerve and contains fibers from L5, S1, and S2.

semitendinosus: from two branches of the tibial portion of the sciatic nerve. Fibers come from L5, S1, and S2.

semimembranosus: branches of the tibial portion of the sciatic nerve. Fibers come from L5, S1, and S2.

gluteus maximus: the inferior gluteal nerve from the femoral plexus; fibers come from L5, S1, and S2.

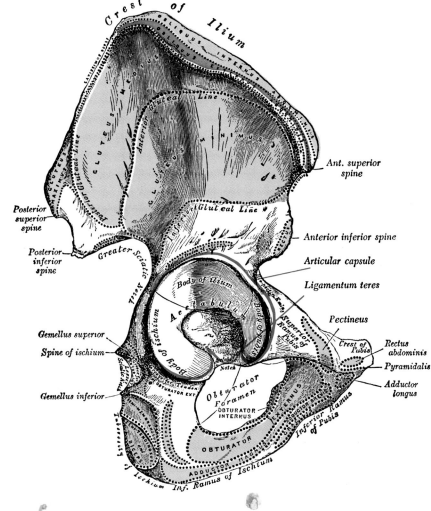

FIG. 12–14.   Right ilium, ischium, and pubis. Lateral surface.

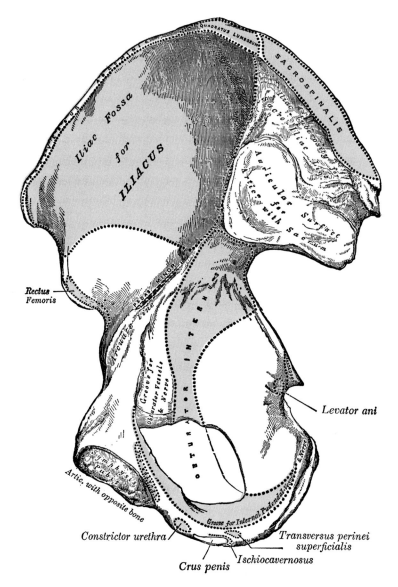

FIG. 12–15.   Right ilium, ischium, and pubis. Medial surface.

gluteus medius: branches of the superior gluteal nerve from fibers from L4, L5, and S1.

gluteus minimus: branches of the superior gluteal nerve from fibers from L4, L5, and S1.

gracilis: a branch from the anterior division of the obturator nerve that contains fibers from L3 and L4.

adductor longus: a branch of the anterior obturator nerve that contains fibers from L3 and L4.

adductor brevis: a branch of the anterior obturator nerve that contains fibers from L3 and L4.

adductor magnus: branches from the posterior division of the obturator nerve, which contains fibers from L3 and L4, and also a branch from the sciatic nerve, which innervates the lower fibers.

pectineus: a branch of the femoral nerve, with fibers from L2, L3, and L4.

tensor fasciae latae: a branch from the superior gluteal nerve from the femoral plexus; it contains fibers from L4, L5, and S1.

piriformis: branches from S1 and S2.

obturator internus: a nerve from the sacral plexus containing fibers from L5, S1, and S2.

obturator externus: a branch of the obturator nerve with fibers from L3 and L4.

quadratus femoris: a nerve from the sacral plexus containing fibers from L4, L5, and S1.

gemellus superior: a nerve from the sacral

plexus containing fibers from the fifth lumbar and first and second sacral nerves.

gemellus inferior: a nerve from the sacral plexus containing fibers from L4, L5, and S1.

STUDY QUESTIONS

1. Using Figures 12–14 and 12–15 generate a list of origins for the muscles acting on the hip joint. Use the diagrams of the femur in Chapter 13 for the insertions of these muscles. Compare your estimated origins and insertions to those from Gray's Anatomy or some other text and, where necessary, make adjustments.

2. Create a list of anatomic and mechanical reasons and mechanisms explaining the incidence of fractures of the anterior superior iliac spine during intense running and jumping.

3. Referring to an anatomy book such as Gray's, discuss the possibility of stretch-related injury to nerves both anterior, posterior, lateral, and medial to the hip joint and identify the mechanism by which such injury could occur during dance aerobics, flexibility exercises, etc.

4. Why can knee flexion combined with hip extension magnify the stretch on the soft tissues falling anterior to the hip joint, such as the femoral nerve and quadriceps femoris?

5. In comparing the pelvic girdle with the shoulder girdle, present both supporting and refuting arguments why the former but not the latter is properly designated as a girdle.

6. In what respects is the biceps femoris similar to the biceps brachii? In what respects is it different?

7. Draw a free body diagram that illustrates how the gluteus medius and gluteus minimus prevent the Trendelenburg sign.

REFERENCES

1. Brinckmann, P., Hoefert, H., and Jongen, H.T.: Sex differences in the skeletal geometry of the human pelvis and hip joint. J. Biomech., 14:427, 1981.
2. Gray, H.: Anatomy of the Human Body. Edited by C.D. Clemente. Philadelphia, Lea & Febiger, 1985.
3. Nordin, M., and Frankel, V.H.: Biomechanics of the hip. In Basic Biomechanics of the Skeletal System. Edited by V.H. Frankel and M. Nordin. Philadelphia, Lea & Febiger, 1980.
4. Basmajian, J.V., and DeLuca, C.J.: Muscles Alive. 5th Ed. Baltimore, Williams & Wilkins, 1985.
5. Joseph, J., and Williams, P.L.: Electromyography of certain hip muscles. J. Anat., 91:286, 1957.
6. Karlsson, E., and Jonsson, B.: Function of the gluteus maximus muscle: an electromyographic study. Acta Morphol. Scand., 6:161, 1965.
7. de Sousa, O.M., and Vitti, M.: Estudio electromiografico de los musculos adductores largo y mayor (abstract). Arch. Mex. Anat., 7:52, 1966.
8. Goto, Y., Kumamoto, M., and Okamoto, T.: Electromyographic study of the function of the muscles participating in thigh elevation in the various planes. Res. J. Phys. Ed., 18:269, 1974.
9. Merchant, A.C.: Hip abductor muscle force. J. Bone Joint Surg., 47A:462, 1965.
10. Soderberg, G.L.: Kinesiology—Application to Pathological Motion. Baltimore, Williams & Wilkins, 1986.
11. Markee, J.E., et al.: Two-joint muscles of the thigh. J. Bone Joint Surg., 37A:125, 1955.
12. Basmajian, J.V., and DeLuca, C.J.: Muscles Alive. 5th Ed. Baltimore, Williams & Wilkins, 1985, pp. 232–239.
13. Gregor, R., Cavanagh, P.R., and LaFortune, M.: Knee flexion moments during propulsion in cycling–a creative solution to Lombard's Paradox. J. Biomech., 18:307, 1985.
14. Elftman, H.: The work done by muscles in running. Am. J. Physiol., 129:672, 1940.
15. Luttgens, K., and Wells, K.F.: Kinesiology. Philadelphia, W.B. Saunders, 1982.
16. Gregiore, L., Veeger, H.E., Huijing, P.A., and van Ingen Schenau, G.J.: Role of mono- and biarticular muscles in explosive movements. Int. J. Sports Med., 5:301, 1984.
17. O'Donoghue, D.H.: Treatment of Athletic Injuries. Philadelphia, W.B. Saunders, 1976.
18. Clark, M., Gosnell, M., Hager, M., and Doherty, S.: The calcium craze. Newsweek, January 27:48, 1986.
19. Farmer, M., White, L.R., Brody, J.A., and Baily, K.R.: Race and sex differences in hip fracture incidence. Am. J. Public Health, 74:1374, 1984.
20. Miller, E.H., and Benedict, F.E.: Stretch of the femoral nerve in a dancer—a case report. J. Bone Joint Surg., 67A, 2:315, 1985.
21. Klein, K.: Muscular strength and the knee. Phys. Sports Med., 2:29, 1974.
22. Rasch, P., and Burke, R.: Kinesiology and Applied Anatomy. 6th Ed. Philadelphia, Lea & Febiger, 1978.
23. Grace, T.G., et al.: Isokinetic muscle imbalance and knee joint injuries. J. Bone Joint Surg., 66A:734, 1984.

13 THE KNEE JOINT

MARK D. GRABINER

ANATOMIC CONSIDERATIONS

The knee joint, typically classified as a diarthrodial hinge joint, is the largest and most complex joint in the body. The knee joint is vulnerable in athletes and presumably also in nonathletes.

Finnish investigators have recently reported that in both men and women the knee joint is the most common site of sports injury that requires surgery, and that the frequency in women is significantly higher than in men.[1] Motion of the knee joint is dominated by flexion and extension but normally occurs in the sagittal, frontal, and transverse planes. Three articulations compose the knee joint: two tibiofemoral joints and the patellofemoral joint. The former two are the sites at which the medial and lateral femoral condyles make contact, through intervening articular cartilage, with the superior articular surface of the tibia (Fig. 13–1). The patellofemoral joint is composed of the posterior surface of the patella and the patellar surface of the femur.

The patella is a sesamoid bone, which is characterized by its development within a tendon, in this case the tendon of the quadriceps femoris muscle. The patella protects the anterior aspect of the knee joint and acts as a sort of pulley by changing the angle of insertion of the patellar ligament on the tibial tuberosity, thus improving the mechanical advantage of the quadriceps muscle group (Fig. 13–2). Most cases of dislocation of the knee are actually a dislocation of the patella. Loss of the patella results in an average loss

of motion of 18° and a 49% loss of strength in the extension mechanism.[2]

Though the most efficient line of pull for the quadriceps muscles is parallel to the femoral shaft, these muscles insert on the tibial tuberosity at a point lateral to the patella. The resulting bowstring effect (Fig. 13–3) tends to draw the patella laterally, perhaps causing chondromalacia in response to chronic stress (as is produced in jogging) or actual dislocation of the patella in response to acute stress (as is produced in football or in landing from jumps).

The lateral drift of the patella is increased by the pull of the vastus lateralis and by the noncontractile iliotibial band and lateral patellar retinaculum. The contraction of the vastus medialis maintains proper patellar alignment. British sports medicine physicians often prescribe static exercises designed to strengthen the vastus medialis as the first approach to the treatment of chondromalacia patellae.

Two factors can accentuate the lateral force on the patellae: relatively wide hips in proportion to stature (characteristic of females) and a habitual position of medial rotation of the femur (tibial torsion, often the result of pronated ankles). In the prevention and assessment of knee injuries, increasingly the Q angle is being measured and evaluated (see Fig. 13–12).

The articular capsule of the knee, unlike in other joints, does not form a complete joint-enveloping structure. The few true capsular ligaments that do connect the bones are as-

208

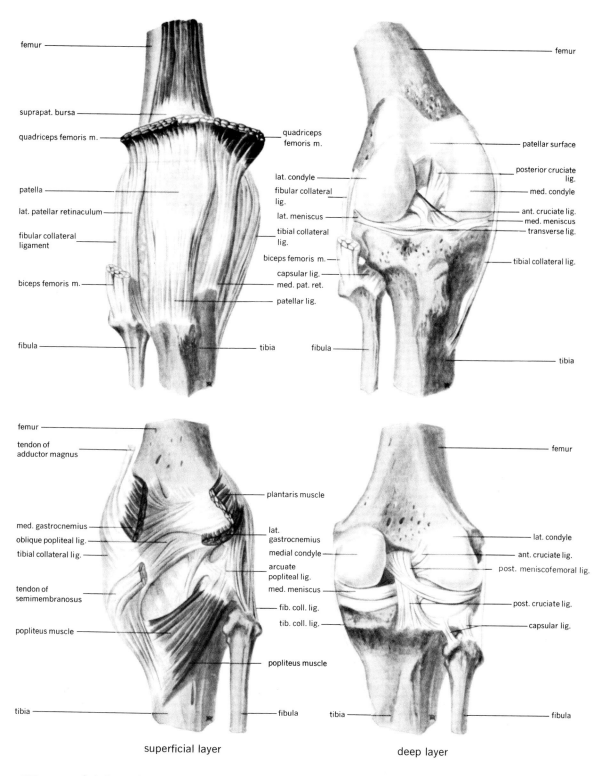

superficial layer

deep layer

FIG. 13–1. Anterior and posterior of right knee joint, showing muscles, ligaments, and bones. (Crouch, J.E., and McClinte, J.R.: Human Anatomy and Physiology. Courtesy John Wiley & Sons, Inc., 1971.)

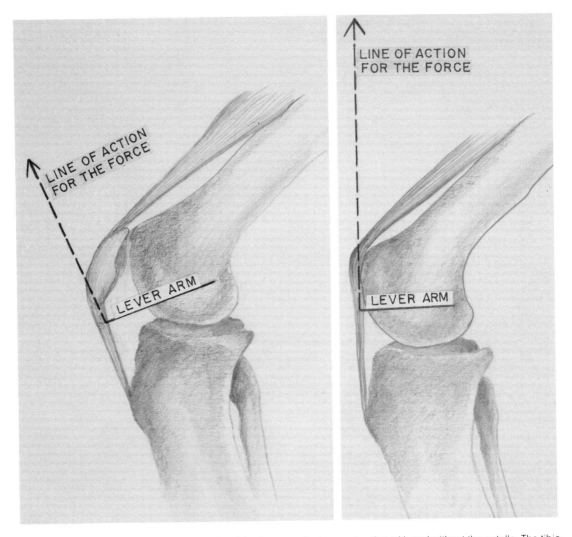

FIG. 13–2.   Illustration of the differing lengths of the lever arm for knee extension with and without the patella. The tibia moves around a center of rotation located between the condyles of the femur. The torque for knee extension is equal to the force in the patellar ligament multiplied by the perpendicular distance from the line of action of the force to the center of rotation. The presence of the patella changes the angle of pull of the patellar tendon and increases the perpendicular distance, thus increasing the torque for a given amount of force.

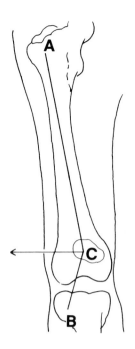

FIG. 13–3. Bowstring effect. As the quadriceps contracts, its origin *(A)* and its insertion *(B)* are drawn toward each other. As a result the patella *(C)* is displaced laterally. (From Pevener, D.N., Johnson, J.R.G., and Blazina, M.E., Phys. Ther., *59*:870, 1979.)

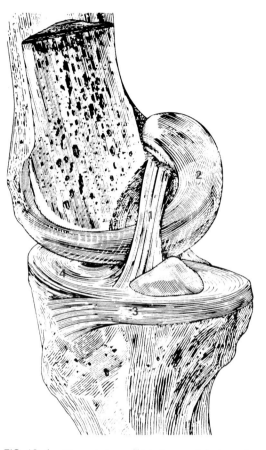

FIG. 13–4.   The anterior cruciate ligament during extension in the right knee joint. Medial view. The lower medial half of the femur, including the medial femoral condyle, has been removed to fully expose the ligament. *1,* Anterior cruciate ligament. *2,* Lateral femoral condyle. *3,* Medial meniscus. *4,* Lateral meniscus. (From Girgis, Marshall and Al-Monajem, 1975.)

sisted by tendinous tissues of the associated knee joint muscles. The patellar ligament is the continuation of the tendon of the quadriceps muscle of the thigh distal to the patella. It is extremely strong and runs from the patella to the tibial tuberosity. It resists the tendency of the superior tibial surface to translate anteriorly with respect to the femur during some types of motion (Fig. 13–1).

Other major ligamentous structures serving to stabilize the knee joint include the oblique popliteal, arcuate popliteal, medial and lateral collateral, and anterior and posterior cruciate ligaments (Fig. 13–1). The oblique and arcuate popliteal ligaments reinforce the knee posteriorly. They help in resisting any tendency for the joint to move beyond its limit of extension (hyperextension). Also, the direction of their fibers suggests that they restrict rotary movement.

The medial (tibial) collateral ligament has been suggested as being more important than the lateral collateral ligament with respect to knee stability.[3] The medial collateral ligament is composed of a superficial portion, the tibial

collateral ligament, and a deep portion, the medial capsular ligament. These structures are important in controlling varus (turned in) and valgus (turned out) angulation, tibial rotation, and anteroposterior tibial displacement.[3]

The cruciate ligaments, which lie in the interior of the knee joint, cross each other in a sagittal plane and provide stability in the sagittal and coronal planes. If either of the cruciates should be severely strained or ruptured, sliding of the tibia with respect to the femur becomes evident, a condition referred to as the drawer sign. The anterior drawer sign is tibial displacement beneath the femur in an anterior direction and reflects the integrity of the anterior cruciate, whereas the pos-

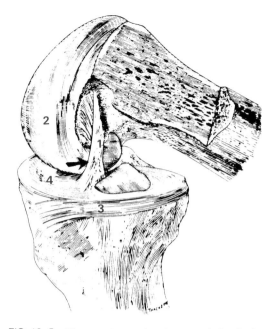

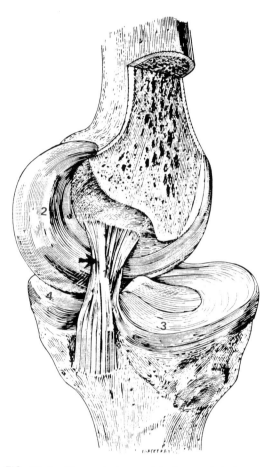

FIG. 13–5. The anterior cruciate ligament during flexion in the right knee joint. Medial view. As in Figure 13–4, the medial femoral condyle has been removed. Note the tightness of the anteromedial band of the anterior cruciate ligament (arrow) during flexion and the looseness of the major part of the ligament. *1*, Anterior cruciate ligament. *2*, Lateral femoral condyle. *3*, Medial meniscus. *4*, Lateral meniscus. (From Girgis, Marshall and Al-Monajem, 1975.)

FIG. 13–6. The posterior cruciate ligament during extension of the right knee joint. Posterolateral view. The lower lateral part of the femur, including the lateral condyle, has been removed to reveal the attachments of the ligament. Only the posterior band of the ligament (arrow) becomes taut during extension. *1*, Posterior cruciate ligament. *2*, Medial femoral condyle. *3*, Lateral meniscus. *4*, Medial meniscus. (From Girgis, Marshall and Al-Monajem, 1975.)

terior drawer sign is posterior tibial displacement and reflects the integrity of the posterior cruciate.[4] Figures 13–4 through 13–7 illustrate how these two ligaments are affected by natural knee movement and range of motion. The effects of high strain rates, loads, or extreme range of motion can be disastrous.

The medial and lateral menisci (semilunar cartilages) play an important role in knee function (Fig. 13–8). They aid directly in stabilizing the joint by deepening the articular surfaces of the tibia, by serving as a source of both shock absorption and transmission of forces by increasing the articular surface area (the tibiofemoral contact area is reduced up to 50% when the menisci are removed), by increasing the efficiency of joint lubrication (meniscectomy can result in up to a 20% increase in the intrajoint coefficient of friction), and by attaching to the bones and other soft tissues of the joints that restrict some types of motion.[2]

Sullivan et al. demonstrated the role of the menisci in transmission of force by noting that

loss of meniscus function, for example through partial or complete removal, can result in significant effects on subchondral bone, on trabecular bone of the proximal tibia, and on the tibial cortex, as well as on the articular cartilage.[4a] The changes produced illustrate one of the features of bone that cause its mechanical properties to change in response to changes in applied forces.[4b] The alterations in the tibial bone result from the medial displacement of the center of pressure when meniscal function becomes impaired. Bourne et al. determined the medial displacement of the center of pressure by the increases in compression on the medial aspect of the

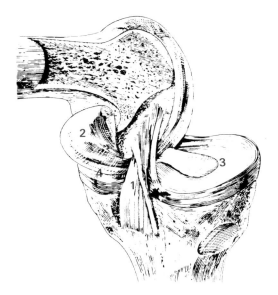

FIG. 13–7.   The posterior cruciate ligament during flexion of the right knee joint. Posterolateral view. The lateral femoral condyle has been removed. During flexion, the small posterior band of the ligament (arrow) is loose while the remaining major portion of the ligament is taut. *1*, Posterior cruciate ligament. *2*, Medial condyle. *3*, Lateral meniscus. *4*, Medial meniscus. (From Girgis, Marshall and Al-Monajem, 1975.)

tibia; compression increased as meniscectomy proceeded from partial to full.[5]

JOINT MOVEMENTS

Motion of the knee joint, although measurable around all three axes, is dominated by flexion and extension in the sagittal plane. The range of motion from full extension (0°) to full flexion is approximately 140°. Motion of the knee in the transverse plane typically accompanies flexion and extension and is referred to as internal and external tibial rotation. Movement in the transverse plane (and sagittal plane) is a function of knee position in the sagittal plane.[5] No rotation of the knee is allowed when the knee is fully extended; however, up to 45° of external rotation and 30° of internal rotation are possible when the knee is flexed to 90°. At full extension the rotation is restricted by the bony architecture of the joint, whereas beyond 90° of flexion the motion is limited by the stretched soft tissues around the joint.

Costigan and Reid[6] reported on the tibial rotation during knee flexion and extension excursions. These simultaneous actions are important in normal knee motion. The radial torque at the knee was measured and found to be a function of foot position (rotated in or rotated out). The least amount of laterally directed torque at the knee was found when the foot was rotated out 17°. Costigan and Reid found that there is indeed a foot position, greater than 17° but less than 50° (one of the experimental positions), at which the radial torque at the knee is reduced to zero; this position varies among individuals. This foot position has implications for exercises such as parallel squats and vertical jumping, which

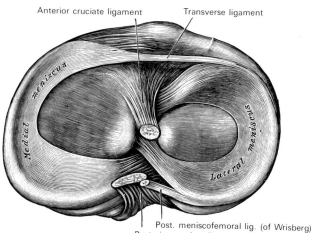

Anterior cruciate ligament   Transverse ligament

Post. meniscofemoral lig. (of Wrisberg)
Posterior cruciate ligament

FIG. 13–8.   Head of right tibia seen from above, showing the menisci and the attachments onto the tibia of the cruciate ligaments. (From Gray's Anatomy, 30th Ed. Philadelphia, Lea & Febiger, 1985, p. 404.)

require knee flexions and extensions of the weight-supporting extremity. In the frontal plane, adduction and abduction of the tibia is limited to only a few degrees.

MUSCLES OF THE KNEE JOINT

Twelve muscles act at the knee joint and may be classified into three groups: the hamstrings, the quadriceps femoris, and the unclassified groups.[7] The hamstrings group (Fig. 13–9) includes the semitendinosus muscle, the semimembranosus muscle, and the biceps femoris (long and short heads). All but the short head of the biceps act as hip extensors, and their roles at that joint are discussed more completely in Chapter 12. Because all of the hamstrings demonstrate a line of pull posterior to the axis of knee rotation, they all serve as knee flexors.

In addition to flexing the knee, the semimembranosus and semitendinosus muscles internally rotate the tibia when the knee is partially flexed. In a weight-bearing condition, these muscles tend to externally rotate the femur on the tibia. These motions are relatively equivalent.

The quadriceps femoris is made up of the rectus femoris and the three vasti muscles, the vastus lateralis, vastus medialis, and vastus intermedius (Fig. 13–10). Only the rectus femoris acts at more than one joint. All of the members, however, unequivocally cause powerful knee extension and also, because of their medial insertion, tend to cause internal rotation of the tibia.

The structure of the quadriceps has long been a matter of curiosity—why are there four separate heads for this muscle? After over 100 years of study (Duchenne studied the group in 1866), the solution has yet to be satisfactorily presented. The vastus medialis, especially, has attracted much attention because of its physical prominence and distinct electrical behavior. Its electrical behavior is related to the decrease in the magnitude of the quadriceps moment arm for knee extension during the final 15° of motion.[8] The increases in the activity of the vastus medialis toward the end of knee extension have been related to its role as a stabilizer of the patella against lateral dislocation.[9] In general, it is still relatively safe

to suggest that all quadriceps muscles are more or less simultaneously active during knee extension, and proportionately active during increases and decreases in extension tension.[10]

The unclassified group of knee joint muscles includes the sartorius, gracilis, popliteus, gastrocnemius, and plantar muscles. The latter two muscles do act predominantly at the ankle joint, although both pass posteriorly to the knee joint and possess some flexion capabilities. The gracilis muscle can be considered as part of the mass of muscle referred to as the hip adductors; however, in crossing the knee joint it tends to cause a torque associated with internal rotation of the tibia as well as with knee flexion.[11] The sartorius, which is the longest muscle in the body, is also associated with internal rotation of the tibia and acts also at the hip as a flexor.

The popliteus is a small, deep muscle posterior to the knee joint (see Fig. 14–13). The orientation of its fibers makes it an internal tibial rotator. The muscle's activity is generally observed at the onset of knee flexion, associated with the unlocking mechanism of the knee, and during walking. During walking, the activity of the popliteus muscle is associated with the period of internal tibial rotation, beginning at mid-swing and continuing until single-limb support.[12] In addition, the popliteus muscle helps stabilize the weight-bearing leg when it is in a flexed-knee position. During these conditions the femur is influenced by forces that tend to displace it anteriorly on the tibia. The popliteus aids the posterior cruciate ligament in restraining this undesired motion.

LOCKING MECHANISM OF THE KNEE

Normally, when the knee is fully extended in a normal upright standing posture, the line of gravity falls anteriorly to the tibiofemoral contact point. Thus, the knee is held in extension by the gravitational torque. Because of a disparity in the diameters of the medial and lateral femoral condyles and the corresponding menisci, continued contraction of the quadriceps femoris can and is required to cause external rotation of the femur on the

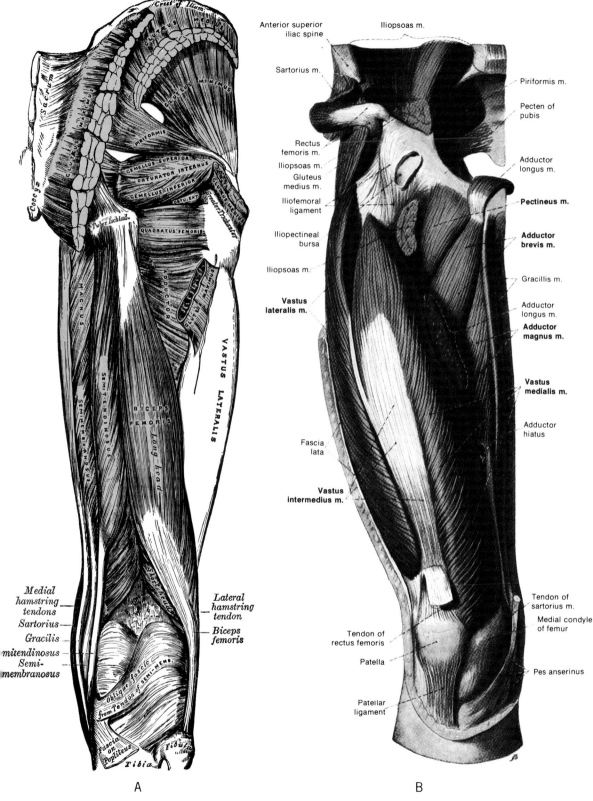

FIG. 13–9.   A, Posterior superficial muscles of the thigh. B, The intermediate layer of anterior and medial thigh muscles. (Sobotta/Figge: Atlas of Human Anatomy. Courtesy Urban & Schwarzenberg, Baltimore-Munich, 1977.)

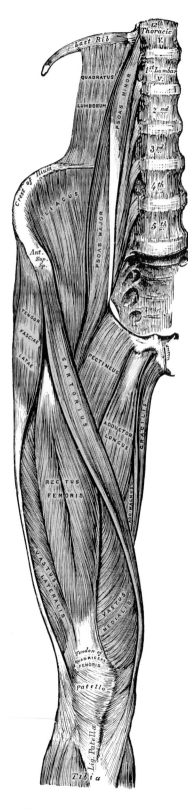

FIG. 13–10.   Muscles of the iliac and anterior femoral regions. (From Gray's Anatomy. 30th Ed. Philadelphia, Lea & Febiger, 1985, p. 558.)

tibia. (Note: internal rotation of the tibia can be accomplished in this fashion if, as in the case of the weight-bearing leg, the tibia resists rotation.) This rotation causes the femur to seat itself more closely into the menisci in what has been called a "screw home" movement.[7]

MECHANICAL CONSIDERATIONS OF INJURY TO THE KNEE

Knee strains result from motion that exceeds the normal limits of the joint. When forced beyond this natural restriction, the ligaments may be stressed beyond their elastic limit (the point after which permanent strain, or deformation, occurs) into the plastic region of their load-extension curve (see Fig. 15–4). The result is a permanent deformation of the ligaments, the magnitude of which depends on the applied force. At the knee, ligamentous strain can occur in any movement direction. In perhaps the most common type of knee injury, often seen on the football field, the foot is fixed and the femur rotates medially with respect to the tibia, which simultaneously rotates laterally (Fig. 13–11). The entire knee is generally displaced medially, resulting in medial ligamentous stress. When the force is continued, the anterior cruciate ligament and, ultimately, the posterior cruciate will become stressed. The "unhappy triad" refers to an injury that affects simultaneously the medial collateral ligament, anterior cruciate ligament, and medial meniscus. Common in athletics, this type of injury has also been reported to occur during lateral impact simulations, not unlike the impact that might occur if one's car were hit broadside.[13]

Severe strain is the precursor to either patellofemoral or tibiofemoral knee dislocation. An anatomic factor that predisposes an individual to patellofemoral dislocation is an abnormal Q-angle. The Q-angle is the deviation between the line of pull of the quadriceps femoris and the patellar ligament. It is usually measured as the angle between the line from the anterior superior iliac spine and the center of the patella and the center of the patella to the tibial tuberosity.[14] A Q-angle of 10° is considered normal.[15] Angles greater than this can result in lateral patellar dislocations when

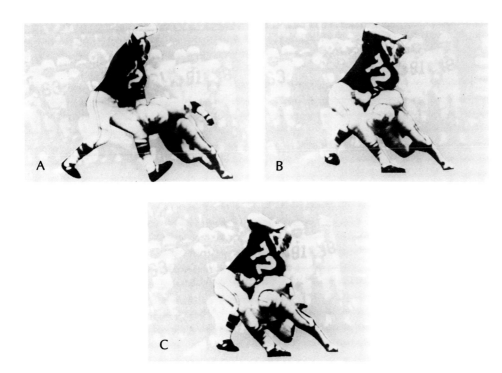

FIG. 13–11. An all-too-familiar sequence on the football field in which damage to the knee joint can be debilitating (Photos J.B. Wang, Journal of Bone and Joint Surgery.)

contraction of the quadriceps reduces the angle. Other anatomic conditions that predispose an individual to this type of injury include the typically wide pelvis of the female, knock knees or genu valgum, and a relatively flat lateral femoral condyle.

Of a far more serious nature, and fortunately less common, is tibiofemoral dislocation. This type of injury is life-threatening. It may occur in any direction but is most common anteriorly and associated with a force causing hyperextension of the knee. Posterior dislocation of the knee is a result of a direct force on the anterior aspect of the tibia with the knee semiflexed. This force causes the tibia to be driven posteriorly, rupturing the posterior cruciate and the posterior portion of the articular capsule. Lateral dislocation occurs when the tibia is forced laterally with respect to the femur, causing damage to the medioposterior aspects of the capsule and the cruciates. Medial dislocation is uncommon, resulting from a force applied to the shank from the lateral to the medial side. This force slides the tibia medially with respect to the femur and ruptures the lateral collateral ligament, cruciates, and posterior aspect of the capsule. In rotary dislocations the femur is rotated with respect to the tibia when the foot is fixed, injuring cruciates, the articular capsule, often the menisci, and any soft tissues crossing the knee.

Meniscus injury is generally concurrent with ligamentous sprain. The mechanisms of injury to the medial and lateral menisci differ. The C-shaped medial meniscus is anchored to the medial collateral ligament by the coronary ligament. When the medial collateral ligament is sprained as a result of a force directed laterally to medially, the distance between the tibia and femur increases, placing stress on the medial meniscus where it is attached to the medial collateral ligament. The damage results from avulsion of the meniscus from either the inferior tibial or the superior femoral attachments. Damage to the O-shaped lateral meniscus is less frequent than damage to the medial meniscus. It is more susceptible to overuse injury than to acute macrotrauma.[15]

Athletes frequently experience pain along the lower leg that they call shin splints. The

American Medical Association has tried to establish a definition of the term, but it remains a "wastebasket" diagnosis. Perhaps because the disorder is not defined, several theories regarding the cause of the disability exist. Shin splints might involve injury to the soft tissues (muscles, tendons, and ligaments); the pain might result from stress fractures, periosteal irritation, or both; shin splints might result from vascular compromise secondary to increased compartmental pressure (a theory now largely discarded); and they might be caused by muscle fatigue and muscle injury resulting from undue stress and leading to periostitis, stress fracture, or even a complete fracture.[16]

Shin splints are said to be epidemic among dancers. In ballet dancers the site of pain is along the anterolateral aspect of the lower leg and along the proximal portion of the anterior tibial muscle. In runners it is usually felt along the posteromedial aspect of the lower leg.[17] In mild cases the symptoms may disappear within 10 to 14 days if the patient switches to light exercise on a softer surface. In more severe cases cessation of the activity appears essential.

Anterior tibial compartmental syndrome can be either acute or recurrent. The former variety requires special mention because permanent paralysis results unless surgery is instituted within a few hours of the occurrence of pain. The anterior tibial compartment is an unyielding cylinder composed of the tibia, the fibula, the interosseous membrane, and the crural fascia, enclosing the anterior tibial and other muscles, with only small openings for the passage of tendons, nerves, and blood vessels. Strenuous exercise (as well as tibial fractures and other conditions unrelated to shin splints) can cause swelling within the compartment, compressing and obstructing the veins and initiating a cycle of increasing internal pressure. If surgical decompression is not performed, necrosis of the enclosed soft tissue occurs. This condition has been reported to occur occasionally in tennis players and soccer players, and it has been observed to result from karate kicks and judo leg sweeps. It may represent an exaggeration of the shin splint syndrome.

In recurrent anterior tibial compartmental

syndrome, high tissue pressure impedes blood flow and causes muscle ischemia during exercise. This syndrome is painful and causes weakness of the involved muscles, but the symptoms disappear after a short rest.[17]

Hairline stress fractures result from a bone's inability to withstand repeated subthreshold bending stresses such as those encountered in such rhythmic repetitive exercises as jogging, running, and marching. Stress fractures have been documented in only three species: humans, race horses, and racing greyhounds. In humans they occur principally in the metatarsals, where the injury is termed a march fracture, and in the fibulae. In the latter case the mechanism may be the forceful contraction of the plantar and long toe flexors drawing the fibula toward the tibia. The fractures occur most frequently near the inferior tibiofibular joint. Strong calf muscles working at their maximum strength also can cause the tibia to bow forward. Tibial fractures are sometimes observed in male ballet dancers.

Ski injuries are common and very instructive to the kinesiologist. They involve two factors—fixation and enhancement—and three motions—external rotation (usually associated with abduction), forward fall, and internal rotation. Injury occurs only if both factors and at least one of the forces are present. Fixation results when a ski becomes fixed, in turn fixing the foot attached to the ski. If the ski bindings do not release and a large amount of kinetic energy is present, a torsion strain is exerted through external rotation. This most common mechanism of ski injuries can result in fracture of the lateral malleolus, spiral fracture of the ankle and/or tibia, or sprains of the knee and ankle.

When a ski tip digs in, sharp deceleration can result, hurling the skier over the top of his boots. A boot-top fracture, tearing of the Achilles tendon, and dislocation of peroneal tendons may follow. Internal rotation is caused by one ski tip's crossing over the other. Ankle sprain, knee injury, fractures of the medial malleolus, and spiral tibial fractures may be the outcomes.[18] Age, speed, and ability do not appear to affect the frequency of injury to the knee ligaments in skiing.

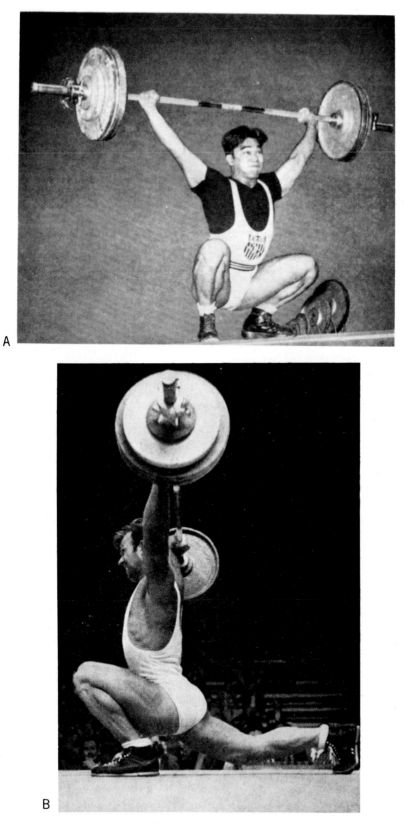

FIG. 13–12. *A* and *B*, Two examples of the weight-bearing knees under extreme loading conditions.

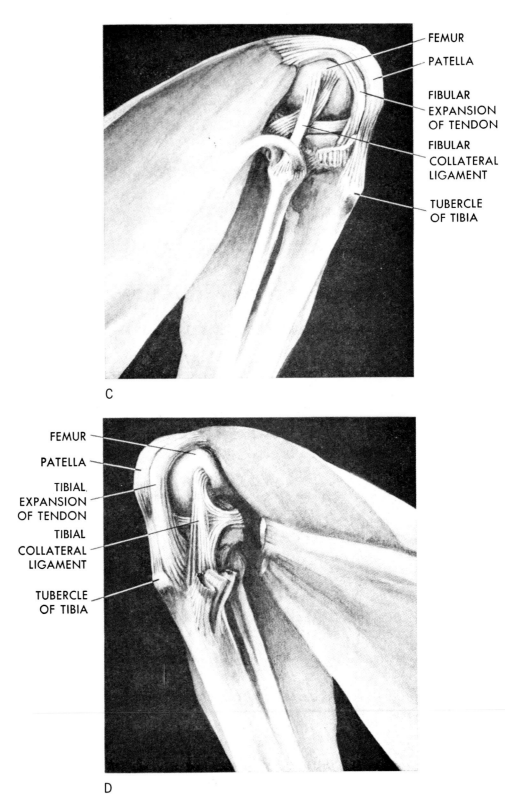

FIG. 13–12.   *C* and *D*, The anatomic manifestations of the conditions.

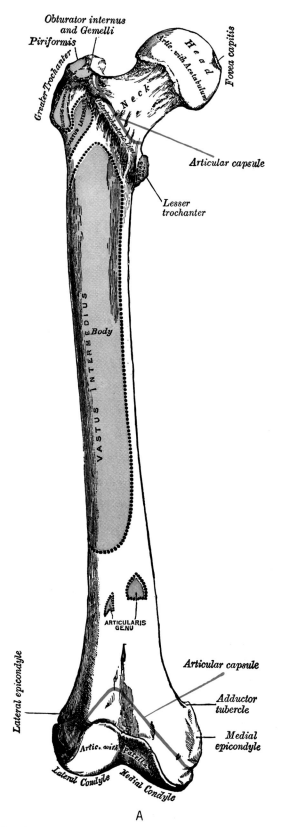

FIG. 13–13.   *A*, Right femur. Anterior surface.

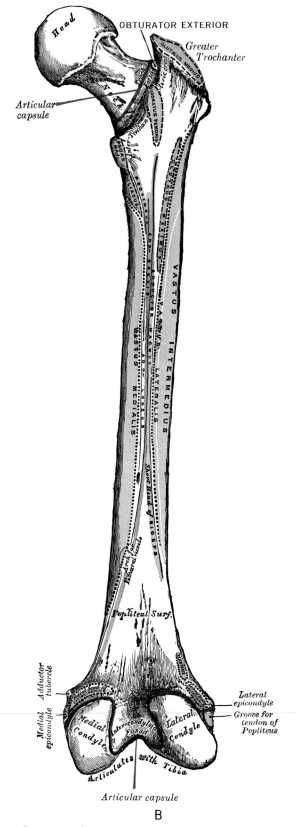

B

FIG. 13–13. *B*, Right femur. Posterior surface.

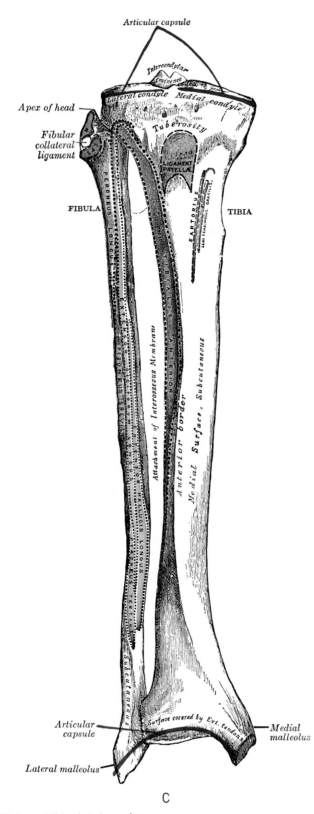

FIG. 13–13. *C*, Right fibula and tibia. Anterior surface.

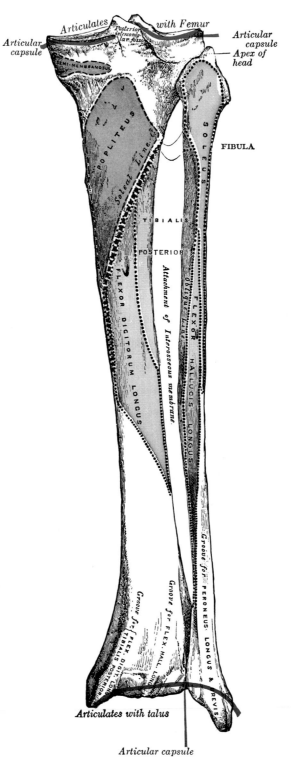

D

FIG. 13–13. *D*, Right tibia and fibula. Posterior surface.

Women tend to injure the medial collateral ligaments more often than do men.[19]

Exercises that cause the weight-bearing knee to become fully flexed have been condemned as potentially dangerous to the supporting structures of the knee (Fig. 13–12).

The preclusion of rotation of the fixed foot under this condition causes increased stress upon knee ligaments and cartilage. The solution to this dangerous practice is to limit the degree of knee flexion such as in parallel squat exercises.

STUDY QUESTIONS

1. Using Figs. 13–13A, B, C, and D, generate a list of origins and insertions for the muscles acting on the knee joint. Compare your estimated origins and insertions to those from Gray's Anatomy or some other text and then, where necessary, make adjustments.

2. Present a discussion regarding the predisposition of the elderly to falls related to weakness in the quadriceps femoris and the general importance of this muscle during locomotion and standing posture.

3. What are the mechanical differences between a leg press exercise using a leg press machine and the parallel squat exercise performed with a barbell? What, if any, training differences would be associated with the two exercises, and why?

4. Answer the previous question but compare exercises using knee flexion-extension machines to free-weight exercises such as the parallel squat.

5. Describe the anatomic/architectural restrictions to knee rotation, internal rotation, and external rotation when the knee is fully flexed.

6. Describe why the quadriceps muscle of the thigh tends to internally rotate the tibia.

7. Discuss the mechanics of the occurrence of the unhappy triad as it might occur in an automobile collision in which the injured person's car was hit broadside.

8. Judges have ruled that for a school to refuse to let girls participate with boys in football constitutes sex discrimination. If the decision were based on kinesiologic factors, how would you rule? Justify your answer. Suggestion: Read Falls, H.B.: Coed football: hazards, implications, and alternatives. Phys. Sportsmed., *14*:207, 1986.

9. A newspaper reporter wrote that as the result of 10 years of intensive practice of figure skating, the body of a former national champion had become knock-kneed and pigeon-toed to such an extent that it was impossible for her to cross her legs. Explain the kinesiology of these disabilities.

REFERENCES

1. Sandelin, J.: Acute sports injuries requiring hospital care. Br. J. Sports Med., 20:99–102, 1986.
2. Sutton, F.S.: The effect of patellectomy on knee functions. J. Bone Joint Surg., 37A:1028, 1976.
3. Distefano, V.: Functional anatomy and biomechanics of the knee. Athletic Training, 13:113–118, 1978.
4. Marshall, J.L., et al.: The anterior drawer sign: what is it?. J. Sports Med., 3:152, 1975.
4a. Sullivan, D., et al.: Medial restraints to anterior-posterior motion of the knee. J. Bone Joint Surg., 66A:930, 1984.
4b. Nordin, M., and Frankel, V.H.: Biomechanics of whole bone and bone tissues. In Basic Biomechanics of the Skeletal System. Edited by V.H. Frankel and M. Nordin. Philadelphia, Lea & Febiger, 1980.
5. Bourne, R.B., Finlay, B., Papadopoulos, P., and Andreae, P.: The effect of medial meniscectomy on strain distribution in the proximal part of the tibia. J. Bone Joint Surg., 66A:1431, 1984.
6. Costigan, P.A., and Reid, J.G.: Radial torque of the tibia during a deep knee bend. In Biomechanics. IX-B. Edited by D.A. Winter, et al. Champaign, IL, Human Kinetics, 1985, p. 420.
7. Rasch, P.J., and Burke, R.K.: Kinesiology and Applied Anatomy. 6th Ed. Philadelphia, Lea & Febiger, 1978.
8. Lieb, F.J., and Perry, J.: Quadriceps function: an anatomical and mechanical study using amputated limbs. J. Bone Joint Surg., 50A:1535, 1968.
9. Basmajian, J.V., and DeLuca, C.J.: Muscles Alive. 5th Ed. Baltimore, Williams & Wilkins, 1985, pp. 324–332.
10. Andres, T.L.: Quadricep function—a brief review. Am. Correct. Ther. J., 31:49, 1977.
11. Basmajian, J.V., and DeLuca, C.J.: Muscles Alive. 5th Ed. Baltimore, Williams & Wilkins, 1985, p. 322.
12. Mann, R.A., and Hagy, J.L.: The popliteus muscle. J. Bone Joint Surg., 59A:924, 1977.
13. Hearon, B.F., Brinkley, J.W., Raddin, J.H., and Fleming, B.W.: Knee ligament injury during lateral impact. Aviat. Space Environ. Med., 56:3–8, 1985.
14. Olerud, C., and Berg, P.: The variation of the Q-

angle with different positions of the foot. Clin. Orthop., *191*:162, 1984.
15. O'Donoghue, D.H.: Treatment of Athletic Injuries.
Philadelphia, W.B. Saunders, 1976.
16. Gans, A.: The relationship of heel contact in ascent
and descent from jumps to the incidence of shin
splints in ballet dancers. Phys. Ther., *65*:192, 1985.

17. Veith, R.G., et al.: Recurrent anterior compartmental
syndrome. Phys. Sportsmed., *8*:80, 1980.
18. Ellison, A.E.: Skiing injuries. Clin. Symp.,
29(1):1–40, 1977.
19. Marshall, J.L., and Johnson, R.J.: Mechanisms of the
most common ski injuries. Phys. Sportsmed., *5*:49,
1977.

14 THE ANKLE AND FOOT

MARK D. GRABINER

ANATOMIC CONSIDERATIONS

The human foot has evolved from a flexible grasping organ to a relatively rigid weight-bearing supportive system. Some claim that the evolution of the foot has been less than successful, or at least incomplete. For example, still present are the functional grasping muscles, which are of reduced importance.

The foot is composed of 33 joints and 26 bones, grouped as the seven tarsal bones (talus, calcaneus, navicular, cuboid, medial cuneiform, intermediate cuneiform, and lateral cuneiform); five metatarsal bones (arranged medial to lateral); and fourteen phalanges (three for each toe, except for the great toe, which has only two) (Figs. 14–1 and 14–2).

The bones of the foot articulate such that they form three structural arches that, along with an extremely complex system of ligaments, and, to a lesser degree, of muscles, provide internal support. These arches, two longitudinal (medial and lateral) and one

transverse, contribute to the strength, stability, mobility, and resilience of the foot.[1] During weight-bearing and other types of loading, the arches serve as shock absorbers, dissipating energy before it is transferred across the ankle joint and to the shank. The joints of the foot (Fig. 14–3) include the ankle (talocrural), transverse tarsal, intertarsals (gliding joints between the seven tarsal bones), tarsometatarsal (gliding joints between the tarsals and the proximal ends of the metatarsals), metatarsophalangeal (condyloid joints between the distal ends of the metatarsals and the proximal phalanges), and interphalangeal joints (hinge joints that allow flexion and extension of the toes).

The plantar fascia (plantar aponeurosis) is found on the plantar aspect of the foot. Running longitudinally, it is divided into central, lateral, and medial portions. It attaches posteriorly on the calcaneus and anteriorly at the base of the first row of phalanges. Plantar

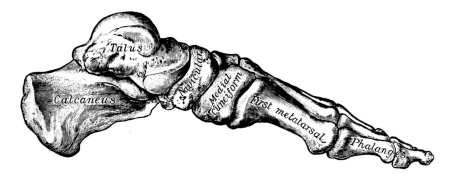

FIG. 14–1. Bones on the medial aspect of the foot. Observe the concave medial longitudinal arch. (From Gray's Anatomy. 30th Ed. Philadelphia, Lea & Febiger, 1985, p. 423.)

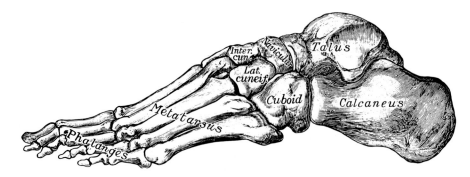

FIG. 14–2. Bones on the lateral aspect of the foot. Observe that the concavity of the lateral longitudinal arch is less pronounced than that of the medial arch shown in Figure 14–1. (From Gray's Anatomy. 30th Ed. Philadelphia, Lea & Febiger, 1985, p. 423.)

fasciitis is a common foot disorder in runners; although the cause remains unknown, anatomic anomalies and overuse are suspected. Sammarco[2] presents the plantar fascia as a truss, which is a rigid structure composed of elements fastened so as to resist changes in its shape by preventing motion between its elements. Its purpose is to support a larger load or span a greater distance than the individual elements could by themselves. The plantar fascia serves as a mechanism by which the tarsal joints may be passively stabilized. As an individual performs heel raises or any activity requiring toe extension, the fascia becomes stretched and tightened because of the change in orientation of its distal attachment. This change then shortens the base of the truss, from the heel to the ball of the foot. The result is tarsal and metatarsal stabilization and an increase in the height of the longitudinal arch (Figs. 14–4, 14–5, and 14–6).

The geometry of the foot and its relationship to function have historically been disputed similarly to the way body somatotyping has; there is general disagreement as to what represents a structurally or functionally normal foot. Stacoff and Luethi[3] suggest that the proper way to evaluate feet is to categorize them during performance.

Typically, a normal foot has a medium-height longitudinal arch, a straight podogram, which is an imprint of the foot not unlike a fingerprint, and a vertically oriented hindfoot, which is the angle that the Achilles tendon makes from the vertical. A flat foot, or pes planus, has a low arch or no arch and is often pronated. Pes cavus, or a highly arched foot, is supported mostly at the fore- and hindfoot.

The manner in which loads are distributed under the foot has been a focus of investigation for decades. In the normal weight-bearing stance, all of the metatarsal heads are in contact with the ground and together bear 50% of the load, the heel being responsible for the remaining 50%. The metatarsal of the great toe in the normal foot is responsible for twice the load of the other metatarsals,[2] although this relationship can be changed by shoes, the changes in the location of the center of gravity during dynamic conditions, and muscular contraction. During gait, as the heel height of shoes increases, the pressures below the heads of the four lateral metatarsals increase while those below the hallux are reduced.[4] Soames[5] reported on the changes in the distribution of pressures below the metatarsals during gait when shoes were worn as opposed to the barefoot condition, illustrating the sensitivity of the distribution of pressure to the conditions under which measurement is performed.

ANKLE JOINT

The ankle joint consists of the tibiotalar, fibulotalar, and distal tibiofibular joints. It is classified as a diarthrodial hinge joint and is inherently stable by virtue of its bony architecture, a medial and lateral collateral ligamentous system, the articular capsule, and the distal aspects of the interosseus membrane.[6] The ankle joint is critical in the transmission of force both toward and away from

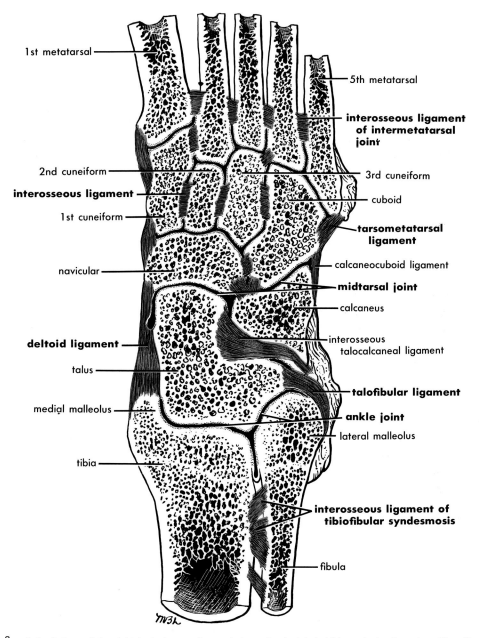

FIG. 14–3.   Articulations of the right foot observed superiorly as the foot is held in a plantar flexed position. Section is in an oblique plane. (From Crouch, J.E.: Functional Human Anatomy. Philadelphia, Lea & Febiger, 1985, p. 172.)

the body during weight-bearing and other loading. The magnitudes of these forces may be so large, up to ten times body weight during some types of running, for example,[7] that even small structural misalignments or damage can lead to chronic and severe orthopedic problems. Transmission of forces occurs at the juncture of the distal end of the tibia and the superior surface of the talus; the fibula plays little role. Architecturally, a mortise, or flanged slot, is formed by the distal malleoli of the tibia and fibula into which the superior aspect of the talus fits. This structure is a major source of stability for the ankle joint.

The major ligaments supporting the joint (Figs. 14–7 and 14–8) include the distal aspect of the interosseous membrane, the articular capsule, the deltoid ligament (medially), the anterior and posterior talofibular ligaments (laterally), and the calcaneofibular ligament

TRUSS

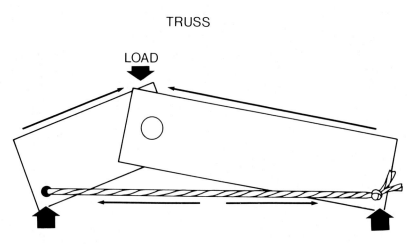

FIG. 14–4. Diagram of a truss. The wooden member is analogous to the bony structures of the foot. The plantar fascia is represented by a tether between the ends of the bone. The shorter the tether, the higher the truss is raised. (From Frankel, V.H., and Nordin, M.: Basic Biomechanics of the Skeletal System. Philadelphia, Lea & Febiger, 1980, p. 209.)

(laterally); the latter four are considered collateral ligaments.[1]

The biaxial hinge joint allows for approximately 45° of flexion known as dorsiflexion, and 45° of extension, known as plantar flexion. Various populations, of course, can demonstrate significantly greater values. Usually the first 10 to 20° is defined as dorsiflexion; the remaining motion is defined as plantar flexion.

SUBTALAR JOINT

The subtalar joint, a gliding diarthritic joint found between the inferior aspect of the talus and the superior aspect of the calcaneus, is considered one of the intertarsal joints. The foot's motion through the subtalar joint can be modeled by representing the ankle (classified anatomically as a hinge) as a ball-and-socket joint. The uniaxial hinge of the ankle

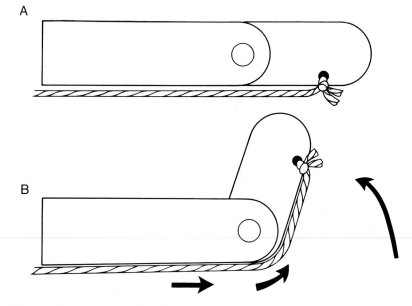

FIG. 14–5. A, Diagram of a Spanish windlass. The metatarsal is represented by the fixed wooden member and the proximal phalanx is represented by the moving member. The rope attached to the moving member represents the attachment of the plantar fascia to the proximal phalanx. B, As the moving member turns, the rope advances. (From Frankel, V.H., and Nordin, M.: Basic Biomechanics of the Skeletal System. Philadelphia, Lea & Febiger, 1980, p. 209.)

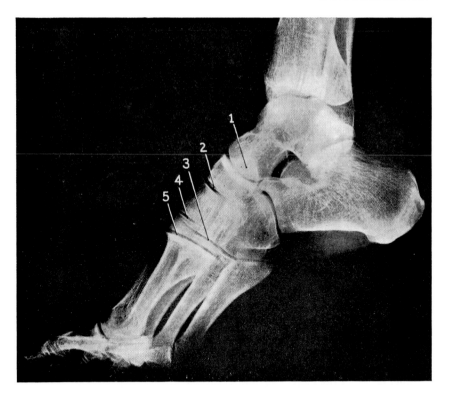

FIG. 14–6. Adult foot. 1, Tuberosity of navicular bone, partly obscured by the shadow of the head of the talus. 2, Cuneonavicular joint. 3, Joint between metatarsal III and the lateral cuneiform bone. 4, Joint between metatarsal II and the intermediate cuneiform bone. 5, Joint between metatarsal I and the medial cuneiform bone. (From Gray's Anatomy. 30th Ed. Philadelphia, Lea & Febiger, 1985, p. 420.)

combined with the axis of the subtalar joint effectively allows the foot three axes of rotation. Sammarco[2] reported that the axis of the subtalar joint is approximately 42° from the heel, directed anteriorly and superiorly (38° from vertical), and 16° medially from the long axis of the foot (Fig. 14–9).

The subtalar joint allows essentially two motions, independent of motion at the ankle joint. Inversion of the foot occurs when the sole of the foot is turned medially. Eversion of the foot occurs when the sole is turned laterally. Eversion and inversion are sometimes referred to as pronation and supination, respectively. Eversion often occurs with dorsiflexion and abduction (outward rotation of foot), whereas inversion can occur with some degree of plantar flexion and adduction (inward rotation). Generally, the range of motion demonstrates a mean of 20° of inversion and 5° of eversion.[8]

TRANSVERSE TARSAL JOINT

The transverse tarsal joint (midtarsal) can be considered the articulation between the tri-axial talonavicular and biaxial calcaneocuboid joints. The navicular and cuboid bones articulate such that they allow only slight movement and hence can be considered as a single segment. Viewed superiorly, the transverse tarsal joint forms an S-shaped line. The joint allows movement of the anterior aspect of the foot with respect to the posterior.

Two types of motion are allowed through two axes.[2] The axis about which inversion and eversion occur is oriented with the long axis of the foot rising posterior to anterior from the foot's plantar surface at an angle of 15° and is directed medially at an angle of 9°. Motion around this axis allows the foot to conform with a variety of surface orientations during locomotion. A second axis rising similarly to the first but at an angle of 52° is directed medially at an angle of 57°. This axis of rotation will augment both dorsi- and plantar flexion. The orientation of the axes and therefore the movement is variable and can be influenced by the architecture of the foot and the status of the musculature crossing the joints.

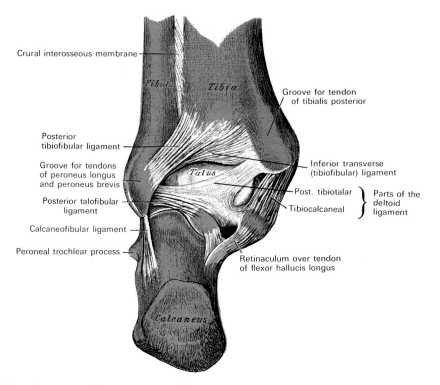

FIG. 14–7. The left ankle joint. Posterior aspect. (From Gray's Anatomy. 30th Ed. Philadelphia, Lea & Febiger, 1985, p. 412.)

Motion of the foot distal to the transverse tarsal joint belongs to the intertarsal and tarsometatarsal joints. In both cases, motion is restricted to nearly negligible dorsiflexion and to 15° of plantar flexion. The toes move in flexion and extension around both the metatarsophalangeal (diarthritic ellipsoid) joints and interphalangeal (diarthritic hinge) joints. Motion about the metatarsophalangeal joints includes abduction and adduction. The hallux, or great toe, has a flexion range of 30° and an extension range of 90°. The small toes have a slightly greater range of flexion, 50°.

MUSCULATURE OF THE ANKLE JOINT AND FOOT

The portion of the lower extremity between the knee and the ankle joint is the site of origin for the muscles causing ankle motion. These muscles are categorized into three groups—the anterior crural, the posterior crural, and lateral crural. Of the muscles associated with the ankle and foot 12 are extrinsic to the foot, and 19 are intrinsic.

Anterior Crural. The anterior crural mus-

cles are associated with the anterior compartment, which is bordered by the tibia and the intermuscular septum (Figs. 14–10 and 14–11). The four muscles enclosed in the anterior compartment are the tibialis anterior, extensor hallucis longus, extensor digitorum longus, and peroneus tertius. The first three muscles are primary agonists for dorsiflexion.[9] Rasch and Burke[10] suggest that the tibialis anterior muscle and extensor digitorum longus provide for an even elevation of the foot. The peroneus tertius is a part of the extensor digitorum longus and is considered its fifth tendon;[11] it has been observed only in humans and the great apes.

The tibialis anterior is generally considered an inverter of the foot (subtalar joint), though some researchers have reported that it is not active during inversion unless dorsiflexion occurs simultaneously.[12] Houtz and Fischer[13] found the tibialis anterior to be active during pedaling of a bicycle even though the ankle is already dorsiflexed. This activity is perhaps related to a function in joint stabilization.

It is fairly well accepted that the tibialis an-

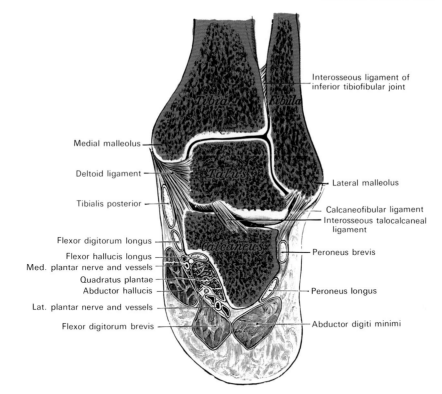

FIG. 14–8.   Coronal section through right talocrural and talocalcaneal joints showing the interosseous talocalcaneal ligament and the relationship of structures coursing beneath the malleoli. (From Gray's Anatomy. 30th Ed. Philadelphia, Lea & Febiger, 1985, p. 414.)

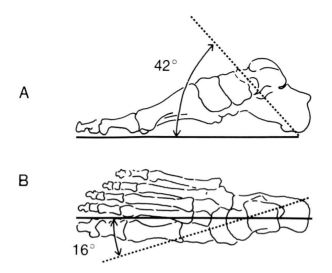

FIG. 14–9.   Simplified axis of rotation of the subtalar joint. A, Sagittal plane (lateral view). B, Transverse plane (top view). (Adapted from Manter, 1941.)

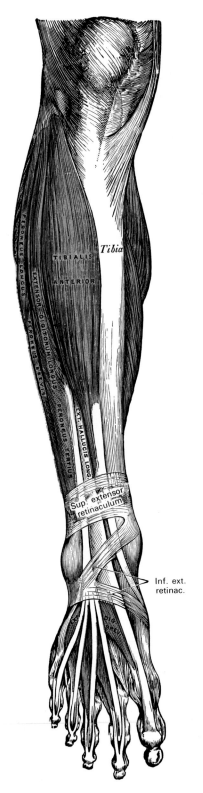

FIG. 14–10. Muscles of the anterior leg. (From Gray's Anatomy. 30th Ed. Philadelphia, Lea & Febiger, 1985, p. 574.)

terior plays no role in the normal static support of the long arch of the foot. During dynamically loaded conditions, however, muscular contraction does assist the primary source of arch support, the osseoligamentous structures. Individuals with flat feet also require muscular support of the arches, especially support by the tibialis anterior.[11]

Posterior Crural. The muscles of the posterior crural group can be further classified as either superficial or deep. The superficial group includes the gastrocnemius, soleus, and plantaris muscles. The deep group is composed of the popliteus muscle, flexor hallucis longus, flexor digitorum longus, and tibialis posterior (Figs. 14–12 and 14–13).

The two heads of the gastrocnemius and the soleus are referred to as the triceps surae. These muscles, along with the plantaris muscle, insert commonly into the calcaneal (Achilles) tendon (tendocalcaneus). The two-headed gastrocnemius is the most superficial, covering the soleus. Although both are strong plantar flexors, the gastrocnemius, being a two-joint muscle, can be affected by the position and movement of the knee (Fig. 14–14). The plantaris muscle, a vestigial, rudimentary muscle,[6,11] is absent in up to 8% of the human population.

The muscles composing the deep group are the popliteus (discussed in Chapter 13), the flexor hallucis longus, flexor digitorum longus, and tibialis posterior. The flexor hallucis longus serves primarily as a flexor of the great toe, inserting at the base of the distal phalanx. The flexor digitorum longus, the tendon of which divides into four separate tendons attaching to the bases of the four distal phalanges (toes two through five), flexes the distal phalanxes of those toes. The tendons of both of these muscles pass behind the medial malleolus and are connected by a strong tendon (Fig. 14–15).

Soderberg's[14] statement that little is known about the ankle and foot is accurate, considering that controversy surrounds the actions of the flexor hallucis longus and the flexor digitorum longus. Gray[11] indicated that the flexor hallucis longus is an important contributor to foot propulsion during gait; however, Frennette and Jackson[15] reported that though the muscle is not essential in this role, it is

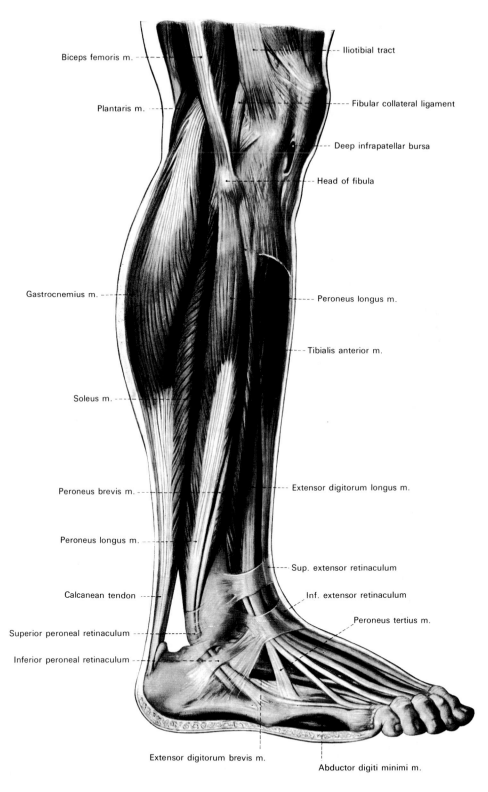

Biceps femoris m.

Plantaris m.

Gastrocnemius m.

Soleus m.

Peroneus brevis m.

Peroneus longus m.

Calcanean tendon

Superior peroneal retinaculum

Inferior peroneal retinaculum

Iliotibial tract

Fibular collateral ligament

Deep infrapatellar bursa

Head of fibula

Peroneus longus m.

Tibialis anterior m.

Extensor digitorum longus m.

Sup. extensor retinaculum

Inf. extensor retinaculum

Peroneus tertius m.

Extensor digitorum brevis m.

Abductor digiti minimi m.

FIG. 14–11.   Muscles of the right leg, viewed from the lateral aspect. (From Benninghoff and Goerttler, Lehrbuch der Anatomie des Menschen. 11th Ed., Vol. 1. Urban & Schwarzenberg, 1975.)

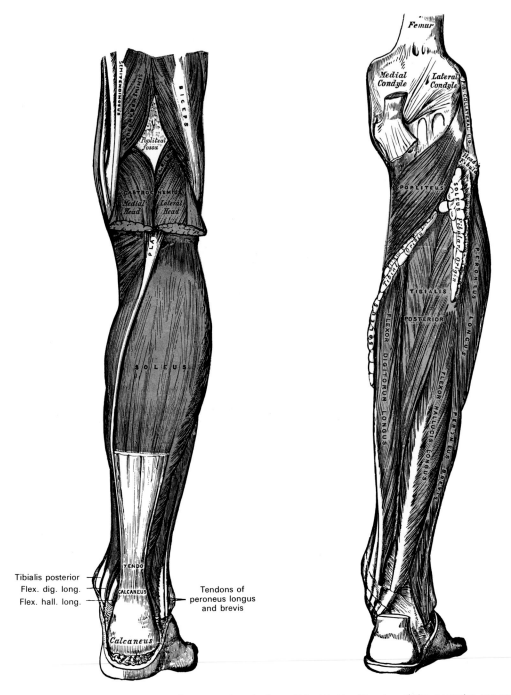

FIG. 14–12. Muscles of the posterior compartment of the leg. Superficial layer. (From Gray's Anatomy. 30th Ed. Philadelphia, Lea & Febiger, 1985, p. 576.)

FIG. 14–13. Muscles of the posterior compartment of the leg. Deep layer. (From Gray's Anatomy. 30th Ed. Philadelphia, Lea & Febiger, 1985, p. 578.)

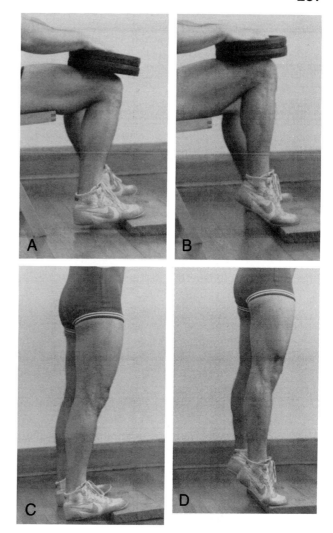

FIG. 14–14. Two exercises used for strengthening the plantar flexors. *A* and *B*, Note how in the sitting posture, the flexed knee joint shortens the gastrocnemius, thereby causing its contribution to motion to be reduced. To lift the same weight as in *C* and *D*, the individual must recruit the soleus to a greater extent.

critical in maintaining equilibrium while standing.

The tibialis posterior lies deep to the triceps surae, and, like the flexor digitorum longus and the flexor hallucis longus, crosses behind the medial malleolus. Because of its insertion on the inferior surface of the navicular bone, the tibialis posterior muscle is a prime mover for inversion and assists in weight-bearing plantar flexion.

Lateral Crural. Two muscles compose the lateral crural group, the peroneus longus and the peroneus brevis muscles. An intermuscular septum separates this group from the anterior and posterior groups. Both muscles pass behind the lateral malleolus to their insertions on the plantar surface of the foot. They both assist in plantar flexion, though

their major contributions are to foot pronation (combined eversion and abduction).

There are 11 muscles intrinsic to the foot, all but one associated with the plantar aspect. Several of those muscles are analogous to those found in the hand. The extensor digitorum brevis is found on the foot's dorsal aspect. The most medial aspect of this muscle is often considered a separate muscle, the extensor hallucis brevis. These muscles extend the toes.

The muscles of the plantar region are divided into medial, lateral, and intermediate groups. The medial group is associated with the great toe and the lateral group with the small toe. The intermediate group is associated with tendons that separate the medial and lateral groups. Despite the anatomic

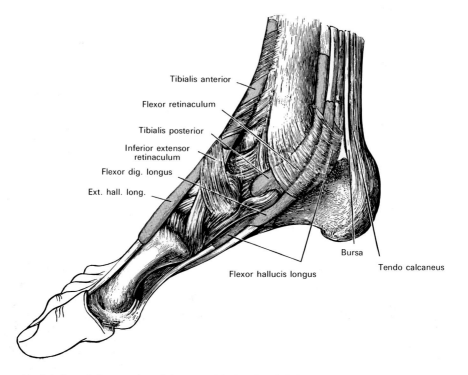

Tibialis anterior

Flexor retinaculum

Tibialis posterior

Inferior extensor retinaculum

Flexor dig. longus

Ext. hall. long.

Bursa

Tendo calcaneus

Flexor hallucis longus

FIG. 14–15. Medial view of the muscles of the synovial sheaths of their tendons around the ankle. (From Gray's Anatomy. 30th Ed. Philadelphia, Lea & Febiger, 1985, p. 583.)

grouping, the muscles of the three groups are more often categorized by their layers, first through fourth, which are apparent during dissection.

The most superficial layer, the first, is found deep to the plantar fascia. It is composed of the abductor hallucis, the flexor digitorum brevis, and the abductor digiti minimi, all of which originate from the calcaneus (Fig. 14–16).

The second layer of plantar muscles is composed of the quadratus plantae and the lumbricals. The former originates on the calcaneus; the latter arise from the tendons of the flexor digitorum longus. The quadratus plantae, which inserts into the tendon of the flexor digitorum longus, aids that muscle in toe flexion by altering its line of pull to more closely approximate the long axis of the foot (Fig. 14–17).

The four lumbricals arise from the tendons of the flexor digitorum longus and aid in the flexion of the proximal phalanges. The foot, like the hand, has an extensor expansion, and the lumbricals, acting through it, also extend the phalanges of the four lateral toes.

The third plantar layer is made up of the flexor hallucis brevis, the flexor digiti minimi brevis, and the adductor hallucis. The flexor hallucis brevis divides into two parts just distal to its origin. Each part, medial and lateral, inserts into the medial and lateral aspect, respectively, of the proximal phalanx and includes a sesamoid bone. This muscle flexes the proximal phalanx of the great toe.

The flexor digiti minimi flexes the little toe. It is superficial to the fifth metatarsal and runs somewhat parallel to it. The adductor hallucis is a two-headed muscle possessing an oblique and transverse aspect. Both heads converge to the insertion at the base of the proximal phalanx. Primarily an adductor of the great toe, it can also flex the proximal phalanx (Fig. 14–18).

The fourth plantar layer consists of the dorsal and plantar interossei. The four dorsal interossei, each having two heads arising from adjacent metatarsals, insert at the base of the proximal phalanges. These muscles abduct the toes and through the extensor expansion help to flex the proximal phalanx and extend the distal phalanges.

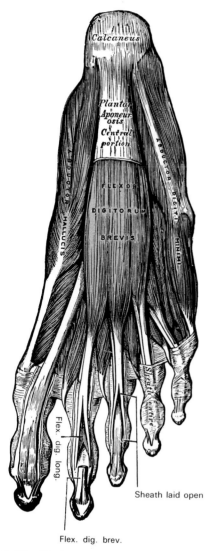

FIG. 14–16.   The first layer of plantar muscles. Right foot. (From Gray's Anatomy. 30th Ed. Philadelphia, Lea & Febiger, 1985, p. 585.)

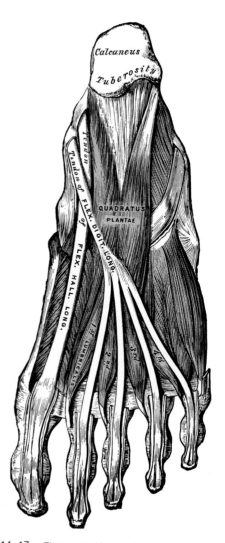

FIG. 14–17.   The second layer of plantar muscles. Right foot. (From Gray's Anatomy. 30th Ed. Philadelphia, Lea & Febiger, 1985, p. 587.)

The three plantar interossei are found along the plantar surface of the metatarsals; each interosseus is connected to only one metatarsal. Their origins and insertions are such that they adduct toes three through five, and through the extensor expansion they flex the proximal and extend the distal phalanges.

MECHANICAL CONSIDERATIONS OF INJURY TO THE ANKLE AND FOOT

Injuries to the ankle joint are the most common trauma in athletics. Functionally, the diarthritic hinge joint permits only dorsiflex-ion and plantar flexion. Extreme motion in either direction can cause injury but does so less frequently than motion caused by laterally directed forces, which result in either inversion or eversion.

Inversion injuries account for 85% of all ankle injuries. Relative to the axis of the shank, inversion injuries also consist of adduction and plantar flexion forces. If the joint displacement is severe enough to partially or completely tear supportive ligaments, the medial aspect of the talus becomes impinged on the medial malleolus, over which it then pivots. The lateral ligaments are thereby stressed, and if the inversion continues, the

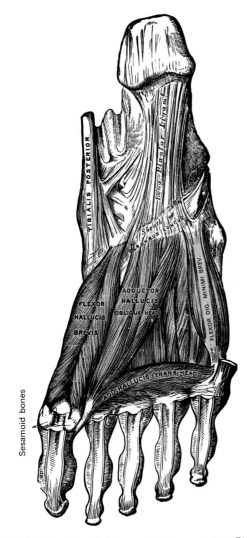

Sesamoid bones

FIG. 14–18. The third layer of plantar muscles. Right foot. (From Gray's Anatomy. 30th Ed. Philadelphia, Lea & Febiger, 1985, p. 588.)

medial malleolus can fracture, usually in a vertical direction.

In eversion injuries, the lateral malleolus, which is longer than its medial counterpart, becomes stressed as the foot moves laterally with respect to the tibia and also abducts and dorsiflexes. The lateral malleolus prevents the talus from pivoting. Rather, the impingement of the talus on the lateral malleolus causes extreme stress on the talus prior to strain on the medial ligaments. A fibular fracture commonly results, sometimes with damage to the medially located deltoid ligament. Damage to the lateral ligaments is possible if joint displacement proceeds.

Johnson, Dowson, and Wright[16] reported on the different influences of high- and low-top shoes on injuries to the ankle joint. High-top shoes, not surprisingly, were found to reduce the stress on the collateral ligaments during inversion and eversion, making those types of shoes safer. Because high-top shoes are heavier, however, they are not used frequently. Low-top shoes were found to have the potential to cause greater ligamentous damage if the material is mechanically stiff because of restriction placed on subtalar joint movement. The authors recommended that if low-top shoes are worn they be as flexible as possible around the ankle joint.

NEURAL INNERVATIONS

tibialis anterior: a branch of the deep peroneal nerve with fibers coming from L4, L5, and S1.

extensor hallicis longus: a branch of the deep peroneal nerve with fibers coming from L4, L5, and S1.

extensor digitorum longus: a branch of the deep peroneal nerve with fibers coming from L4, L5, and S1.

peroneus tertius: a branch of the deep peroneal nerve with fibers coming from L4, L5, and S1.

gastrocnemius: branches of the tibial nerve that contain fibers from S1 and S2.

soleus: branch of the tibial nerve containing fibers from L4, L5, and S1.

plantaris: branch of the tibial nerve containing fibers from L4, L5, and S1.

popliteus: branch of the tibial nerve containing fibers from L4, L5, and S1.

flexor hallicis longus: a branch of the tibial nerve with fibers from L1, S1, and S2.

flexor digitorum longus: a branch of the tibial nerve with fibers from L5 and S1.

tibialis posterior: a branch of the tibial nerve with fibers from L5 and S1.

peroneus longus: the superficial peroneal nerve with fibers from L4, L5, and S1.

peroneus brevis: the superficial peroneal nerve with fibers from L4, L5, and S1.

extensor digitorum brevis: the deep peroneal nerve containing fibers from L5, and S1.

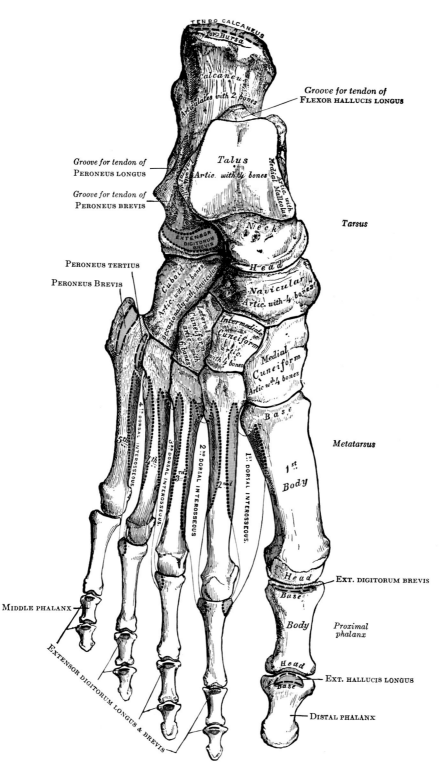

FIG. 14–19.   Bones of right foot. Dorsal surface.

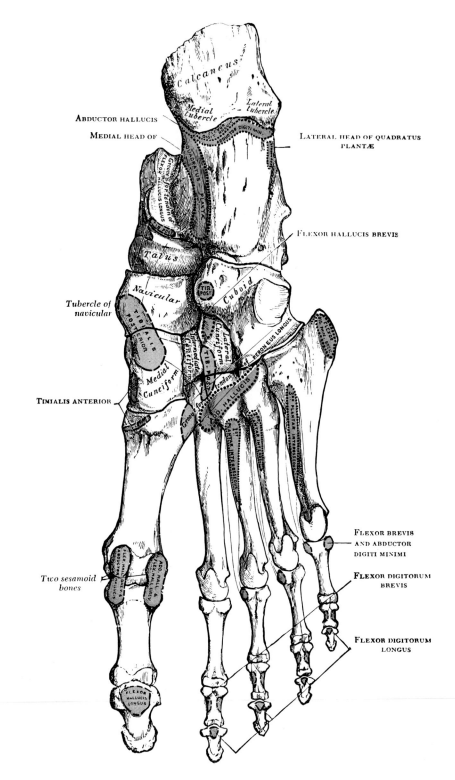

FIG. 14–20. Bones of right foot. Plantar surface.

extensor hallicis brevis: the deep peroneal nerve containing fibers from L5 and S1.

abductor hallucis: the medial plantar nerve with fibers from L4 and L5.

flexor digitorum brevis: a branch of the medial plantar nerve with fibers from L4 and L5.

abductor digiti minimi: the lateral plantar nerve containing fibers from S1 and S2.

quadratus plantae: the lateral plantar nerve containing fibers from S1 and S2.

lumbricals: the first by a branch of the medial plantar nerve containing fibers from L4 and L5; the remaining three by the lateral plantar nerve containing fibers from S1 and S2.

flexor hallucis brevis: the medial plantar nerve containing fibers from L4, L5, and S1.

flexor digiti minimi brevis: a branch of the lateral plantar nerve containing fibers from S2 and S3.

adductor hallucis: the lateral plantar nerve containing fibers from S1 and S2.

dorsal interossei: the lateral plantar nerve containing fibers from S1 and S2.

plantar interossei: the lateral plantar nerve containing fibers from S1 and S2.

STUDY QUESTIONS

1. Using Figures 14–19 and 14–20, generate a list of origins and insertions for the intrinsic muscles of the foot and insertions for the extrinsic muscles. Use Figure 13–14 for the origin of the extrinsic muscles. Compare your estimated origins and insertions to those from Gray's Anatomy or some other text and where necessary make adjustments to your responses.

2. Using the diagram of a truss and the corresponding radiograph of the foot (Figs. 14–13 and 14–14), describe how the forces are acting in such a way as to require stabilization of the metatarsals and tarsals.

3. Describe the relative importance of varying ranges of plantar and dorsiflexion to a variety of athletic populations.

4. Why would individuals accustomed to high-heeled shoes experience discomfort when wearing low-heeled shoes? Where might the discomfort be found and what are some possible anatomic and mechanical reasons?

5. Draw a free-body diagram of the leg and foot to explain why the actions of the tibialis anterior and the extensor digitorum longus can cause an even elevation of the foot.

6. Draw a free-body diagram of the flexor hallucis longus, the flexor digitorum longus, and tibialis posterior if their tendons, rather than taking the normal course behind the medial malleolus, cross anterior to it. How and why would the actions be significantly altered?

REFERENCES

1. Crouch, J.E: Functional Human Anatomy. Philadelphia, Lea & Febiger, 1985.
2. Sammarco, G.J.: Biomechanics of the foot. *In* Basic Biomechanics of the Skeletal System. Edited by V.H. Frankel and M. Nordin. Philadelphia, Lea & Febiger, 1980.
3. Stacoff, A., and Luethi, S.: Special aspects of shoe construction and foot anatomy. *In* Biomechanics of Running Shoes. Edited by B. Nigg. Champaign, Ill., Human Kinetics, 1986.
4. Soames, R.W., and Clark, C.: Heel height induced changes in metatarsal loading patterns during gait. *In* Biomechanics IX-A. Edited by D.A. Winter, et al. Champaign, Human Kinetics, 1985, pp. 446–450.
5. Soames, R.W.: Foot pressure patterns during gait. J. Biomed. Eng., 7:120, 1985.
6. Frankel, V.H., and Nordin, M.: Biomechanics of the ankle. *In* Basic Biomechanics of the Skeletal System. Edited by V.H. Frankel and M. Nordin. Philadelphia, Lea & Febiger, 1980.
7. Vaughan, C.L.: Biomechanics of running gait. CRC Crit. Rev. Biomed. Eng., 12:1, 1984.
8. Dul, J., and Johnson, G.E.: A kinematic model of the human ankle. J. Biomed. Eng., 7:137, 1985.
9. O'Connell, A.L.: Electromyographic study of certain leg muscles during movements of the free foot and during standing. Am. J. Phys. Med., 37:289, 1958.
10. Rasch, P., and Burke, R.: Kinesiology and Applied Anatomy. Philadelphia, Lea & Febiger, 1978, pp. 311–332.
11. Gray, E.R., and Basmajian, J.V.: Electromyography and cinematography of the leg and foot ("normal" and flat) during walking. Anat. Rec., 161:1, 1958.
12. Basmajian, J.V., and DeLuca, C.V.: Muscles Alive. Baltimore, Williams & Wilkins, 1985, pp. 310–353.

13. Houtz, S.J., and Fischer, F.J.: An analysis of muscle action and joint excursion during exercise on a stationary bicycle. J. Bone Joint Surg., *41A*:123, 1959.
14. Soderberg, G.L.: Kinesiology. Baltimore, Williams & Wilkins, 1986, pp. 243–266.
15. Frennette, J.P., and Jackson, D.W.: Lacerations of the flexor hallicus longus in the young athlete. J. Bone Joint Surg., *59A*:673, 1977.
16. Johnson, Dowson, and Wright: A biomechanical approach to the design of football shoes. J. Biomech., 9:581, 1976.

III APPLIED KINESIOLOGY

15 ANALYSIS AND ASSESSMENT OF HUMAN MOVEMENT PERFORMANCE

MARK D. GRABINER
JOHN GARHAMMER

Biomechanics is defined as the application of engineering principles to biologic systems, or the study of internal and external forces generated by and acting on biologic systems and of the effects of these forces. The components of biomechanics include those factors associated with the biologic and mechanical aspects of motion. The analysis and assessment of human motion, however, does not necessarily include contributions by all of these factors. A diagram of many of the cognate areas of biomechanics is presented in Figure 15–1. As an interdisciplinary area of study, biomechanics exemplifies the adage "the sum is greater than the individual parts."

In many respects, whether one is dealing directly with individual cells or with complex systems such as the moving animal or human, a major objective of biomechanics is the improvement of performance. Such improvement, whether that of an elite athlete or of an individual recovering from a traumatic injury, can be accomplished in at least three manners: by improving the individual (for example, by increasing muscle function and interaction), by improving performance equipment (such as modifying protective gear for contact sports, aerodynamic design of bobsleds, and wheelchair design); or improving the execution of the task itself, perhaps to better meet the physiologic or structural constraints of the individual.

Improvement of any or all of the above occurs as a function of some type of analysis following some type of a measurement. Measurement may be done by visual inspection, such as a physical educator, physical therapist, or coach performs. Other measurement must be made in a controlled laboratory environment using computer-controlled measurement devices.

Following measurement, analysis of the data, which in this case is performance, occurs by breaking down the performance into some number of critical performance skills. For example, the time it takes for a cross-country skier to complete a course can be broken down into the time spent going uphill, going downhill, and traveling on the flats. Because the techniques for each of these skills differ, they can be further analyzed or broken down into individual segmental contributions, such as the contribution to performance of the upper compared to the lower extremities.

After data collection, measurement, and analysis comes assessment or evaluation, during which are made judgments regarding the presence or absence of the variables that are deemed crucial to improved performance. An example might be a gymnast's loss of vertical height when dismounting from an apparatus to the benefit of increased horizontal distance. In a triple somersault this loss can lead to injury in the worst scenario, or to loss of points in a less devastating situation. Similarly, a wheelchair athlete might find that his efficiency is decreased by the position of the wheels with respect to the seat itself.

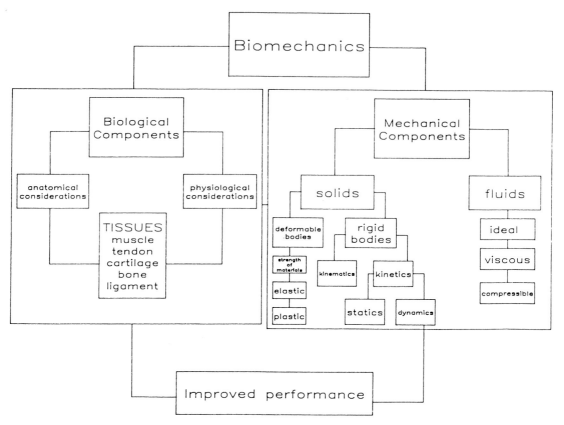

FIG. 15–1. Schematic diagram of the major components of the biomechanics study.

The term efficiency can be used physiologically, mechanically, or in both manners. From a mechanical standpoint, efficiency relates to the mechanical energy put into a system compared to the mechanical energy generated by the system. A task that increases the energy demand without concomitantly increasing the performance decreases efficiency. Effective motion, by definition, is independent of efficiency and relates only to the success or failure of the involved task. For example, a sprinter finds it advantageous to minimize the vertical oscillations of his center of gravity because these oscillations require that work be done against the force of gravity, work that is actually perpendicular to the direction of the desired motion. Any vertical change in the height of the center of gravity that is not directly related to the proper projection of the sprinter along a parabolic trajectory is both inefficient (from an energy standpoint) and ineffective (because to travel the extra vertical distance requires extra time). Similar cases can be made for the hurdler, long jumper, and high jumper.

JOINT AND MUSCULAR ANALYSIS

One of the fundamental types of human motion analysis is often referred to as a joint and muscular analysis. This deductive type of analysis answers the question "What are the anatomic bases of execution of this movement task?" This type of analysis begins with a specific movement task, identifies specific characteristics of the task, and ultimately assesses the performance with respect to some criterion. If the analysis is being performed on one who has sustained an injury, the criterion might be the performance of a normal individual. The performance of an elite athlete might be used when analyzing a lesser skilled athlete. In either case, the comparison is made against what is commonly referred to as a model.

The various approaches to joint and muscular analysis have some common elements. Three fundamental procedural steps include:

1. Describing the movement and, where

appropriate, dividing it into important segments, or phases.
2. Subjecting each phase to the joint and muscular analysis.
3. Subjecting the analyzed data to the selected criteria.

The description of the movement consists primarily of taking a simple or complex motor skill and defining it as a series of individual movements that ultimately are kinematically and kinetically linked. Hay and Reid[1] indicate that a performance represents only a discrete execution of the skill. This interpretation suggests that analysis of just one performance of a complex skill (state) might not reflect overall ability (trait). Every dive, leap, or lift, for example, consists of so many integrated segments that a coach, scientist, or casual observer must be fairly knowledgeable not only with respect to the skill itself but also with respect to the performer.

In a simple exercise such as a parallel bar dip, the general description might include merely the initial position, the movement phase, the return phase, and the terminal position. For a complex skill such as swimming, however, one must consider a variety of aspects. Further, competitive swimming could be broken down into the start, stroke, and turns.

The second step, the joint and muscular analysis, is performed for each defined phase of the particular movement or skill. First, one must identify the specific joint action that is occurring. For example, in the elapsed time from heel strike to full foot support during human locomotion, the joint action observed at the ankle joint is plantar flexion. Similarly, the joint action observed at the knee is flexion. Though by themselves these observations do not provide a great deal of relevant information because of the numerous other factors that must be considered, they are a point of departure and also illuminate an important point: standard biomechanical terminology must be adhered to at all times. A person evaluating a particular analysis should be able to determine precisely the motion taking place merely by its description.

After the joint action is identified, the tendency of external forces to cause motion at

that joint should be listed. These external forces are treated as simple vectors with magnitude and direction. For example, using Figure 9–9, the effect of gravity acting through the center of gravity of the forearm-wrist-hand-weight segment creates an external torque that tends to cause elbow extension. An exception to this case is observed when the elbow is flexed to an angle such that it moves beyond the vertical, in which case the external force tends to cause elbow flexion.

Following the identification of these external forces and their associated tendencies at the joint of interest, the next step is to identify the general muscle group that most likely is active. The active muscle group is determined as a function of both the effect of the external forces and the classification of the movement with respect to the angular velocity (technically, the acceleration) of the involved joints or segments. These decisions become intuitive after practice and using a set of simple rules. One of the techniques that is useful at this point of analysis is to draw a free-body diagram of the system.

The initial question to be answered is whether the observed joint action is in the same or the opposite direction as the external forces. If the particular joint under analysis does not display movement in either the same or the opposite direction as the external force tendency, the forces and torques are equivalent and the contraction of the muscles can be classified as isometric. If the joint displays movement in an opposite direction to the external force, the muscular contraction is concentric.

If the observed joint action is in the direction of the external forces, subsequent questions regarding the kinematics of the motion must be answered. Using Newton's laws of motion, one must determine whether the angular velocity of the joint or segment is greater than or less than the angular velocity that would be associated with the external forces.

Gravity, the fundamental external force, causes accelerated motion toward the earth at 9.8 m/sec². The velocity of a particular body falling under the influence of gravity is determined using the simple equations associated with constant acceleration. The equation $V_f = V_i + a \times t$ indicates that the final velocity, v_f, can be calculated by multiplying the value for its acceleration, a, by the time, t, during which it was accelerated and adding to it the initial velocity, v_i. A ball released from 0 initial velocity and allowed to fall freely for 2.3 sec, therefore, will have velocity $V_f = 0 + 9.8$ m/sec² × 2.3 sec, which is 22.54 m/sec. The only condition that will prevent this velocity from being attained if the gravity function remains constant is the effect of external forces, such as air drag, on the system.

An example of this analysis with respect to determining the type of muscular contraction associated with a particular joint action can be made using an exercise called the parallel squat. The parallel squat is performed with a barbell placed across the shoulders. The performer begins in the erect upright position, flexes the hips and knees until the thighs are parallel to the ground, then reverses the motion. The final position is the same as the beginning position.

Using the knees for this example, the observed joint action is flexion. The tendency of the external force, represented by the vector of gravity acting through the mass of the weight and barbell, is to cause the knees to flex. The tendency is greater as the knees become more flexed and the vector of gravity moves farther from the axis of knee rotation. Using the angular analogue of the equation to determine what the velocity of knee flexion should be after some elapsed time, or simply by observing that the task is generally performed more slowly than would be expected if only gravity were acting on the system, one may proceed with the analysis. Because the observed knee flexion is associated with movement in the direction of the external force but is slower than what would be expected by virtue of the external force, the knee flexion is attributed to eccentric contraction of the knee extensors. If in the unlikely and perhaps unfortunate case that the knee flexion is actually faster than would be associated with gravity, the knee flexion is a function of knee flexor activity and the type of contraction is concentric.

Joint and muscular analyses, although extremely simple, are fundamental in the qualitative analysis of movement. Analysis of this kind, perhaps informally, will precede more complex analyses and modeling procedures. Because the process is simple, its usefulness is limited. Naturally, the more steps that are considered, the more complex the process. The steps previously outlined represent what can be performed reasonably well without the need for extreme supposition or extrapolation, or without the use of laboratory-oriented instrumentation.

Important factors that are not generally addressed in the joint and muscular analysis include the activation and action of multijoint muscles, cocontraction of synergists and antagonists, and contributions to segmental kinetics by passive sources, that is, elastic energy from stretched muscles and passive joint torques arising from ligaments, cartilage, and joint capsules.

Cocontraction of synergists is beneficial to effective and efficient movement in that the torques generated by their contraction tend to contribute to the desired motion and simultaneously stabilize a necessary body segment, or the torques directly neutralize any undesired joint action of one of the agonists or synergists.

Cocontraction can be either detrimental or critical to performance, depending on the situation. If cocontraction is associated with the initial stages of learning a novel skill or pathologic spasticity, it involves mechanical and physiologic inefficiency. During a ballistic motion and locomotion, however, simultaneous activation of agonists, synergists, and antagonists are required. If in a qualitative analysis neither the magnitude of a muscular contraction with respect to its maximum, nor the moment arms through which the muscles act are known, the addition of the above neuromuscular considerations to joint and muscular function would probably cause the entire muscular system to contract isometrically in even the simplest of tasks.

Another aspect not considered in the joint and muscular analysis relates to the muscular properties of extensibility and elasticity. Extensibility is the muscle's ability to lengthen, whether the muscle is active or at rest. Elasticity is the muscle's ability to restore itself to its original (pre-stress) shape (configuration). Elasticity is an internally generated force, as is the tension that a muscle generates. During the initial description of a movement phase, a joint position can be defined with respect to the anatomic position. This deviation, which will cause certain muscles to be lengthened, has important implications for the subsequent motion. The stretch-shorten cycle[2] is the combination of eccentric and concentric contractions that allows for greater force and velocity outputs and efficiencies than if the movement were initiated from a concentric contraction not preceded by the lengthening.

MUSCLE ELASTICITY AND ELASTIC ENERGY CONTRIBUTIONS TO MOVEMENT

The force-velocity relationship illustrates that eccentric muscular contraction can result in a force output greater than the maximal isometric force. This force output is a result of chemical and mechanical influences, the latter being associated with muscle elasticity. Muscle elasticity has been associated with such anatomic structures as the tendons, cell membranes, fascia, and the cross-bridges.

Muscle is often modeled as consisting of three functional components (Fig. 15–2), the contractile element, the parallel elastic component (PEC), and the series elastic component (SEC). The contractile element is responsible for the active generation of muscular force, "active" indicating that it requires metabolic energy. This component represents in reality the actin-myosin interaction. The PEC is parallel with the contractile element and is said to reside in the sarcolemma and other fascial tissues surrounding the muscle fibers, bundles, and groups. The SEC is in series with the contractile element and is said to reside mainly in the tendons and cross-bridges.

Figure 15–2 implies that if the muscle were lengthened while at rest or active, both the PEC and SEC would extend and thus exert a spring-like restoring force, somewhat proportionate to the amount of displacement. The restoring force sums linearly with the force generated by the contractile component. When a muscle contracts the PEC remains uninvolved; the SEC is lengthened before tension can be transmitted through the tendon to the insertion. The SEC serves a number purposes.[3] It serves as a buffer between a muscle and its insertion, protecting the insertion from damage during the abrupt transition from the resting to the active state. The SEC also stores the mechanical (potential, elastic) energy that allows the muscle to contract faster than it could if the muscle depended on only the contractile component.

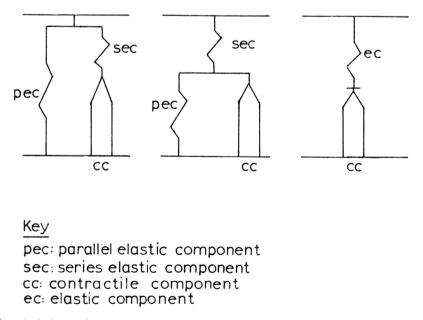

Key

pec: parallel elastic component
sec: series elastic component
cc: contractile component
ec: elastic component

FIG. 15–2.   Three typical representations of the three-component model of muscle. Each has its own set of elastic and extensibility properties based on the configuration of components.

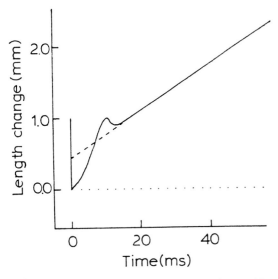

FIG. 15–3.   The biphasic shortening curve observed for isolated muscle. The two distinct phases represent shortening of the SEC (steep slope) and the contractile component (shallow slope). The transition period between the two phases is considered an effect of the measurement system.

The accumulation of elastic energy and its subsequent recovery and addition to the system is the basis for the stretch-shorten cycle. A biphasic shortening curve illustrates the mechanics of the SEC and contractile component interaction (Fig. 15–3).

Experiments of this type are performed with excised muscle that is stimulated maximally at a constant length, and in an isometric contraction, and then allowed to shorten without resistance. At time t_0, the resistance to the muscle is reduced or eliminated. Two distinct phases of shortening are observed. The first, having a relatively steep slope, is associated with the recoil of the SEC. A transition period is then followed by a period of shortening with a relatively shallow slope associated with the shortening of the contractile component.

Average velocity may be calculated as

$$V_{avg} = .5 \times (v_1 + v_2)$$

Because the slope of the time-displacement function is greater for the SEC than for the contractile element, the velocities differ in the same way. The average velocity for the shortening period is greater as a result of the contribution by the recoiling elastic element. The elasticity of ligaments and cartilage can also contribute to movement. An example of this contribution is flexion relaxation in which the reduction of the erector spinae excitation might be attributed to the elastic contribution to extensor torque by the muscle itself, as well as to the joint capsules of the facet joints.

Elasticity of biologic tissues and other materials can be tested by placing the tissue under a known load and measuring its deformation. Results are plotted in a load deformation curve (Fig. 15–4).

The results of a load deformation test can reveal to a researcher a number of important qualities and quantities of the material being tested. The area from point A to point B is called the elastic region. When applied forces cause deformation in this region and are subsequently reduced, the material will regain its normal shape—that is, there will be no permanent deformation. The same cannot be said when a material is deformed into the region marked by points B and C, the plastic region. When the deforming force is removed the material will not return to its normal shape because it has incurred structural damage. Point D represents the failure point at which the material has become so deformed that complete mechanical failure will occur. Tests of this type done on bone, cartilage, and ligaments can be crucial in understanding the mechanics of injury.

Another purpose for these tests is associated with developing synthetic materials whose mechanical properties are similar to the natural materials. By drawing perpendicular lines from the point of failure to both the X and Y axes, one can determine three other qualities of the material: the total load that a material can withstand (its strength); the total deformation the material can undergo before failing; and the total amount of energy (elastic or potential) stored in the material which is determined by calculating the area between the curve and the X axis.

It should be clear that the study of biomechanics covers a spectrum, from single cells to complex movement, from individuals recovering from traumatic injury to elite athletes. It should also be noted that even though a biomechanist might be interested in the biologic aspects of motion, the tools prerequi-

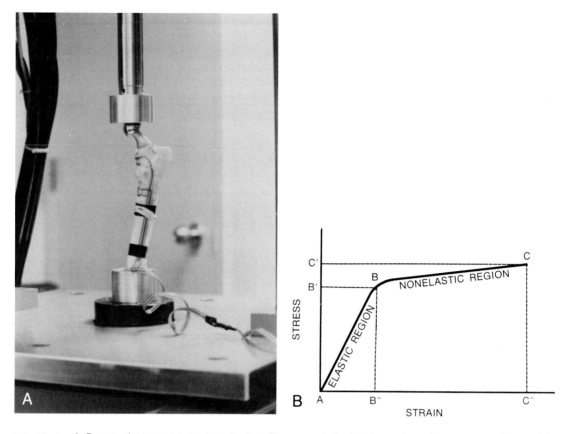

FIG. **15–4.** *A,* Picture of a materials-testing situation. The computerized instrument can be programmed to provide any sequence of compression, tensile and rotary forces, at a range of magnitudes and frequencies. *B,* Load deformation curve for cortical bone tested in tension.

Yield point (B)—point past which some permanent deformation of the bone occurred.

Yield stress (B')—load per unit area that the bone sample sustained before nonelastic deformation took place.

Yield strain (B")—amount of deformation that the sample sustained before nonelastic deformation occurred. The strain at any point in the elastic region of the curve is proportional to the stress at that point.

Ultimate failure point (C)—the point past which failure of the sample occurred.

Ultimate stress (C')—load per unit area that the sample sustained before failure.

Ultimate strain (C")—amount of deformation that the sample sustained before failure.

(From Frankel, V.H., and Nordin, M.: Basic Biomechanics of the Skeletal System. Philadelphia, Lea & Febiger, 1980, p. 18.)

site for study are those found under the mechanical components of motion.

BIOMECHANICAL CONSIDERATIONS FOR LIFTING TASKS

The need to lift objects occurs at home, at work, during exercise, and during certain sports competitions. Such lifting efforts often result in or aggravate low-back injuries and even cause disability. Disability, which often is paid for by insurance companies and has another cost associated with nonproductive

time off, is a large financial burden all over the world. In the United States, for example, eight million back injuries occur per year, each one associated with an average $18,000 in medical costs and $22,000 in compensation. Many of the problems associated with low-back pain result from high-magnitude forces generated in the structures of the lumbar and sacral regions as a result of faulty lifting mechanics, excessive loads, or both. Structural damage and the resulting pain is frequently caused by repeated minor overloading of the area over a long period of time rather than by a single traumatic event. The probability of suffering injury and pain in the low back might be reduced by performing proper strengthening exercises for the lower torso musculature, by practicing appropriate lifting mechanics, and by exercising caution regarding the magnitude and frequency of load lifting. Only the mechanics of lifting objects from the floor will be considered in this section.

What constitutes appropriate lifting mechanics depends on the required lifting task. Generally, lifting should be done with the legs (in the leg or squat-style lift with the torso remaining quasi-erect), rather than with the back (in the back or stoop-style lift) (Fig. 15–5). The most notable exception is the situation of lifting from the floor an object that is too large to be straddled between the legs. When the object is small enough to be lifted between the legs, the line of gravitational pull on its center of gravity passes relatively close to the lumbosacral joint. The moment arm of the resistance is therefore kept relatively

short, and the muscular effort required to provide the extensor torque, acting through a substantially smaller moment arm, is subsequently reduced. It is this muscle force, such as that created by the erector spinae muscle, that when excessive generates large compression forces on the lumbar vertebrae. The magnitude of these muscle forces can be many times that of the resistance. Lifting a 450-N (100-lb) load can result in a compression force at the base of the vertebral column in excess of 4000 N. This magnitude is considered hazardous to some workers, according to the standards established by the National Institute of Occupational Safety and Health.

Any attempt to use a squat lifting style for an object too large to be lifted between the legs will cause the object's center of gravity to pass relatively far away from the axis of rotation (considered here to the lumbosacral joint) because the larger object must pass an-

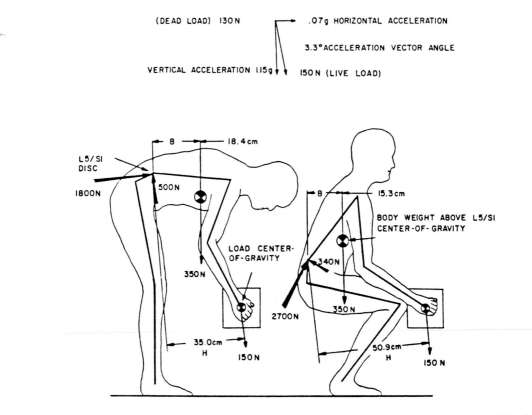

FIG. 15–5. Forces generated at the lumbosacral joint for stoop- and squat-style lift of 150 N, as predicted using biomechanical modeling techniques. (From Chaffin, D.B., and Andersson, G.B.J.: Occupational Biomechanics. New York, John Wiley & Sons, 1984, p. 205.)

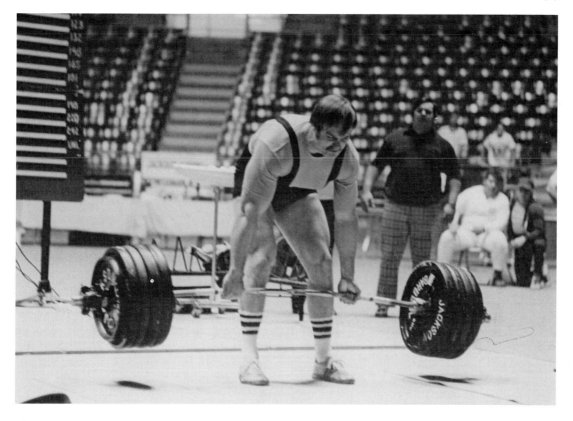

FIG. 15–6.   Early phase of the dead lift with 815 lb as performed in competitive powerlifting by John Kuc. Note the stoop lift position. (Photo by B. Klemens.)

teriorly to the knee joints during the initial part of the lift, making the distance to its center of gravity a function (sine of the hip angle) of the length of the thigh and the object's width. In such situations, biomechanical modeling techniques have indicated that the stoop-style lift will result in lower compressional forces at the lumbar vertebrae and disks because the object's center of gravity can be kept closer to the lumbosacral joint than with the squat-style lift.[4] Such a comparison is illustrated in Figure 15–5, where a 150-N (33-lb) load is being lifted. Shear forces are greater using the stoop technique. Shear forces are necessitated primarily by the facet joints rather than by the intervertebral disks, which are affected more by compression forces.

Based on the type of information presented here and other research using electromyography and intradiskal and intra-abdominal pressure measurements, the best and safest method for lifting is as yet unclear but de-

pends on several factors. Some of these factors, such as muscular strength and the exact size and shape of the individual motion units of the vertebral column, are subject specific. Perhaps the best advice is to avoid asymmetric loading patterns, that is, lifts that occur outside of the sagittal plane; to be conservative in lifting efforts; and to establish lifting limits through gradual increases and attention to bodily feedback such as pain and soreness.

An interesting observation relative to lifting styles can be made with competitive strength and power athletes. In competitive power lifting, very heavy loads, frequently in excess of 800 lb in the upper weight categories, are lifted from the floor in the dead lift. Figure 15–6 illustrates such a lift shortly after its initiation. Note the stoop or back lift position with the heavy weight.

In contrast, note the squat or leg lift positions that are maintained during a clean lift (Fig. 15–7). In this lift it is not uncommon for

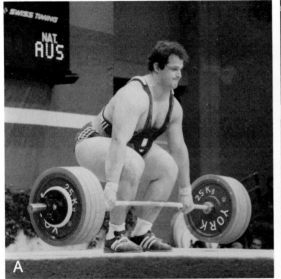
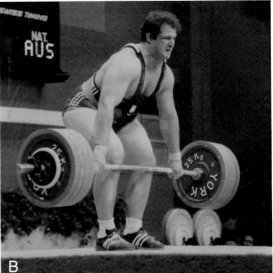
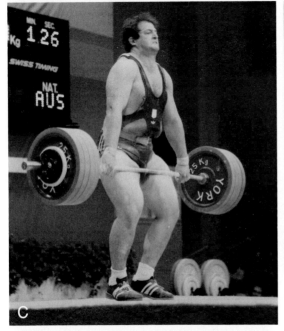
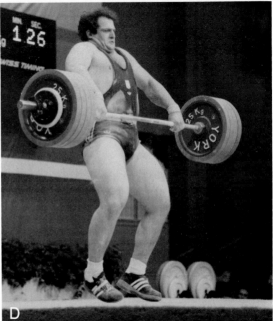
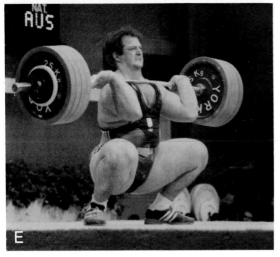

FIG. 15–7. Sequence of positions in performing the clean phase of the winning clean and jerk (528 lb) in the super heavyweight division at the 1984 Olympic games in Los Angeles. *A,* Liftoff. *B,* End of the first pull. *C,* Start of the second pull (note the shift of body position to bring the barbell closer to the lumbosacral joint). *D,* End of the second pull, or jump, start of the movement under the bar. *E,* Catch position. (Photo by B. Klemens.)

500 lb or more to be lifted in the upper weight categories. The reasons for these technique differences in competitive lifting style are not clearly understood. Part of the differences may be due to genetic factors such as segment lengths and the structure of bone and joints. Specific methods of training and training adaptation are other considerations. Finally, the goal of each lift must also be considered. The dead lift is a slow lift to a terminal position with the bar at about midthigh level (see Fig. 6–7). The clean lift is a much faster lift, particularly the second pull, after the bar reaches knee height and must be lifted to the shoulders. Note in Figure 15–7 that the lifter moves the bar as close to the hip and lumbosacral joint as possible for the second pull. At this point the bar reaches maximal acceleration, and the resulting forces exerted on body segments such as the lower back reach values far in excess of the barbell weight.

REFERENCES

1. Hay, J.G., and Reid, J.G.: The Anatomical and Mechanical Bases of Human Motion. Englewood Cliffs, Prentice-Hall, 1982.
2. Komi, P.: The stretch-shorten cycle and human power output. *In* Human Muscle Power. Edited by N.L. Jones, N. McCartney, and A.J. McComas. Champaign, Human Kinetics, Publishers, 1986.
3. Hill, A.V.: The series elastic component of muscle. Proc. R. Soc. Lond., B, *137*:273, 1950.
4. Chaffin, D.B., and Andersson, G.B.J.: Occupational Biomechanical Models. New York, John Wiley, 1984. Chapter 6.

16 PRINCIPLES OF TRAINING AND DEVELOPMENT

JOHN GARHAMMER

Organized exercise programs are formulated for many specific purposes. Among these are general health and physical fitness, improvement of performance in various work tasks and sports, rehabilitation, and therapeutic treatment. For each individual and his specific objective, the details of the exercise program will be different. This disparity makes it virtually impossible to specify a standard program suitable for everyone or anyone, although the literature abounds with examples of such attempts. Many books and articles, for instance, list specific exercises for various purposes, sometimes even specifying the exact number of repetitions.

The viewpoint of this chapter is that any specific exercise program should be formulated by informed judgment and should apply established general principles. It is the purpose of this chapter to identify *general principles*, on the basis of which a trained professional can create an appropriate exercise program or evaluate an existing program.

THE NATURE OF PERFORMANCE

Any human performance can be viewed as the expression of a number of components called performance factors, some of which are general factors and some of which are specific factors. Historically, some comprehensive human capabilities have been suggested, such as general intelligence, physical fitness, and general athletic ability. These concepts are so complex and inclusive as to be unwieldy and almost undefinable.

In practice, it is more useful to analyze them into component factors. A factor such as strength contributes to so many different kinds of motor performance that it is usually considered to be a relatively general factor. At the other extreme, certain coordinated movements such as hitting a high backhand drop shot in badminton are so specialized as to be very specific factors. The statistical technique of factor analysis has been used to identify the component factors in many kinds of motor performance. Those factors most often identified include muscular strength and cardiovascular-respiratory endurance as relatively general factors and specific coordinations and joint flexibilities as factors that are highly specific to the performance under consideration.

Any performance might be formally or informally analyzed to determine its components in terms of general or specific factors. Once these are identified, developmental or training efforts can be formulated, and it is at this point that the principles listed in this chapter become helpful, especially when pursuing the more general factors.

It seems easy to conceive of supposedly general factors. On analysis, however, these often are shown to be composed of more specific subfactors. For example, strength may be subdivided into discrete subfactors of dynamic, static, and explosive strength (power). Studies on effects of various training methods confirm the idea that these are separate subfactors that can be developed differentially.

Muscular endurance can be defined as the ability of a muscle to sustain an isometric contraction or to continue dynamic contractions. Muscular endurance can best be discussed relative to maximum muscular strength. As an individual's muscular strength increases, the number of times an absolute weight, say 50 lb, can be lifted in a given movement will increase. This increase in absolute muscular endurance is valuable to a gymnast who must pull up her (constant) body weight many times in a competitive event or to a laborer who must lift similar objects repeatedly during each work day. As an individual's muscular strength increases, however, he may or may not experience much of an increase in relative muscular endurance, that is, the number of times a weight requiring a fixed percentage of maximum strength, say 60%, can be lifted. The exact training effect would depend on the method used to develop the increased strength—for example, lifting weights for higher repetitions (10 to 15+) versus lower repetitions (3 to 6), as discussed later in this chapter.

THE NATURE OF PHYSICAL FITNESS

Although "physical fitness" is frequently chosen as a desirable goal, the concept seems to have no completely satisfactory definition. The President's Council on Physical Fitness and Sports defined it as "the ability to carry out daily tasks with vigor and alertness, without undue fatigue, and with ample energy to enjoy leisure time pursuits and to meet unforeseen emergencies."[1] In order to create an operational definition of physical fitness, a special committee of physical educators suggested that a physical fitness test should (1) measure a component that extends from severely limited dysfunction to high levels of functional capacity, (2) have improved results with appropriate physical activity, and (3) reflect changes in functional capacity accurately.[2]

Three areas of positive health that meet these criteria for physical fitness testing were identified: cardiovascular endurance, obesity (body composition), and musculoskeletal function. Physical fitness is thus associated with functional health and is distinguished from its traditional association relating performance primarily to athletic ability, which should more appropriately be designated as "motor fitness." The committee found that "pure" factors of strength, endurance, and power were not measured by traditional motor performance tests. Therefore, they recommended a separate battery of motor fitness tests, evaluating the ability to (1) move or support the body against the pull of gravity, (2) run with speed over short distances, (3) start, stop, and turn rapidly while running, and (4) expend energy in one explosive self-propelling act.

MASTER PRINCIPLES

Master principles are those that apply pervasively to more than one of the identifiable performance factors—strength, cardiovascular-respiratory endurance, flexibility, and speed of movement. Because some principles are relatively specific to individual performance factors, they are listed in a separate section following the master principles, but this does not imply that they are less important.

1. The Overload Principle. Beneficial human performance adaptations occur in response to demands applied to the body at levels beyond a certain threshold value (overload) but within the limits of tolerance and safety. Low-level demands, to which the body has already adapted, are not sufficient to induce a further training adaptation. In the useful range, an adequate training stimulus normally causes some disruption of tissues or of biochemical balance. During the interval between training bouts, repair and restoration occur, accompanied by some overcompensation that raises the person's capability to a new level. The nature of the training stimulus varies for each specific factor or quality of performance, and the exact threshold value varies with the immediate state of training and with other individual characteristics.

Overload during exercise can be quantified in terms of training volume (amount of work done) and training intensity (rate of doing work). For strength, training volume is the number of lifting repetitions done in a workout, and intensity is the average weight lifted.

Strength training studies by Berger[3] and O'Shea[4] in the 1960s indicated that three sets of five to six repetitions (after warm-up) resulted in the greatest specific strength gains over a short-term training period. Thus, the volume would be 15 to 18 repetitions (3 × 5 or 3 × 6) per exercise, and the intensity would be the average weight used for the exercises, which should be heavy enough to produce some fatigue by the end of each set. More-recent research by Stone, et al.,[5,6] however, indicated that cycling sets and repetitions over a period of months from high volume (5 × 10) to medium volume (5 × 5) to low volume (3 × 3) produces even greater strength gains. Varying the intensity from workout to workout can also increase gains, particularly for more advanced athletes.[7,8] To improve muscular endurance to a greater extent and deemphasize strength gains, higher repetition sets (10 to 15) can be used, resulting in lower intensity work but at a higher volume. Some skills that *use* strength for optimal performance are poor *developers* of strength. Thus, although strength is helpful in batting a softball, the skill can be repeated consecutively an almost unlimited number of times, indicating that the amount of resistance is inadequate for efficient development of strength. With weight training equipment, the amount of resistance, the number of repetitions, and the number of sets of exercise can be regulated precisely to bring efficient strength adaptation.

For *cardiovascular respiratory* conditioning, overload can be evaluated by measuring heart rate or, with laboratory equipment, oxygen uptake in milliliters per kilogram of body weight per minute.[9] The maximum achievable human heart rate depends on age, sex, and individual variables. For sedentary individuals, achieving pulse rates as low as 120 beats per minute may possess some training value. For persons in better physical condition, pulse rates above 150 beats per minute are necessary to produce a training effect. Experienced athletes in serious training may exceed 90% of their maximum heart rates in training bouts. However, at higher rates the action of the heart becomes inefficient, as it does not have time to fill with blood between beats.

Cardiovascular-respiratory overload is generally created by continuous endurance-oriented activities such as running, cycling, swimming, rowing, and cross-country skiing.[9] The training volume in running, for example, is the total distance covered, while the intensity is the average speed or pace—usually measured in minutes per mile. As with strength training, some variation in running volume and intensity from workout to workout, week to week, and month to month is conducive to progress.

Another productive method to increase intensity is interval training.[10,11] With this method, the athlete runs a given distance in segments or work intervals separated by rest intervals, permitting a much higher average intensity than a continuous run allows by preventing the build-up of excessive levels of catabolites. As with strength training, intensity must be adjusted to produce enough stimulus to elicit a favorable adaptation (training effect) in the body. Some individuals run long distances regularly but at such a slow pace that no improvement occurs, although they maintain their fitness level. Conversely, sprinting a short distance will not provide cardiovascular-respiratory conditioning, even though it is of high intensity. A proper combination of volume and intensity is required to produce desired adaptations.

The development and maintenance of bone strength and joint flexibility also depends on the types of demands made on the body. Bones require compression, shear, and bending forces, whose magnitudes are expressed as force per unit area of bone. During growth, physical activities such as running, jumping, and climbing create adequate forces to develop strong bones. In adulthood, physical activities and excercise must be sufficient to maintain or develop specialized bone strengths for specific activities such as skiing or tennis. *Osteoporosis* (increased porosity and decalcification of bone) has been thought to be an inevitable symptom of aging, but its occurrence in younger bedridden patients and astronauts suggests that inactivity, rather than aging per se, is the causative factor. Specifically, the longitudinal forces of weight-bearing are required to prevent the loss of calcium from long bones like the femur.

To develop joint flexibility a joint must be moved slightly beyond its normal range of motion (to the point of minor discomfort) and held for a few seconds. To maintain flexibility, joints must regularly be moved through their full range of motion. The connection between flexibility and overall physical fitness is questioned by some, but its relationship to performance and injury reduction is generally accepted.[12,13]

2. The Frequency Principle. Training workouts should be sufficiently spaced to allow tissue growth, nutritional replenishment, and biochemical resynthesis to take place and should be sufficiently frequent to provide for physiologic development.

For developing strength, empirical and experimental evidence indicates that workouts 3 days per week yield excellent progress for beginners, with even 2 workouts per week being productive. A slightly more advanced program is the "split routine" in which upper-body exercises are done twice a week and lower-body exercises on alternate days. More advanced trainees can work each body area 3 days per week. Competitive weight-lifters and athletes in strength-oriented sports may also workout 5 or 6 days per week with weights but with a less clear distinction between body areas. However, they will use a great deal of variation in their programs relative to the exercises, sets, repetitions, and intensity. One or two weight-lifting workouts per week will usually be sufficient to maintain strength levels for several weeks, such as during periods of frequent sport competition, with or without traveling.

Strength and cardiovascular-respiratory conditioning can be accomplished by most individuals (not those highly trained in either factor) through the use of circuit weight training, in which the continuous alternation of exercises and activated muscle groups maintains elevated heart rates. Though either factor might be better developed with specialized training for that factor, circuit training is an effective and economical method (especially for large groups) to improve both[14] and can be used for short periods for variety a few times a year.

For cardiovascular-respiratory endurance, flexibility, and bone strength development

and maintenance, frequent exercise periods are desirable. Even daily workouts are feasible, if time permits, provided proper variation of volume and intensity is used.

3. The Transfer Principle. The factors (strength, endurance, etc.) of human performance are basically independent. Training for the development of one factor will improve performance only to the extent that previous performance ability was limited by that factor. The desired performance should be analyzed for its requirements with respect to each factor; the performer's capabilities should be assessed to determine his existing status in light of the performance requirements; and training exercises should be selected in a proper mix to bring performance capabilities up to the requirements. An individual can train efficiently for more than one performance to the extent that the performances require the same mix of factors.

4. The Specificity Principle. This principle is one of the most important in designing a training program. Simply stated, a specific demand (e.g., exercise) made on the body will result in a specific response by the body; furthermore, that response will depend on the condition of the trainee (novice versus expert) and on his status when the demand is made (fatigued versus well rested).

It is not possible to train in a manner exactly specific for any performance, except perhaps by performing the activity itself, but the exercises should relate closely to the requirements of the performance in terms of the muscle groups used, pattern and range of motion at specific joints, speed of motion, and repetition of movements. For example, a shot-putter can do upper-body pressing exercises with a barbell or dumbbells so that the arm makes an angle with the torso similar to that which occurs during throwing. The training movements can be less specific when an athlete is training months before any competition but should become more specific as the competition draws closer. This approach provides variety in the long-term training program. Similarly, a distance runner, swimmer, or cyclist can work out with considerable "over-distance" in the months before a meet but emphasizes the distances closer to that of the competition as it approaches.

Specificity in exercise and conditioning is important and should be a major consideration in designing a training program, but it need not be carried to the extreme. Although for physical activities such as a dance performance or occupational tasks the conditioning can vary less from the demands of the actual activity, some variety is still desirable.

Examples of the specificity of bodily adaptations to specific training are almost countless. Cardiovascular-respiratory endurance developed by distance swimming will not of itself transfer to performance in distance running or cycling, and may even hinder it. This lack of transference is due partly to biomechanical factors such as how the body's weight is supported and which muscles are active through various joint ranges of motion. Endurance exercise has also been shown to inhibit strength-power development.[15]

Flexibility enhanced through one particular activity might not indicate the presence of the flexibility required for other activities. This nontransference of flexibility may be not just for different joints, but also for a given joint for slightly different movement pattern requirements (Fig. 16–1).

Bone growth and development are well known to result in architectural and density patterns that directly relate to the types (compression, shear, bending), magnitudes, and directions of forces imposed regularly over time (Wolff's law).

5. The Trainability Principle. The more extensively the body is trained with respect to a given factor, the less its remaining trainability. The trainability principle is an expression of the concepts of limits and of diminishing returns. It applies to all performance factors.

6. The Voluntary Stimulation Principle. In keeping with the principles of transfer and of specificity, development of all performance factors proceeds best when training results from normal, voluntary neural stimulation.

For strength, development is optimal when achieved through voluntary neural stimulation. Direct electrical stimulation of muscles by artificial means is often of value in pathologic conditions and in rehabilitation under medical supervision. Passive exercise, massage, manipulation, and application of external forces may be of value for recuperation from heavy exercise but affect contraction

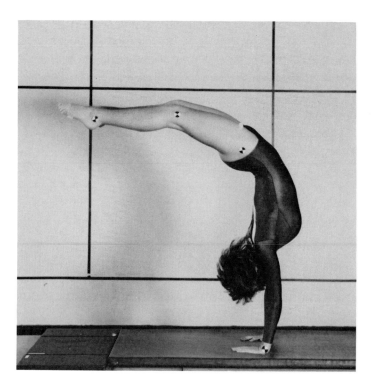

FIG. 16–1. Gymnast showing specific low-back flexibility, wearing joint markers for biomechanical analyses. (Reproduced with permission from A.V.S. and the Department of Physical Education and Sports Sciences, Loughborough University of Technology, and the British Journal of Sports Medicine.)

only through the possible activation of natural reflexes, without otherwise causing strength development in normal subjects. Methods and devices claiming effortless development of strength are fraudulent. Much evidence suggests that strength development is primarily neural (and to some extent motivational) in its genesis, and that peripheral biochemical and morphologic changes in muscle are important secondary derivatives. For endurance, similar principles apply.

Flexibility can be gained by any exercise that forces the joint beyond the range of motion to which it has been adapted, whether this exercise be passive, assistive, or resistive. Even here, there are advantages to stretching by voluntary neural stimulation. A passive or ballistic stretch can initiate a stretch reflex within the muscles being stretched. Minor injury is then more likely to occur, because the muscles stretched are not fully relaxed. If, however, the stretch is powered by slow concentric contraction of the antagonists, the stretched muscles presumably will be relaxed through the mechanism of reciprocal innervation, and the contractile fibers themselves are less susceptible to trauma. At the same time, strength and tonus are developed in the antagonists, tending more or less permanently to counterbalance the residual tension in the muscles that need to be stretched. The generalization is that slow, controlled stretch is preferable to passive or "bouncing" ballistic stretching.

7. The Progression Principle. Because the absolute value of a minimal training stimulus, with respect to any of the factors, tends to change regularly as progress is made, the amount of overload should be increased gradually but persistently over a long period of training. If this is not done, the training stimulus (although remaining the same in absolute value) soon becomes subminimal; if increments are made in very large steps the exercise becomes either impossible or dangerous.

For strength and cardiovascular-respiratory endurance, the statement of the progression principle can be extended by noting that the trainee must, progressively, do either more work in the same time or the same work in a shorter time. Progression is made by increas-

ing the volume of the overload, the intensity of the overload, or both. This is a fundamental concept in designing training programs.

For flexibility, it is the extent of stretching, rather than the intensity, that is subjected to gradual and progressive increase.

8. The Overtraining Principle. Overtraining, which can occur with respect to both strength and endurance development, is a state of chronic fatigue leading to undesirable morphologic, systemic, and psychologic changes. The treatment for overtraining is temporary cessation of training or decrease in the volume and intensity of the training regimen, together with recreational relaxation. Overtraining is more hazardous than undertraining.

9. The Motivation Principle. The motivational acceptance of fatigue, effort expenditure, discomfort, and boredom of training is an important factor in the development of strength, endurance, and sometimes other factors. Some commercial advertisements to the contrary, there is no easy way to train seriously with fun and enjoyment. However, most normal humans find unique rewards in the pure psychophysiologic euphoria that follows a session of training or vigorous performance. In fact, an antidote to the fatigue of prolonged sedentary work is an exercise bout that reaches well into the realm of physiologic fatigue, followed by a shower, a meal, and a period of relaxation.

10. The Compatibility Principle. This principle can also be called the individuality principle. Simply stated, any exercise program should be compatible with the goals and abilities of the trainee. The program should be neither too easy nor too stressful but it must stimulate adaptation. Consideration must be given to a person's age; weeks, months, or years of training experience; types of exercise used in the past; type of training used in the immediate past; and short- and long-term goals relative to exercise and fitness, sport competition, etc. Although general guidelines can be found for most situations and practical experience is valuable, it must never be forgotten that each individual responds differently to a given training stimulus. Close observation of the effects of any training program allows "fine tuning" of the program to produce the best possible results in any given situation.

SUMMARY

The master principles just discussed apply to the improvement of all or most of the factors generally involved in motor performance. Their correct application in conditioning programs is vital to success. The exercises used in any program should for the most part satisfy the principles of specificity, transfer, and voluntary stimulation. The exercises or components making up the entire program should also be chosen to develop a reasonable balance in fitness/performance factors—for example, all major muscle groups should be conditioned even though some may need emphasis. Likewise, other factors such as cardiovascular-respiratory endurance and flexibility should not be ignored if strength development is of prime importance in a program. All workouts should begin with a short period of warm-up activities (e.g., jogging in place, jumping jacks, or jumping rope) that involve many muscle groups to raise heart rate, respiration rate, and muscle temperature. Stretching exercises can easily be incorporated into a warm-up period.

Another key to progress is to have progression in a long-term program. A program is made progressive by varying the components of overload—volume and intensity—so that the trend over time is toward increases in one or both. Increasing the frequency of workouts is another method of adding to the demands of a conditioning program. As years of training go by, the trainability of an individual decreases, and smaller increments of improvement should be expected from the ever-growing value of overload. Excessive overload, however, cannot be tolerated by either novice or experienced trainees and will lead to overtraining and the need for greatly reduced overload and rest. Hence, any conditioning program must be compatible with and adjusted according to the trainee's ability to recuperate from and adapt to the program's demands (compatibility). Motivation can be maintained only if reasonable progress is made, which requires an intelligently designed training program. Thus, positive feed-back increases motivation, which can further stimulate training drive and additional progress.

PRINCIPLES PERTAINING TO INDIVIDUAL PERFORMANCE FACTORS

STRENGTH

1. The Range of Motion Principle. A strength exercise should begin from a position in which the muscle is fully stretched and end in a position in which it is fully shortened if flexibility, maximum tension, and strength throughout the range are desired as outcomes.

2. The Recovery Principle. Moving or massaging a fatigued muscle during rest pauses will increase its speed of recovery; general body position also can influence circulation and prevent stagnation of metabolites in a muscle.

ENDURANCE

1. Muscular endurance and cardiovascular-respiratory endurance are separate factors in human performance; development of one does not necessarily accompany development of the other.

2. Increased strength and skill contribute significantly to muscular endurance, primarily by increasing the efficiency and reducing the energy cost and fatigue decrement associated with a given task.

3. The development of endurance depends largely on training the oxygen uptake and transport mechanisms. The ability of the heart to pump blood is the most common limiting factor in cardiovascular-respiratory endurance, but not the only important one.

FLEXIBILITY

1. Flexibility is related to body type, sex, age, bone and joint structure, and other factors beyond the individual's control.

2. Flexibility is predominantly a function of habits of movement, activity, and inactivity.

3. Work or exercise that constrains a joint

within a restricted range of motion tends to reduce flexibility.

4. Lack of normal flexibility constrains the extent and quality of performance and may be responsible for specific ailments.

5. The decrease in flexibility normally accompanying aging is caused by failure to maintain movement through a complete range of motion.

SPEED OF MOVEMENT

1. Maximal speed of movement is partly an innate individual characteristic.

2. Speed of movement is influenced by reaction and response times, which are partly innate individual characteristics, but which can be minimized by training in attention, mental set, and skills.

3. Speed of movement is reduced by failure of antagonistic muscles to relax appropriately; to some extent this is a skill and is subject to training influences.

BONE GROWTH AND DEVELOPMENT

1. The ability of bone to adapt healthfully to imposed loads depends not just on the frequency and absolute magnitude of externally applied forces, but also on the bony area through which the force is transmitted, and on the magnitude of tensile, compressive, shear, and bending components of that force.

2. Optimal growth and development of the skeleton depends critically on the consistent, uninterrupted operation of the general factors in a healthful life regimen—freedom from debilitating disease, noxious drugs, and chemicals, adequate intermittent periods of sleep and relaxation, and balanced nutrition. These conditions are particularly important in the period between conception and maturity and again during old age.

TRAINING INJURIES

Muscle injuries as a result of strenuous physical activity cannot be entirely eliminated, but with proper training techniques their frequency can be greatly reduced. Solomon and Micheli state that one principle cannot be repeated too often: the repetitive use of body mechanics that strengthen compensatory muscles and thereby produce musculoskeletal balance tends to reduce the number of injuries, while the repetition of any techniques that create muscle imbalance tends to increase the number of injuries. In the latter case, the body usually breaks down at its weakest point.[16]

REFERENCES

1. Clarke, H.H.: Basic understanding of physical fitness. Phys. Fit. Res. Dig., 1:1, 1971.
2. Jackson, A.S.: Special Committee for Revision of the AAHPER Youth Fitness Test: Second Working Draft, Mimeographed.
3. Berger, R.: Effect of varied weight training programs on strength. Res. Quar., 33:168, 1962.
4. O'Shea, J.P.: Effect of selected weight training programs on the development of strength and muscular hypertrophy. Res. Quar., 37:95, 1966.
5. Stone, M., O'Bryant, H., and Garhammer, J.: A hypothetical model for strength training. J. Sports Med. Phys. Fitness, 21:342, 1981.
6. Stone, M., et al.: A theoretical model of strength training. Nat. Strength Cond. Assoc. J., 4:36, 1982.
7. Garhammer, J.: Sports Illustrated—Strength Training. New York, Time, Inc., 1987.
8. Stone, M., and O'Bryant, H.: Weight Training—A Scientific Approach. Minneapolis, Burgess Publishing Co., 1987.
9. Cooper, J.: The new aerobics. New York, Bantam Books, 1970.
10. Fleck, S.: Interval training—physical basis. Nat. Strength Cond. Assoc. J., 5:40, 1983.
11. MacDougall, D., and Sale, D.: Continuous vs. interval training. Can. J. Appl. Sport Sci., 6:93, 1981.
12. Roundtable: Understanding injury in its relationship to strength and flexibility. Part 1. Nat. Strength Cond. Assoc. J., 8(1):14, 1986.
13. Roundtable: Understanding injury in its relationship to strength and flexibility. Part 2. Nat. Strength Cond. Assoc. J., 8(2):14, 1986.
14. Gettman, L.R., and Pollock, M.L.: Circuit weight training: A critical review of its physical benefits. Phys. Sportsmed., 9:44, June, 1981.
15. Hickson, R.C.: Interference of strength development by simultaneously training for strength and endurance. Euro. J. Appl. Physiol., 45:255, 1980.
16. Solomon, R.L., and Micheli, L.J.: Technique as a consideration in modern dance injuries. Phys. Sportsmed., 14:88, August 1986.

RECOMMENDED READING

Rasch, P.J.: Weight Training. 5th Ed. Dubuque, William C. Brown, 1983.
Wilmore, J.H.: Athletic Training and Physical Fitness. Boston, Allyn and Bacon, 1976.

17 KINESIOLOGY IN DAILY LIVING

PHILIP J. RASCH

LIFTING

Because the levers of the human body are adapted for range, speed, and precision of movement, rather than for handling weight, it is not surprising that the incidence of back injuries attributed to lifting is extremely high. Such trauma may be due to acute injury, such as is sustained by the industrial worker, or to a continual mild overstretching of the muscles and ligaments, such as is experienced by the homemaker. They may result from the "nut-cracker" effect of compression forces or from lesions of the soft tissues. These conditions are especially apt to occur in elderly individuals, whose intervertebral discs and muscles have lost their strength and elasticity.

To offset the mechanical disadvantages inherent in the human machine requires the use of the most efficient techniques of body mechanics. General rules are difficult to apply, because the way burdens are lifted depends on their size, shape, and position in space and the habits of the person lifting them. In dead lifting, seven cardinal principles are observed:

1. The feet are kept flat on the floor. The lifter does not balance himself on his toes, as is sometimes shown in shop posters depicting the techniques of lifting.

2. The legs are spread a comfortable distance apart to increase the stability of the body. If the stance is exceptionally wide, the muscles of the groin are more easily strained.

3. The weight is kept as close to the lifter as is convenient.

4. The spine is kept as straight as possible.

5. The actual lifting is done by the largest and strongest muscles which can be utilized for the purpose—usually the extensors of the knees and hips. In most cases the knees are bent, and the object is grasped in the hands and then lifted by forcefully contracting the extensors of the knee and hips, not by pulling upward with the arms and back (Figs. 17–1 and 17–2).

6. The lifter faces in the direction in which he intends to move so that he does not have to turn while holding the weight and thus generate forces that may result in injury. In many cases, however, the lifter can take advantage of the counterbalancing of the body and of follow-through to perform in one smooth motion what might otherwise be accomplished in a series of inefficient discrete movements.

7. When the lifter comes erect from the squat position (Fig. 17–2), any attempt to lift a heavy weight should be stopped immediately if the hips cannot be kept below the level of the torso.

Almost all forms of work are performed most efficiently when these principles are kept in mind. In using the wringer on a mop bucket, for example, the worker will profit by facing in the direction in which the wringer handle moves so that the weight of the body can be applied on the downstroke and the strength of the legs employed on the upstroke. At the other extreme, one acute witness of the hard-rock drilling contests of the early Southwestern miners noted that the man swinging the hammer bent forward as much at the hip and knee as at the elbow and

266

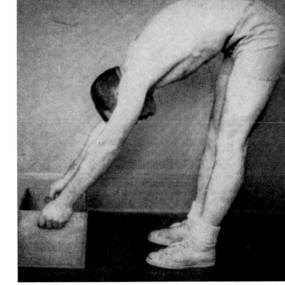

FIG. 17–1. Incorrect technique of lifting. In this position, the principal stresses will come on the muscles of the spinal column, which, in this position, is literally "hanging from its ligaments." This is termed the cantilever position and is responsible for many back strains. (Photo by Pierson.)

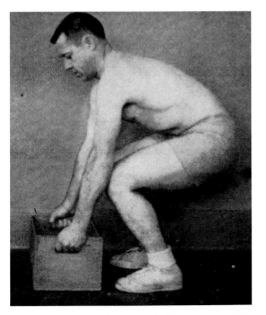

FIG. 17–2. Usually recommended technique of lifting. In this position, the principal stresses will come on the quadriceps muscle of the thigh, the largest and strongest muscles in the body. Leskinen et al.[11] point out that this method requires a greater expenditure of energy because of the vertical displacement of a greater proportion of the body weight and is of value only if the load can be lifted close to the body, but the peak spinal compression is lower. (Photo by Pierson.)

shoulder, caught the elbow of the lower arm on the forward thigh, and threw it back up into the air by the upward jerk of the leg.[2] The two types of work are very different, but the principles involved are exactly the same.

MOVING WEIGHTS

The principles for the most efficient method of pushing are very similar to those for lifting:

1. The feet are placed a comfortable distance apart, with one foot near the object to be pushed and the other extended to the rear.

2. The spine is kept straight and the hips are kept low.

3. The hands are placed at the level of the object's center of gravity. If they are placed above it, the object will tend to tip forward rather than slide forward.

4. The object is moved by contracting the extensors of the hip, knee, and ankle and straightening the legs, not by extending the arms.

Variations of the principle of pushing can be found in the use of the shovel, in which the advanced hand, or hand and thigh, can be used as a fulcrum and the weight lifted by pushing down on the shovel, and in canoeing, in which the principal effort is made by a push of the arm whose hand and fingers grasp the top of the paddle. It should be noted that in both cases first-class leverage is involved and force is produced because the force arm is longer than the resistance arm.

HANDLING AN OBJECT OVERHEAD

The problem of handling an object overhead, as in removing a box from a closet shelf, is rendered more severe by the fact that moving the object builds up a horizontal momentum and raises the center of gravity of the mover, thus decreasing his stability and rendering him more likely to be tipped in the direction in which the object is moving or to suffer a strain in trying to prevent undesired movement. A solution is to place one foot in advance of the other. The object is first moved with the body's center of gravity supported by the advanced foot. As the object comes forward, the body weight is shifted to the support of the back foot, which can be moved still farther backward if necessary. In effect, this maneuver sacrifices space to gain a reduction of momentum. The inability to make this sacrifice and the dangers attendant on loss of stability make lifting an object overhead while standing on a kitchen stool or similar support potentially hazardous. In all overhead lifting an effort should be made to avoid thrusting the hips forward or increasing the lordotic curve of the back.

CARRYING WEIGHTS

If the weight must be carried, the normal erect posture is modified so that the center of gravity of the lifter plus the load approximates the center of gravity of the lifter alone. This modification explains the high efficiency (Table 17–1) of carrying loads on the head (Fig. 17–3). The trunk apparently functions as a counterbalance, altering its inclination so that the projection of the center of gravity at the feet remains relatively constant. The most common cause of accidents in carrying loads is loss of balance resulting in the placement of insupportable muscular strains on the body. Observation of the following principles will assist in carrying loads safely and efficiently:

1. If possible, the load is divided into two

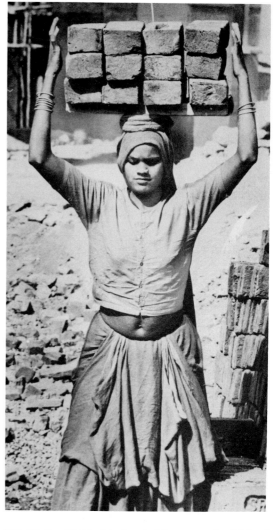

FIG. 17–3. East Indian female laborer carrying 70 lb of bricks on her head. (Los Angeles Times photo by Tyler Marshall.) Note that the gravital line of the worker plus the load approximates the gravital line of the worker alone. A study of Nigerian women, who carry similar burdens on their heads, concluded that this method is made possible by extremely erect posture and by a technique of walking that eliminates the bobbing and dipping apparent in Figure 6–2. There appear to be no reports of studies of the effects of this compression on the spine.

equal parcels and one is carried in each hand, so that the spine is kept straight.

2. If the load is a single bundle, the free arm can be raised sideward to assist in keeping the spine erect.

3. The weight is carried close to the body. This reduces unbalancing leverage to a minimum and lessens the moments required to turn the body.

4. The most efficient handle to use on a bundle is the one that exerts the least concentrated pressure on the hands. For example, carrying pails is less fatiguing if the wire bail is covered with a handle.

5. When carrying packages in the hands, the elbows are slightly flexed to take some of the strain off the elbow joint. Normally only the ligamentous structure of the elbow prevents distraction of the loaded joint unless the muscles are voluntarily contracted.

A study sponsored by the U.S. Air Force recommended the following weight limits be placed on equipment that must be lifted by short (5 ft 6 in. and under) men:[3]

To knee level (18 in.) . . . . 61.66 lb
To waist level (42 in.) . . . . 37.91 lb
To shoulder level (62.5 in.) . . . . 27.19 lb

Taller men are normally heavier and can lift somewhat greater amounts.

For women the most economical load appears to be about 35% of the body weight. A load of about 45 lb would appear to be the optimum for continous carriage, although the average woman should be able to handle 50 lb without strain. A possible 20% additional load might be allowed when the burden is compact and easily handled. The optimal load for men is also about 35% of body weight and the optimal rate of carrying about 85 to 95 yd/min. Faster rates of carrying increase the energy consumption to a greater degree than does a 20% increase in the weight.[4]

When a worker must carry sacks, the weight of the sack should not exceed 132 lb on the level and 120 lb on stairs.[5] The recommended maximum load for men is 130 lb, although the amount of weight that can be safely handled is so affected by constitution, strength, age, experience, compactness of load, and other factors that wide variations from this figure can be acceptable. In practice these concepts are often violated. It is almost universally agreed that an infantryman should not carry in excess of 40 lb; however, the American soldier actually carries about 73 lb.[6]

Datta and Ramanathan investigated seven different ways of carrying a load of 30 kg for 1 km at a speed of 5 km/hr.[7] They found that there were significant physiologic differences between the various methods (Table 17–1). An unusual method of carrying loads common until recently among peasant women in Scotland is shown in Figure 17–4.

DELAYED MUSCLE SORENESS

Nearly every physical activity is a combination of concentric and eccentric contractions. One who lifts a weight (through concentric contraction) must produce the same amount of force to control its lowering (through eccentric contraction). Though any form of unaccustomed exercise can produce muscle soreness, in untrained individuals the eccentric part of the exercise can result in soreness whose appearance is delayed for several hours after cessation of the work. This soreness is believed to result from the tearing of sarcomeres in the Z bands and the movement of fluid into the muscle cells. Regular eccentric training prevents this form of soreness.[8]

SITTING AND RISING

In Western cultures it is assumed that an individual accepting an invitation to be seated will sit on a chair or davenport, but this is not necessarily true elsewhere.

Body position reflects anatomic, psychologic, cultural, kinesiologic, and environmental factors. The relative advantages and disadvantages of different positions in general use in various parts of the world have never been studied and offer the kinesiologist a fascinating field of exploration.

In sitting down and rising one is confronted with the problem of supporting the body while the center of gravity moves backward and downward or forward and upward, as the case may be. In sitting down on a chair the individual stands with his back to the chair, places one foot slightly to the rear, inclines the body forward from the hips to keep the center of gravity over the base of support, and lowers the body by relaxing the knee extensors and permitting the joint to bend. In arising from a chair the individual places one foot slightly under the chair, bends forward from the hips, and rises by contracting the knee extensors, transferring the center of

Table 17–1. Selected Physiologic Parameters in Subjects Carrying a Standard Load in Seven Different Modes

Mode	O₂ L/min	Energy kcal/min	Heart Rate beats/min	Min. Ventilation L/min
Double Pack........................... Load divided equally into two packs, one in front and one in back.	1.010	4.83	56.0	18.08
Head .... Load in basket on head.	1.038	4.90	63.8	27.54
Rucksack	1.106	5.27	62.1	30.18
Sherpa............................. Load carried on back supported by head strap.	1.158	5.54	56.7	31.11
Rice Bag............................. Load on back with upper corners held.	1.221	5.93	60.2	33.04
Yoke .... Load carried on bamboo pole across shoulders.	1.301	6.22	65.7	35.29
Hands .... Load carried in two canvas bags.	1.464	6.96	81.5	39.58

gravity forward so that it is supported by the forward foot.

In sitting on or arising from a straight-backed chair, one does not normally require the aid of the hands. In some deep chairs the center of gravity is thrown so far backward that it is difficult to sit down or rise, and in such cases the arms are used to assist in the movement. Schools for fashion models and actors usually teach that it is ungraceful to employ the arms in rising.

Older persons might find it difficult to sit in comfort or to arise after being seated for long periods. Poorly designed chairs cause an excessive decrease in the pull of the thigh-trunk muscles. This decrease permits the lumbar curve to flatten, and the hydraulic pressure resulting from anterior wedging within the fourth or fifth intervertebral disc can force a degenerated piece to protrude, causing a painful stretching of the sensitive posterior longitudinal ligament of the disc.

When the vasti are paralyzed or weakened, the weight of the body may be too great to be withstood by the knee extensors and the individual may be able to stabilize his body in the erect position only by hyperextending the knees to throw the center of gravity forward of the normal line of body weight. A person so afflicted can sometimes be seen to place his hands on his knees and assist himself to rise by pushing the knees backward as he leans forward.

When the seated individual is required to operate foot pedals of some kind, the amount of thrust that can be exerted by the legs may be important. The thrust exerted by the legs is at a maximum when the knees are bent at an angle of approximately 165°. At this point the mean thrust is about 227 kg. If the knees are bent at a smaller angle, the upper part of the body tends to be pushed backward; if they are bent at a greater angle, the body tends to be tilted forward.

SQUATTING

Squatting is the normal resting position in large areas of the world. In the Western culture it is considered undignified and its use is largely restricted to athletes, who have traditionally included squats, duck walks, and similar exercises in their training programs. As has been stated previously, it is now generally agreed that this position predisposes the knee to injury from trauma. Gardeners and others who may work in this position should be careful to avoid twists of the joint when the knee is flexed, as the medial cartilage may be torn or detached.

STAIR CLIMBING

Stair climbing is a special case of locomotion. Raising the body onto the next tread is accomplished by contraction of the soleus,

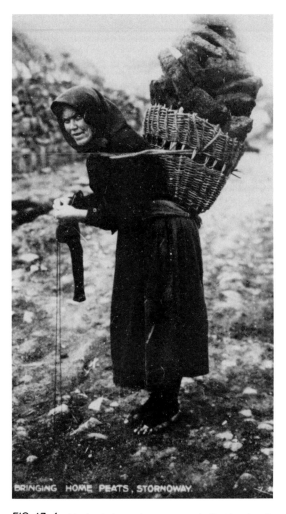

FIG. 17–4. Method of carrying common in Scotland until the 1930s. The load of peat in the creel in the photograph is estimated to be about 40 lb, but women selling fish are said to have carried well over 100 lb, in addition to small baskets over their arms. (Photo courtesy the Country Life Archive, National Museum of Antiquities of Scotland, Edinburgh.) What are the advantages and disadvantages of this technique from the kinesiological standpoint? (Suggestion: Review Farfan, H.F.: Muscular mechanism of the lumbar spine and the position of power and efficiency. Orthop. Clin. North Am., 6:135–144, 1975.)

quadriceps femoris, hamstrings, and gluteus maximus. At the same time the middle gluteal muscle contracts to prevent the body from falling to the unsupported side. The tibialis anterior dorsiflexes the foot and helps the limb clear the stair on which the supporting limb rests. The hamstrings flex the knee and control the terminal part of the knee extension. The erector spinae contract to control the forward bending of the torso. The same muscles are active in eccentric contraction while descending stairs. The average energy cost of ascending stairs, regardless of type, has been reported as 12.1 cal/kg/m of vertical distance covered; the cost of descending is 7.1 cal/kg/m, or about 59% of the cost of ascending.[9]

Placing the ball of the foot on the tread of the stair and then lifting the body by contraction of the gastrocnemius (plantar flexion) is considerably more fatiguing than in placing the entire sole of the foot on the tread and raising the body by extension of the knee joint. By keeping the center of gravity forward, the effect of the resistance arm of the thigh lever is reduced and energy is conserved. Over 50 years ago it was determined that the most efficient rate of stair climbing is about 1.3 sec/step. Elderly people can be observed to grasp the hand rail for support and to lean well forward. The increased flexion of the hip thus obtained enables them to employ the gluteus maximus to better advantage in extending the hip joint.

When descending stairs, the body is kept more erect in order to prevent the center of gravity from getting too far forward. The hip of the swinging leg is flexed slightly, the amount depending on the width of the tread, and the knee and ankle are extended. The extensors of the hip, knee, and ankle of the supporting leg gradually reduce the force that they are exerting and permit a slow flexion. This is a typical "lengthening contraction," or "negative work" in which gravity does work and the extensors resist it. The body is lowered until the ball of the foot of the swinging leg makes contact with the step. The weight is then transferred to this leg, the knee of the other leg is flexed, the foot is lifted and swung forward, and when the knee is extended, the cycle is repeated. The ratio of oxygen costs for ascending and descending stairs at 160 steps/min is about 4.7:1 for males and 5.7:1 for females.[10] Even descending stairs requires a greater energy expenditure than does horizontal walking. Much of this energy appears to be expended in maintaining the body posture while moving from one step to another. The simple act of going down a flight of stairs has been the inspiration for a major work of modern art (Figure 17–5).

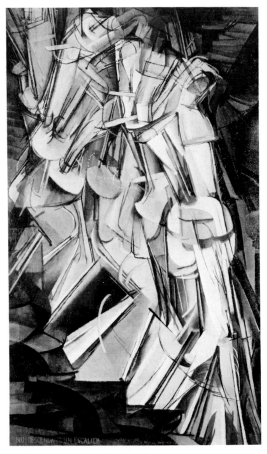

FIG. 17-5. "Nude Descending a Staircase" by Duchamp (1887-1968). This is the most famous attempt in modern art to depict kinesiological action in an essentially static medium. It is said to have been inspired by Marey's multiple exposure photography of moving figures. By the repetition of form, Duchamp endeavored to indicate time and thus add a fourth dimension to art. (Philadelphia Museum of Art, Loise and Walter Arensberg Collection.) The Duchamp painting in turn inspired Gjon Mili to undertake the same theme in a multiple exposure photograph (see A. Feininger, The Complete Photographer, p. 89).

WORKING SPACE ARRANGEMENTS

No worker can hope to function efficiently unless the arrangement of the equipment he is required to use has been designed with a full consideration of anatomic and kinesiologic principles. Each job has its own peculiarities and can involve such details as determining the optimal load for a miner's shovel or the optimal length of a tuna fisherman's pole. The goals of human factors engineering are (1) to make it possible for any worker to operate any machine, and (2) to avoid limiting the performance of the machine by human failure. Here only the barest and most general outline can be given.

1. Work benches and tables should be at the elbow height of the user, whether he is sitting or standing.

2. The height of work chairs should be adjustable. They are in proper position when the operator's feet rest on the floor or on a support. For the average American male the distance from the floor to the top of the chair seat should be about 18 in.

3. Levers to which maximum force must be applied should be at shoulder level for standing operators, at elbow level for seated operators.

4. Controls that must be used often should be between elbow and shoulder height.

5. Convenient arm reach is about 28 in; controls more distant will probably require the average operator to bend his body.

6. Horizontal movements of the hand are faster than vertical movements.

7. Flexion movements of the arm are faster than extension movements.

REST PAUSES

When Taylor made his classic study of the application of kinesiologic principles to the carrying of billets of pig iron, he nearly quadrupled work output by using three basic techniques: (1) motivation (promising the worker an increased wage), (2) selection of the physical type best suited to the work, and (3) introduction of rest pauses. The question of rest pauses has received insufficient attention from kinesiologists. Unlike its mechanical counterparts, the human machine cannot work continuously without a decided loss in efficiency. During World War I the British found that the weekly output for a 55½-hour week was 13% greater than that for a 74½-hour week. During World War II American students determined that hours beyond 48 to 50 a week resulted in higher absenteeism, high injury rates, and lower output per man-hour.[11]

Numerous studies of the energy costs of various industrial, sports, and domestic activities have been made. The energy output

Table 17–2. Classification of Occupational Levels by Energy Expenditure

Work Level	Gross kcal/m²/hr	Gross kcal/min	Pulmonary Ventilation L/kg/min
Sedentary	40–70	1.1–2.0	<0.12
Light	70–110	2.0–3.0	0.12–0.20
Moderate	110–180	3.0–5.0	0.20–0.30
Heavy	180–300	5.0–8.0	0.30–0.50
Very heavy	300 +	8.0 +	0.50 +

reqired is generally expressed in terms of calories used per minute. The British Ministry of Labour has developed the so-called Slough Scales to classify different occupations in terms of energy expenditure required (Table 17–2).[12]

Apparently easy work may be strenuous if it is done by relatively weak muscles, is predominantly static, is performed in an awkward position, or is carried out under extreme environmental conditions. For jobs requiring a large amount of fairly continuous effort, the maximum daily energy expenditure on the job should not exceed 2000 kcal for men and 1500 kcal for women.[13]

If left to himself, the worker will take voluntary rest pauses, perhaps as an unconscious means of self-protection. The frequency and duration of these will vary with the severity of the work being done, but for manual labor rest periods approximate 10 min out of every hour. A British ergometrist has proposed that rest pauses should be the same for men and women when the average work output is below 300 watts; when it is in excess of that figure, women should be given extra rest allowances.

RHYTHM

Rhythm may be an important factor affecting the efficiency with which movements are made. Each individual has his own preferred speed of movement. The ease and efficiency of movement may be increased if it is done to a distinct rhythm. Perhaps one of the factors making for success in a famous backfield, such as the Four Horsemen of Notre Dame, or in a dancing group is the combination of individuals whose preferred movement speed is identical. On the other hand, an as-

sembly line worker whose preferred speed of movement clashes with that imposed on him by his work may find that he is subjected to stresses that render him both inefficient and unhappy.

AVOIDANCE OF INDUSTRIAL FATIGUE

Perrott has suggested five practical ways in which a worker can avoid unnecessary fatigue and trauma:[14]

1. Eliminate unnecessary movements. Repetition of even minute movements can be damaging.

2. Use gravity to accomplish work, as by leaning on a handle to depress it rather than by moving it by arm strength.

3. Position the body so that the prime movers, synergists, fixators, and antagonists can each play their proper roles. In general, work performed at or above the facial level, below the knees, or within an inadequate space is to be avoided.

4. Properly balance the body, as in employing it as a counterweight in lifting a heavy object, in flexing the knees and lifting with the legs rather than with the back (Figs. 17–1 and 17–2), and in employing the strength of the legs rather than of the arms in pushing.

5. Minimize shearing stresses. In pronation of the forearm, for example, the radius rotates across the ulna, whereas in supination they lie side by side. By making a given movement in supination rather than in pronation, much torsion of the soft tissue around the joint can be avoided. The industrial physician must give careful consideration to the possibility of improper body mechanics as an etiologic factor if he hopes to be successful in the diagnosis and treatment of such trauma, but careful attention to the kinesiologic aspects of work can do much to prevent the development of such conditions in the first place.

REFERENCES

1. Leskinen, T.P.J., et al.: A dynamic analysis of spinal compression with different lifting techniques. Ergonomics, 26:595, 1983.
2. Chisholm, J.: Brewery Gulch. San Antonio, Naylor Company, 1949, pp. 113–114.

3. Switzer, S.A.: Weight-Lifting Capabilities of a Selected Sample of Human Males. Aerospace Medical Laboratories Report, MRL-TDR-62-67, June, 1962.
4. Teeple, J.B.: Work of Carrying Loads. Percept. Mot. Skills, 7:60, 1957.
5. Glasow, W., and Miller, E.A.: Carrying heavy sacks on the level and on stairs. Arbeits., 14:322–327, 1951. Abstracted in Index & Abstracts of Foreign Physical Education Literature. Indianapolis, Phi Epsilon Kappa Fraternity, 1955, 1:56–57.
6. United States Army Combat Developments Command: A Study to Conserve the Energy of the Combat Infantryman. Alexandria, Documentation Center, 5 February, 1964.
7. Datta, S.R., and Ramanathan, N.L.: Ergonomic comparison of seven modes of carrying loads on the horizontal plane. Ergonomics, 14:269, 1971.
8. Evans, W.J.: Exercise-induced skeletal muscle damage. Phys. Sportsmed., 15:81, January 1987.
9. Richardson, M. Physiological responses and energy expenditure of women using stairs of three designs. J. Appl. Physiol., 21:1078, 1966.
10. Hesser, C.M.: Energy cost of alternating positive and negative work. Acta Physiol. Scand., 63:84, 1965.
11. Kossoris, M.D.: The facts about hours of work vs. output. Reprinted from Fac. Manag., 1951, p. 275.
12. Brown, J.R., and Crowden, G.P.: Energy expenditure ranges and muscular work grades. Br. J. Ind. Med., 23:277, 1963.
13. Floyd, W.F., and Slade, I.M.: Fitting the job to the worker. Ergonomics, 2:305, 1959.
14. Perrott, J.W.: Anatomical factors in occupational trauma. Med. J. Aust., 1:73, 1961.

RECOMMENDED READING

Ramanathan, N.L., et al.: Biomechanics of various modes of load transport on level ground. Indian J. Med. Res., 60:1702, 1972.

Appendix A

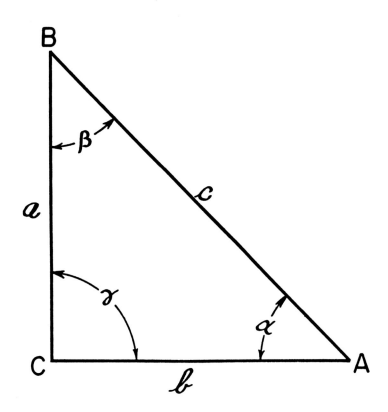

Fig. A–1. Relationships of sides and angles in a right triangle.

TRIGONOMETRIC RELATIONSHIPS FOR RIGHT ANGLES

For the convenience of students in dealing with problems of bone-muscle leverage, some of the elementary trigonometric relationships for right triangles are summarized below.

A, B, and C are the points of a triangle; a and b are the sides opposite angles α and β, respectively; c is the hypotenuse, opposite angle γ, the right angle (Fig. A–1).

1. The sum of the angles of any triangle is equal to 180°.

$$\alpha + \beta + \gamma = 180°$$

2. Two angles are called complementary when their sum is equal to 90°. In a right triangle the two angles between the hypotenuse and the adjacent sides are complementary.

$$\alpha + \beta = 90°$$

3. The sum of the squares of the sides of a right triangle is equal to the square of the hypotenuse (Pythagorean theorem).

$$a^2 + b^2 = c^2 \qquad a^2 = c^2 - b^2$$

$$\sqrt{a^2 + b^2} = c \qquad a = \sqrt{c^2 - b^2}$$

4. The sine of an angle of a right triangle is equal to the side opposite divided by the hypotenuse, and is equal to the cosine of the complementary angle.

$$\sin \alpha = \frac{a}{c} = \cos \beta = \cos (90° - \alpha)$$

5. The cosine of an angle of a right triangle is equal to the side adjacent divided by the hypotenuse, and is equal to the sine of the complementary angle.

$$\cos \alpha = \frac{b}{c} = \sin \beta = \sin (90° - \alpha)$$

Following is a table of sines of the whole angles from 0° to 180°. The cosines of the angles may be found by taking the sine of the complementary angle, according to 5, above.

Degrees	Sines	Degrees	Sines	Degrees	Sines	Degrees	Sines
0 or 180	.00000	23 or 157	.39073	46 or 134	.71934	69 or 111	.93358
1 or 179	.01745	24 or 156	.40674	47 or 133	.73135	70 or 110	.93969
2 or 178	.03490	25 or 155	.42262	48 or 132	.74314	71 or 109	.94552
3 or 177	.05234	26 or 154	.43837	49 or 131	.75471	72 or 108	.95106
4 or 176	.06976	27 or 153	.45399	50 or 130	.76604	73 or 107	.95630
5 or 175	.08716	28 or 152	.46947	51 or 129	.77715	74 or 106	.96126
6 or 174	.10453	29 or 151	.48481	52 or 128	.78801	75 or 105	.96593
7 or 173	.12187	30 or 150	.50000	53 or 127	.79864	76 or 104	.97030
8 or 172	.13917	31 or 149	.51504	54 or 126	.80902	77 or 103	.97437
9 or 171	.15643	32 or 148	.52992	55 or 125	.81915	78 or 102	.97815
10 or 170	.17365	33 or 147	.54464	56 or 124	.82904	79 or 101	.98163
11 or 169	.19081	34 or 146	.55919	57 or 123	.83867	80 or 100	.98481
12 or 168	.20791	35 or 145	.57358	58 or 122	.84805	81 or 99	.98769
13 or 167	.22495	36 or 144	.58779	59 or 121	.85817	82 or 98	.99027
14 or 166	.24192	37 or 143	.60182	60 or 120	.86603	83 or 97	.99255
15 or 165	.25882	38 or 142	.61566	61 or 119	.87462	84 or 96	.99452
16 or 164	.27564	39 or 141	.62932	62 or 118	.88295	85 or 95	.99619
17 or 163	.29237	40 or 140	.64279	63 or 117	.89101	86 or 94	.99756
18 or 162	.30902	41 or 139	.65606	64 or 116	.89879	87 or 93	.99863
19 or 161	.32557	42 or 138	.66913	65 or 115	.90631	88 or 92	.99939
20 or 160	.34202	43 or 137	.68200	66 or 114	.91355	89 or 91	.99985
21 or 159	.35837	44 or 136	.69466	67 or 113	.92050	90	1.00000
22 or 158	.37461	45 or 135	.70711	68 or 112	.92718		

Appendix B

Table for Conversion of English Measures to the International System of Units

When you Know	Multiply by	To Find
Inches	25.4	Millimeters
Feet	0.3048	Meters
Yards	0.9144	Meters
Miles	1.609	Kilometers
Pounds*	0.454	Kilograms
Quarts	0.946	Liters
Millimeters	0.039	Inches
Meters	3.281	Feet
Meters	1.094	Yards
Kilometers	0.621	Miles
Kilograms	2.205	Pounds
Liters	1.056	Quarts

* The currently listed conversion of pounds to Kg and vice versa is questionable since Kg is a mass unit and pounds is a force unit. The use of Kg as a weight (force) unit is still popular in physiology and sport. (See force below.)

Angular: degrees $\times$ 0.01745 = radians / radians $\times$ 57.3 = degrees
Mass: slugs $\times$ 14.59 = kilograms / kilograms $\times$ 0.0685 = slugs
Speed: ft/sec $\times$ 0.682 = mph / mph $\times$ 1.467 = ft/sec
ft/sec $\times$ 1.097 = km/hr / km/hr $\times$ 0.911 = ft/sec
m/sec $\times$ 2.237 = mph / mph $\times$ 0.447 = m/s
m/sec $\times$ 3.281 ft/sec / ft/sec pts 0.3048 m/sec
Force: pounds $\times$ 4.45 = newtons / newtons $\times$ 0.225 = pounds
Work, Energy: ft-lbs $\times$ 1.356 = joules / joules $\times$ 0.738 = ft-lbs
calories $\times$ 3.087 = ft-lbs / ft-lbs $\times$ 0.324 = calories[1]
Power: ft-lb/sec $\times$ 0.00182 = hp / hp $\times$ 550 = ft-lb/sec
ft-lb/sec $\times$ 1.356 watts / watts $\times$ 0.7376 ft-lb/sec

[1] NOTE: 1 "food" calorie = 1 Kcal = 1000 calories

RECOMMENDED READING

Knuttgen, R.G.: Quantifying exercise performance with SI units. Phys. Sportsmed., *14*:167, December 1986.

Index

Page numbers in *italics* indicate figures; numbers followed by "t" indicate tables.